AF522262

GENERAL ANIMAL SURGERY AND ANESTHESIOLOGY

GENERAL ANIMAL SURGERY AND ANESTHESIOLOGY

(VSR-411)

(As per Syllabus Approved by VCI)

by:

A.K. Gangwar

Naveen Kumar

Kh. Sangeeta Devi

New India Publishing Agency

Pitam Pura, New Delhi-110 088

Published by
Sumit Pal Jain *for*

New India Publishing Agency

101, Vikas Surya Plaza, CU Block, L.S.C. Mkt.,
Pitam Pura, New Delhi- 110 088, (India)
Phone: 011-27341717, Fax: 011-27341616
Mobile : 09717133558
E-mail: newindiapublishingagency@gmail.com
Web: www.bookfactoryindia.com

ISBN : 978-93-80235-17-2

Composed and Designed by NIPA

FOREWORD

This gives me immense pleasure to know that Teaching Veterinary Clinical Complex, College of Veterinary Science & Animal Husbandry is going to publish a book for the course No. VSR-411 "General Animal Surgery and Anesthesia" for IV Year B.V.Sc. & A.H. students. The status of Veterinary Surgery has been changing considerably in the past few years. The authors cover various practical approaches as required for the academic programme of students. A number of illustrations and photographs have added to the quality and usefulness of the book.

I think that this book will help to the students to be practically strong.

I congratulate the Dean of Veterinary College and authors for their sincere and innovative efforts.

Basant Ram
Vice-Chancellor
N.D.U.A. & T., Kumarganj
Faizabad (U.P.)

Date : October, 2009

PREFACE

Authors feel a great privileged in bringing out the first edition of course VSR-411 "General Animal Surgery and Anesthesia". The exercises in this book have been arranged to provide a sequential knowledge of the subject. The course content of this book is totally based as per the guidelines set up by the Veterinary Council of India. This book is prepared by consulting several standard textbooks and journals of related field. A number of illustrations and photographs have been incorporatd at places to make the text more meaningful.

Authors are grateful to Dr. D.N. Verma, Ex. Dean and Prof. J.P. Misra, Dean, College of Veterinary Sciences and Animal Husbandary for his resolute guidance, sagacious advice and constructive criticism during the preparation of this book.

Authors are hopeful that this book will serve the intended purpose. We will be grateful to the professionals and colleagues if any suggestions are suggested for the betterment of this book.

A.K. Gangwar
Naveen Kumar
Kh. Sangeeta Devi

PROLOGUE

The level of sophistication of Veterinary Surgery has been changing considerably in the past few years. The knowledge of basic principles of surgery and anesthesiology is very essential for a veterinarian. This book provides adequate information about general surgery and anesthesiology.

The Veterinary College has taken responsibility to help the students to acquire in depth knowledge of the basics of surgery and anaesthesia in different species of animals. In this context, this book has been prepared by the Department of Teaching Veterinary Clinical Complex for the courses VSR-411 "General Animal Surgery and Anesthesia". I am pleased to go through the contents and this will covers the whole syllabus in a systematic manner. The authors deserve appreciation for brining out this book in such a nice form.

Sd-
D.N. Verma
Dean

CONTENTS

Section-I
THEORY

Part-A : General Surgery
(Page 1-177)

Part-B : Anesthesiology
(Page 179-330)

Part-A
GENERAL SURGERY

Chapter 1

Historical Aspects and Introduction

Surgery : The branch of medical science which deals with the treatment of injuries, deformities or disease condition by manipulation or operations with the hand. The term surgery is derived from a Greek word - Chirurgia.

Cheir - Hand

Ergon - Work

Veterinary surgery : Veterinary surgery is the surgery which is practiced on animals.

History

- Vedas contains abundant information on the treatment of animals. Salihotra and Palakapya were the greatest of ancient Indian veterinarians.
- Salihotra treated horses and Palakapya elephants.
- The earliest known work on medicine is in 'Atharvaveda' (1000 B.C.).
- A treatise on medicine with a few passages on surgery is called 'Caraka Samhita'
- "Susruta Samhita' is the earliest known work dealing with the medical science especially surgery.

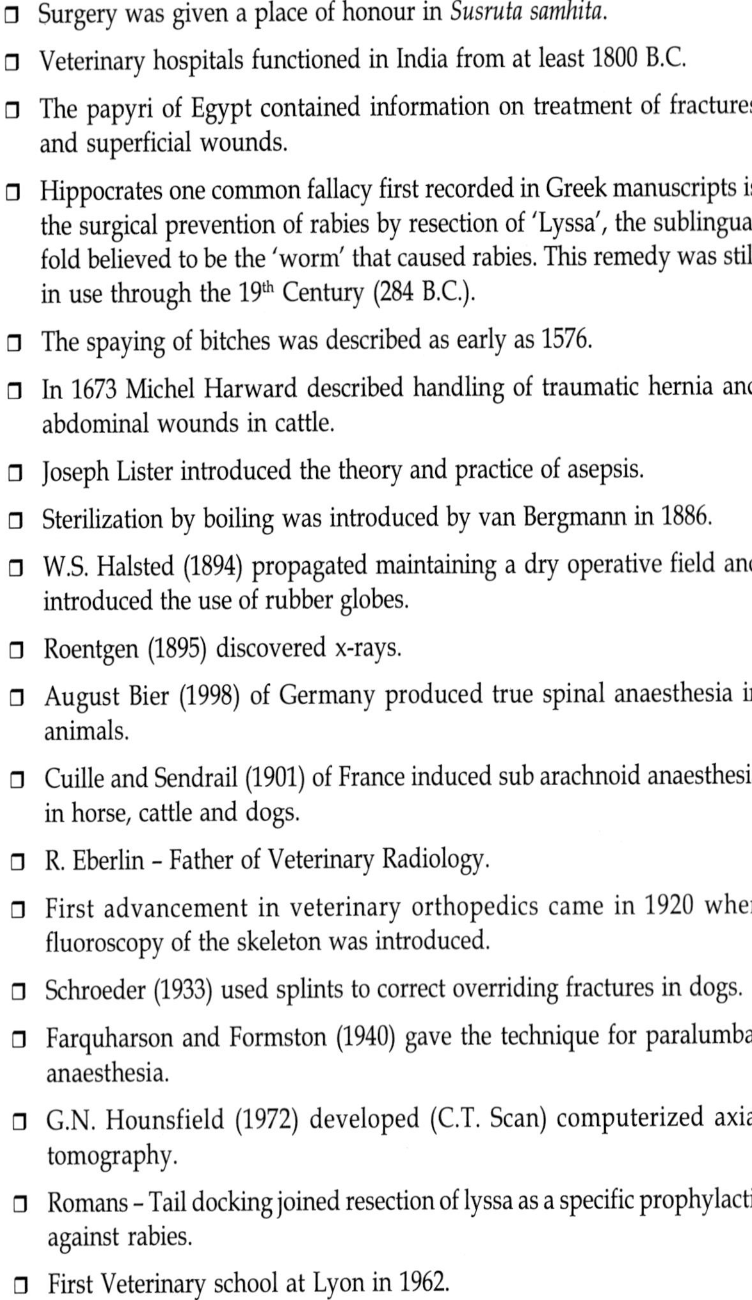

- Surgery was given a place of honour in *Susruta samhita.*
- Veterinary hospitals functioned in India from at least 1800 B.C.
- The papyri of Egypt contained information on treatment of fractures and superficial wounds.
- Hippocrates one common fallacy first recorded in Greek manuscripts is the surgical prevention of rabies by resection of 'Lyssa', the sublingual fold believed to be the 'worm' that caused rabies. This remedy was still in use through the 19th Century (284 B.C.).
- The spaying of bitches was described as early as 1576.
- In 1673 Michel Harward described handling of traumatic hernia and abdominal wounds in cattle.
- Joseph Lister introduced the theory and practice of asepsis.
- Sterilization by boiling was introduced by van Bergmann in 1886.
- W.S. Halsted (1894) propagated maintaining a dry operative field and introduced the use of rubber globes.
- Roentgen (1895) discovered x-rays.
- August Bier (1998) of Germany produced true spinal anaesthesia in animals.
- Cuille and Sendrail (1901) of France induced sub arachnoid anaesthesia in horse, cattle and dogs.
- R. Eberlin - Father of Veterinary Radiology.
- First advancement in veterinary orthopedics came in 1920 when fluoroscopy of the skeleton was introduced.
- Schroeder (1933) used splints to correct overriding fractures in dogs.
- Farquharson and Formston (1940) gave the technique for paralumbar anaesthesia.
- G.N. Hounsfield (1972) developed (C.T. Scan) computerized axial tomography.
- Romans – Tail docking joined resection of lyssa as a specific prophylactic against rabies.
- First Veterinary school at Lyon in 1962.
- F.T.G. Hobday - wrote the first comprehensive text on surgical diseases of the dog and cat.

Classification of surgery : Surgery can be classified on the basis of :

A. Nature of surgery
B. Region/ system involved
C. Instruments /appliances used

A. Nature of Surgery

1. *Aseptic surgery* – Surgery which is conducted in absolute asepsis (free of bacterial contamination).
2. *Antiseptic surgery* – Surgery conducted with the use of antiseptic agents to control bacterial contamination.
3. *Conservative surgery* – Surgery wherein attempt is made to preserve or restore a disabled part, rather than its removal e.g. correction and immobilization of a fracture in a limb rather than amputation of limb.
4. *Radical surgery* – It involves gross removal of a diseased organ from the body for therapeutic purposes e.g. radical surgery of neoplasm.
5. *Major surgery* – A surgical procedure is considered major when the duration of surgery is expected to be more than 30-45 minutes and patient has graded physical status 4 or 5. Major surgery is relatively more difficult to perform than minor surgery. This type of surgery is time consuming, involves risk on the life of patient and requires the help of an assistant and anesthetists also.
6. *Replacement surgery* – Replacement of diseased part by a living tissue (vascular graft), non-living material (heart valve) or dead tissue (corneal or bone graft).
7. *Physiological surgery* – Alterations in the normal physiological mechanisms for the benefits of whole body e.g. vascular shunts.
8. *Experimental surgery* – Done solely for the purpose of experiments e.g. Caesarean section, Thoracic surgery, etc.
9. *Minor surgery* – A surgical procedure is considered minor when the duration of surgery is expected to be not more than 30-45 minutes and patient has graded physical status 1, 2 or 3. Minor surgery is relatively simple to perform having no risk on the life of the patient and does not requires the services of assistant e.g. wound dressing, opening of superficial abscess, superficial neurectomies and tenotomies.
10. *Emergency surgery* – Surgery which is to be performed urgently to avoid further complication of the disease process.

11. *Elective surgery* – Surgery which can be postponed without endangering the life of the patient.

12. *Cosmetic surgery* – Surgery done to improve the appearance of an animal e.g. trimming of the ears, docking of tail etc.

13. *Plastic surgery* – It is done on aesthetic grounds or to restore disturbed function. It includes :

    i. *Reconstructive surgery* – a structure is reconstituted i.e. repair of recto-vaginal fistula, surgery of cleft palate etc.

    ii. *Cosmetic surgery* – when a surgical procedure is used on an otherwise normal organ e.g. removal of a supernumerary teat.

14. *Exploratory surgery* – for confirmation of diagnosis e.g. exploratory laparotomy, paracentesis, biopsy etc.

B. Region / System Involved

1. Thoracic surgery
2. Orthopedic surgery
3. Cardiovascular surgery
4. Opthalmic surgery
5. Neuro surgery
6. Urogenital surgery
7. Head and neck surgery

C. Instruments/ Appliances Used

1. General surgery - when common surgical instruments are used.
2. Microsurgery - magnification facilities are used.
3. Cryosurgery - Liquid N_2 (-196°C) and gaseous N_2O (-70°C) Liquid N_2O (-80°C) are used.
4. Electro surgery - electricity is converted into heat to incise a tissue.
5. Laser surgery - Laser beams are used to cut or destroy the disease tissue.
6. Ultrasonic surgery - high frequency waves are used to destroy the diseased tissue.
7. Fluoroscopic /endoscope surgery.

Halsted's Principles of Surgery

1. Gentle tissue handling
2. Accurate haemostasis
3. Preservation of adequate blood supply
4. Strict asepsis
5. No tension on tissues
6. Careful approximation of tissues
7. Obliteration of dead space
8. Minimum use of suture material

Surgical technique that adheres to Halsted's principles results in significantly lower infection rates.

Chapter 2

Pre-Operative, Intra-Operative & Post-Operative Consideration of a Surgical Patient

Surgical Plan

i. Pre-operative Course of Action

a. Client communication.

b. Clinical laboratory evaluation, radiograph, treatment for fluid or blood volume deficits.

ii. Intra-operative Plan of Action

a. Surgical approach

b. Material and equipment needed

c. Technical and support personnel

iii. Post-operative Requirements

a. O_2 cage

b. Nutritional and fluid support

c. Radiographs

d. Bandages

Pre-operative considerations : A surgeon must keep certain considerations in mind before undertaken surgery. Pre-operative considerations which relate to the owner, patient and surgeon have been described.

1. *Client communication* : An important pre-operative consideration is the presurgical discussion with the client.
   i. The owner must be convinced that every thing being done is in the interest of the animal patient.
   ii. Both emotional and financial aspect of a proposed surgical operation must be taken in to account.
   iii. The surgeon should discuss with the owner the reasons for the surgery, its benefits, degree of operative risk, possible complications, prognosis, operative and post-operative courses and financial responsibilities of the owner.
2. *Surgeon* : The assessment of operative risk is a significant part of the surgeon's pre-operative evaluation.
   - Surgical risk is subtle line between the good and bad outcome of surgery. It can only be minimized and can not be entirely eliminated. In poor surgical risk, chances of death or complications are more.
   - Assessment of surgical risk :

S.No.	Surgical risk	Description
1.	Excellent	Surgery will resolve the problem.
2.	Good	High probability of successful outcome and low potential for complications resulting from surgery.
3.	Fair	Serious but manageable problems. Moderate possibilities of complications.
4.	Poor	Unsuccessful outcome of surgery. Significant chances of complications.

   - Major organ systems that influence the degree of operation risk include the cardiovascular, respiration, renal and gastrointestinal system.
   - Clinical or surgical judgment : Judgment means rational analysis which leads to rational decision. It is mainly gained through experience, is inherent in assessing the operative risk. Whether to operate or not and when to operate form the first part of surgical judgment
   - A surgeon should not undertake a surgical procedure that is beyond his capabilities.

3. Patient assessment and preoperative patient stabilization :
   i. *Identification of patient* : e.g. Patient age, breed, sex, body weight, colour etc.
   ii. *History of the patient* : To eliminate the possibility of many diseases.
   iii. Physical status of surgical patient.
   iv. *Laboratory screening* : Pack cell volume, differential leucocyte count, blood urea nitrogen, alkaline phosphatase, SGPT, total plasma proteins, glucose, serum Na, K, Ca, SGOT, SGPT, urinalysis etc.
   v. *Clinical consideration* : Colour of mucous membrane, capillary refill time, rectal temperature, pulse and respiration rate. In febrile state surgery should be postponed. Paracentesis of swellings and cavities aid for diffentral diagnosis in specific cases.
   vi. *Additional tests* : ECG and thoracic radiograph is indicated in vehicle accidents or the patient with preexisting cardiac abnormalities.
   vii. *Physiological consideration.*

Grade	Definition	Example	Prognosis
1	Animals that are clinically healthy or that have only a localized problem without any clinically detectable systemic effects	Elective procedures e.g. castration, ovariohysterectomy, ear trim and caudectomy, minor wound laceration.	Excellent
2	Animal with pre-existing disease that does not interfere with normal activity or cause any systemic effects. i.e. Diseases with mild systemic disturbances	Skin tumour, obesity, simple fracture, minimal pneumothorax, uncomplicated hernias	Excellent
3	Animal with pre-existing disease that is detectable and could affect ability to physiologically respond to a surgical procedure. i.e. Diseases with moderate systemic disturbances	Low fiver, slight to mild dehydration, polydipsia/ polyurea, respiratory distress, anemia, jaundice, weight loss, cardiac murmurs, moderate hypovolemia and occasional arrhythmia.	Good
4	Animal with pre-existing disease with significant disturbance that would be life threatening if not corrected. i.e. Diseases with severe systemic disturbances	Severe dehydration, high fever, significant anemia, uremia, toxemia, cyanosis.	Guarded
5	Animal in a moribund or comatose condition	Patients not expected to live 24 hours with or without surgery.	Poor

A. Blood Transfusion

If the blood loss is significant i.e. packed cell volume (PCV) is less than 25%, blood should be transfused to the animal. Cross matching of the patient and donor blood is recommended for all transfusions, particularly when multiple transfusions are required.

- Patients can be intravenously transfused @ 25 –90 ml/kg body weight over a period of 15-30 minutes.
- Acute hypovolemia and chronic anemia are most commonly encountered blood volume deficits requiring pre-operative management.
- Normal blood volume of the dog and cat is approximately 90 and 70 ml/kg, respectively.
- The most commonly used crystalloid fluid for blood volume support in the hypovolemic patient is lactated Ringer's solution.
- Minimum arterial blood pressure i.e. 70 mm of Hg should be maintained before surgery.
- A PCV of 27-30% and a haemoglobin concentration of at least 7 to 10 gm/dl should be attained in the anemic patient prior to surgery.
- Plasma protein content of 3.5 gram should also be maintained.
- The amount of donor blood needed.

$$\text{Blood needed (ml)} = \text{Recipient's weight (kg)} \times \frac{\text{Desired PCV} - \text{Recipients PCV}}{\text{Donor's PCV}} \times 70 \text{ (cat) or } 90 \text{ (dog)}$$

$$\text{Blood needed (ml)} = \frac{\text{Recipient wt (kg)} \times \text{Hb rise (gm/dl)} \times 70}{\text{Donor's Hb concentration (gm/dl)}}$$

- For each 1% increase in PCV, 2.2 ml whole blood/ kg body weight may be administered.

B. Fluid and Electrolytes Therapy

Surgical patient require a fluid and electrolyte balance before surgery. The volume of fluid administered is the sum of replacement needs and maintenance requirement.

Dehydration may be

i. Isotonic – (the loss of water and sodium are equal) dehydration can be observed in soft tissue injures, intestinal obstruction, peritonitis.

ii. Hypotonic – (loss of sodium is greater than the loss of water) detected in adrenocorticoid insufficiency and when a hypotonic solution is used to treat an isotonic loss.

iii. Hypertonic – (the loss of water is greater than the loss of sodium) detected in diabetes incipidus, hyperosmolar diabetes mellitus and heat stroke.

- Sodium is the major extracellular cation and chloride is the major extracellular anion. Deficits of sodium and chloride are rectified by isotonic electrolyte solution.
- Fluid may be administered @ up to 100ml/kg/hr to hypovolemic patient that do not have cardiovascular disease.
- *Assessment of fluid deficit and dehydration :*
  1. The degree of dehydration is estimated clinically by assessing skin pliability and elasticity (skin turgor or tinting), dryness of oral mucosa, and the amount of ocular orbital depression (sunken eye).
  2. Packed cell volume (PCV) and total plasma protein (TPP) can be used for fluid assessment.
- *Replacement needs :*
  1. Fluid deficit (Liters) = Degree of dehydration (%) x Patient body wt (kg)

     5% : indicating mild degree of dehydration

     12% : approaching shock or death.
  2. Replacement needs (Liter) = Dehydration (%) X b. wt. X 1L + Losses from vomiting and diarrhea + Maintenance (40-60ml/kg b. wt.).
  3. Deficit (m Eq) = 0.3 X b.wt. (kg) X (Desired - Actual)

Body weight loss (%)	**Sunken eye**	**Skin fold test persists for (Seconds)**	**PCV (%)**	**Total serum solids (g/L)**	**Fluid required to replace volume deficit (ml/kg b. wt)**
4-6	Barely detectable	-	40-45	70-80	20-25
6-8	+	2-4	50	80-90	30-50
8-10	++	6-10	55	90-100	50-80
10-12	+++	20-45	60	120	80-120

C. Disturbances in Acid Base Status

The bicarbonate buffer system is used to determine the acid-base status and hence variation in plasma pH, HCO_3^- and $PaCO_2$ constitute disturbances in acid-base balances.

Acidemia : It refers to reduced plasma pH (H^+ >45mEq/L). Sodium bicarbonate therapy should be considered with a marked acidemia (pH < 7.2).

Alkalemia : It refers to increased plasma pH (H^+ <35mEq/L).

Anion gap : Difference between the total concentration of measured cations(Na^+ and K^+) and that of measured anions (Cl^- and HCO_3^-) is known as anion gap. It is helpful in clinical assessment of acid base disorders.

There are four primary disturbances of Acid-base balance.

Respiratory acidosis : Means a primary increase in plasma $PaCO_2$ (>45mm Hg) and a decrease in pH. Respiratory acidosis is caused by CNS diseases, thoracic lesion, lung disease etc. and characterized by hypoventilation. Compensatory response is seen by production of HCO_3^-. The renal mechanism tries to compensate by generating more HCO_3^- and retained by the kidney.

Respiratory alkalosis : Means a primary decrease in plasma $PaCO_2$ (<35mm Hg) and an increase in pH. Respiratory alkalosis is characterized by hyperventilation e.g. exercise, fever, pain, stress (thermal). Carbonic acid decreased in blood and ratio of bicarbonate to carbonic acid is increased which results in elevation of pH. The renal mechanism tries to compensate by increasing the urinary excretion of HCO_3^-.

Metabolic acidosis : If excess of bicarbonates are removed, a primary decrease in plasma HCO_3^- (<22mEq/L) and a decrease in pH is observed. It leads to base deficit or metabolic acidosis. HCO_3^- is removed through kidney or intestine following diarrhea. Metabolic acidosis is associated with hypokalemia. The amount of bicarbonate needed in the treatment of metabolic acidosis is calculated from the base deficit.

$$\text{Base deficit} = \text{Body wt. (kg)} \times 0.3 \times (\text{Desired} - \text{Observed plasma } HCO_3^-)$$

Metabolic alkalosis : Characterized by primary elevation of HCO_3^- (>33mEq/L) and increase in pH with reciprocal reduction in plasma chloride. This may occur due to excessive vomiting (loss of H^+) or an excessive intake of $NaHCO_3^-$.

Nutritional Status

- The daily maintenance caloric requirement of the normal adult dog ranges between 66-110 K Cal/kg b.wt.
- Normal gastric volume of the dog is 10-20 ml/kg.

Pre-operative Antibiotics (Antibiotic umbrella)

- Use of prophylactic preoperative antibiotics is known as antibiotic umbrella. However, their use should not be considered a substitute for good surgical technique.

Special Consideration

a. Cardiovascular System

- Cardiac murmur, jugular pulse, ascites, pulse deficit and resting heart rate below 70 or above 160 beats/minute may cause suspicion.
- Electrocardiographic examination should be done to evaluate the heart and a thoracic radiographic examination to evaluate pulmonary vasculature, lung parenchyma and heart size.
- Great Dane has a high incidence of cardiomyopathy.

b. Respiratory System

Evaluation of patients with respiratory disease is limited to radiographic examination of the thorax and arterial-blood gas analysis (O_2 and CO_2).

c. Urinary System

- Blood urea nitrogen (BUN) and complete urinalysis, should be done.
- Serum creatinine concentration is a better indicator of GFR.
- Urine specific gravity is also an important indicator of kidney function.
- Urine specific gravity of 1.008–1.012 indicate the early sign of renal failure without significant BUN elevation.

d. Musculoskeletal System

- A complete neurological examination must be conducted to detect possible peripheral or spinal cord trauma, especially in those patients with distal humeral (radial nerve) or pelvic (nerves from lumbo-sacral plexus) fractures.
- Urinary bladder ruptures and urethral tears must be ruled out.
- If a urinary bladder or tear urethral is suspected, a positive contrast urethrogram and cystogram should be performed.

Preparation of Surgical Patient

Dietary Restrictions

- In small animals food intake is generally restricted 6 to 12 hours prior to anesthesia. Water is generally allowed until the anesthetic premeditation is administered.
- Withholding of food for 24-48 hours and water for 6 to12 hours is usually sufficient in large ruminants. The use of purgatives to empty the bowel is not generally recommended in ruminants.

Excretions

- Enemas can be given every two hours up to 1 h before surgery.

Surgical site preparation : it entails

1. Hair removal
2. Skin antisepsis
3. Proper surgical draping

1. Hair Removal

This procedure should be performed in the patient preparation room.

- The animal should be cleaned to remove hair, debris, dust and external parasites and washed with soap and water.
- Hair removal enhances the removal of pathogens.
- Increases visibility at the surgical site.
- Improves skin apposition during closure.
- Decreases the foreign material deposition at the surgical wound.
- A general guideline is to clip 20 cm on each side of the incision to allow for extension of the incision during surgery.
- Dull blades may pull hair out of their follicles and cause what is commonly called *clipper burn.*
- Open wounds should be covered with saline moistened gauze to minimize wound contamination with loose hair or debris.
- Increase in interval between hair removal and surgery increases the incidence of post surgical wound infections. So the hairs should be removed immediately before surgery.
- Methods of hair removal are clipping, shaving and depilators. Clipping causes least trauma. Depilators are rarely used because of their expense and poor action on the animal hair.

2. Skin Preparation

- After removal of hair the operative site should be scrubbed vigorously using centrifugal technique at least 4 times with an antiseptic solution like savlon (1 :30) or chlorxylenol (1 :4 dilution).
- Commonly used scrubbing solutions are hexachlorophene, iodophors (povidone iodine), chlorhexidine, alcohols and quaternary ammonium salts.
- Povidone iodine is not effective against *clostridium* spp.
- Resident canine skin flora (live on superficial cornified layers and outer hair follicles) – *Staphylococcus epidermidis, Corynebacterium* spp., *Pityrosporon* spp.
- Transient bacteria (secondary invaders) can not multiply on skin– *Staphylococcus aureus, E. coli, Streptococcus* spp., *Enterobacter* spp., *Clostridium* spp.

3. Draping

The purpose of drapes is to create and maintain a sterile field around the operative site during surgery.

- Drapes should be placed at the junction of clipped and non-clipped area.
- The draping material must remain impermeable.
- Both reusable and disposable drapes are used in veterinary surgery.
- Polyethylene adhesive incise drapes are useful where extensive lavage is required.
- Orthopaedic stockinetes : If access to the animals paw is not required, it should be covered by orthopaedic stockinet to prevent gross contamination of the surgical site.

Preparation of Surgical Team

- Scrub suits.
- Surgical head covers – to cover the hair to prevent falling of dust and sweat from the head.
- Shoe covers – exclude bacteria from street shoes.
- Face masks – major function is to protect the wound from droplets of saliva expelled by the surgical team members when talking.

- Surgical gowns.
- Surgical gloves.
- Finger nails should always be short and free from dirt.
- Routinely, 7 to 10 minutes thorough scrubbing of hands and arms with liquid soap followed by a rinse in an antiseptic solution is usually sufficient.
- Three surgical scrub solutions used are hexachlorophene, povidone-iodine and chlorhexidine gluconate.

Intra-operative Consideration

- Blood pressure monitoring either by direct monitoring (by catheterization of artery connected to a aneroid manometer) or by indirect monitoring (doppler ultrasonography and oscillometery).
- *Measurement of heart rate* : Heart rate should be monitored at regular interval because it varies during operation. This variation may be due to anesthetic used and the surgical procedure.
- Regular monitoring of heart and lung sounds is essential. These sounds can be noted by esophageal and precordial stethoscopes. Esophageal stethoscope can be made by attaching a ryle's tube at the place of chest piece of a normal stethoscope. This ryles tube is placed in to the esophagus up to the level of the base of the heart.
- *Pulse oximetery* : It gives extra strength to the anesthetist. Percent saturation of the hemoglobin by oxygen is displayed on the screen.

Post-operative Consideration

- The patient should be closely watched till recovery from anesthesia. Recovery from anesthesia can be hastened by warming the animal either by blankets or by administration of warm intravenous fluids.
- Animal should always be extubated as laryngeal reflexes return to maintain a patent airway. If the animal regurgitated during anesthesia, the laryngeal area should be evacuated before extubation.
- Administration of analgesics specially the opioid analgesics which also decrease the cough reflexes.
- The patient should be kept in clean areas.
- Clinical parameters should be noted routinely

- Rectal temperature, respiration rate, pulse rate.
- Appetite, condition of the operative site

- Daily dressing of the surgical wound.
- The sutures or dressing should be protected by Elizabeth collar or side stick.
- Laxative diet, rest, parentral fluid for 3-4 days.
- Antibiotic therapy
- In case of dehydration - fluid therapy
- Skin sutures generally removed 8 to 10 days after complete healing has taken place.

Chapter 3

Sterilization

Sterilization is a process of killing all microorganisms, including bacteria, fungi and their spores, and viruses from animate or inanimate surfaces with the use of either physical or chemical agents. Joseph Lister first gave antiseptic principle in 1867.

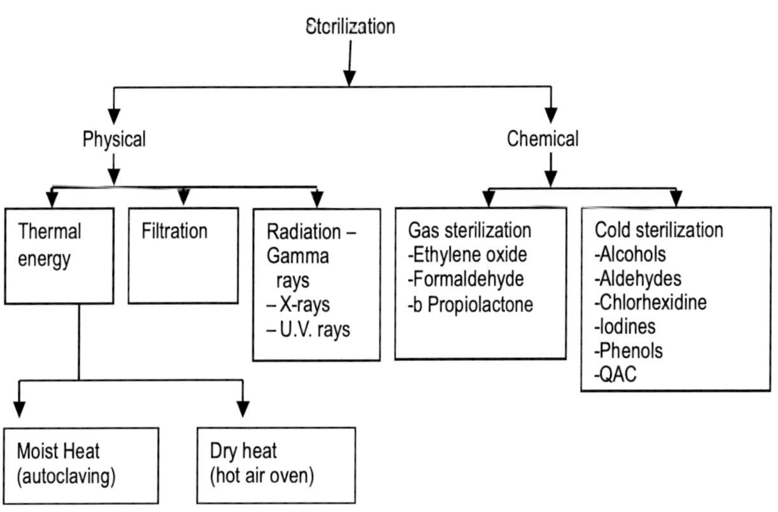

A. Physical Sterilization

Thermal energy, filtration and radiation are the most commonly used physical methods of sterilization.

1. Sterilization by Thermal Energy

It causes denaturation or destruction of cellular proteins of microorganism. Moist heat causes death by coagulation of cellular proteins where as death by dry heat is primarily an oxidation process.

i. Moist Heat/ Steam Under Pressure (Autoclaving)

- More reliable because of its power of penetration, antimicrobial efficiency, ease of control and economy of operation.
- Materials are autoclaved at 121°C under 15 pounds pressure for 30 minutes.
- In emergency 100°C for 10-15 minutes.
- 2% sodium carbonate (Na_2CO_3) (washing soda) or 0.1% sodium hydroxide (NaOH) is added to water used for sterilization. Use of these chemicals has the following advantage:
    a. Both the chemicals slightly raise the boiling point of water hence used at high altitude.
    b. Spores show maximum resistance to heat at neutral pH. Increased acidity and alkalinity decreases this resistance.
    c. It also reduces blunting and rusting of instruments.

Preparation of Surgical Pack

- Proper cleaning of surgical supplies prior to sterilization.
    1. By manual cleaning with moderately alkaline low sudsing detergents.
    2. By ultrasonic cleaners.
- All the towels gowns etc. must be folded as accordion fashion.
- Locks and joints of instruments should be opened.
- Instruments must be free from oil and grease.
- Instrument packs are positioned vertically and longitudinally in the autoclave/sterilizer.
- *Indicators of sterilization* : Colour change at certain temperature

i. *Chemical indicators:* paper strips.

ii. *Biological indictor:* Heat resistant organism that is many more times resistant to the sterilization process than the organisms likely to be present as natural contaminant e.g. spores of *Bacillus stearothermophilus*.

- Sterile packs should be stored in closed cabinets or shelves to increase shelf life of the pack.
- Sterilized pack wrapped in a double layer of muslin pack (four layer of muslin) remains sterilized on open shelves for 3 weeks and in closed cabinets for 7 weeks.
- Sterilized pack should be dated and periodically resterilized if unused.
- In absence of autoclave pressure cooker can be used for 45 minutes.

ii. Dry Heat Sterilization

Dry heat sterilization is commonly used for glassware or materials that resist penetration by steam, such as petroleum jelly, fats and oils, powders and sealed containers etc.

- This method includes direct exposure of instruments to flame and the use of hot air oven.
- Destroys microbes by oxidation process.
- Is a slow process and long exposure time at a high temperature is required as spores are relatively resistant to dry heat.

  170°C - 40 minutes

  160°C - 60 minutes
- Selection of temperature depends upon the resistance of material to heat.

2. Sterilization by Filtration

The mechanism by which microorganisms or other particles are removed from filtered materials depends on the filter type.

1. Screen filters - Collects all particles larger than their pore size on the surface of the filter.
2. Depth filters - are composed of matrix of porous materials. Microorganism retained by these filters may be much smaller than the pore size of the filter e.g. Pharmaceuticals are commonly sterilized by filtration.

3. Sterilization by Radiation

Gamma, X-rays and ultra violet rays are used for sterilization. Certain chemicals sensitive to heat or chemicals are sterilized by radiation.

- Radiation kills organisms by producing ionization in or near the organism.
- Because of heat sensitization, many pharmaceuticals are sterilized by this method
- Surgical materials such as tissues grafts are sterilized by gamma radiation.
- Non-ionizing radiation e.g. ultra violet radiation (Generated by germicidal lamp) is used to destroy airborne microorganisms in operation theatres.
- Used to sterilize repacked items like disposable syringes, catheters, endotrachial tubes, intravenous sets etc.

B. Chemical Sterilization

Chemical sterilization refers to the use of gaseous or liquid chemicals. Chemical methods of sterilization were developed to sterilize materials that are damaged by wet or dry heat.

1. Gas Sterilization

Gas sterilization is used for delicate surgical instruments, rubber or plastic tubing, plastic syringes, hypodermic needles etc. The common gaseous agents used for sterilization are

i. Ethylene oxide
ii. Formaldehyde
iii. β-Propiolactone

Ethylene Oxide

- Capable of destroying all known microorganisms including bacteria virus, spores, fungi by alkylation.
- The effectiveness of ethylene oxide depends on

1. Gas concentration- 450–1500 mg/L
2. Temperature - 21-60°C
3. Exposure time - 48 minutes to several hours

   i. 12 h at room temperature
   ii. 4 h at 55°C

4. Relative humidity – Moisture in necessary for lethal action.
   i. Optimum relative humidity is ≈ 40%
   ii. Minimum relative humidity is 33%
   - Sterilization by using ethylene oxide can be considered as an alterative to autoclaving but is expensive.
   - Sterilization indicators are spores of *Bacillus subtilis var. globigii* because these spores are more resistant to ethylene oxide than other organisms.
   - Ethylene oxide is toxic and irritating to skin and mucous membrane.
   - Continued exposure leads to olfactory fatigue.
   - Clinical sign of human toxicity are nausea, vomiting and mental disorientation.
   - Any object, especially made from polyvinyl chloride, previously sterilized by radiation should not be resterilized with ethylene oxide as this may result in the formation of highly toxic ethylene chlorhydrins.

Formaldehyde

- 1-2% vegetative bacteria are killed in 1-2 h.
- Up to 12 h is required to kill bacterial spores.
- After sterilization with formaldehyde, prolonged airing is necessary.
- Formaldehyde is highly irritating so instruments sterilized by this method must be rinsed in sterile normal saline before use.
- It is used to sterilize surgical equipments and bedding.
- 2% Glutaraldehyde also used for sterilization.

β-Propiolactone

- Used to sterilize hospital room and animal housing buildings.
- Acts more rapidly than does either ethylene oxide or formaldehyde.
- *Disadvantages*
  i. It damage painted and plastic surface.
  ii. Highly toxic and carcinogenic.

2. Cold Sterilization

- Cold sterilization refers to the soaking of instruments in disinfectant solutions.

- A disinfectant is an agent which destroys pathogenic organism on inanimate objects.
- Not effective against tubercle bacillus.
- Spores and viruses may not be destroyed. For this reason critical instruments should not be sterilized by this method.
- It is recommended that $NaNO_2$ (4g/L) should be added to the sterilizing solution to prevent rusting of instruments.
- Commercially prepared disinfectant solution are Cidex and Sterisol.
- For disinfection of endotracheal tubes, plastic sheets and drainage catheters.

Commonly Used Cold Sterilants

Alcohols

- Ethyl alcohol and isopropyl alcohol kills bacteria by the *coagulation* of protein.
- 70% ethyl or isopropyl alcohol has maximum germicidal action because of presence of water which easily denaturates the protein. So 70% alcohol is more germicidal than absolute alcohol.
- Isopropyl alcohol is more bactericidal than ethyl alcohol but former is more irritating to the skin.
- Alcohols are slightly less effective than chlorhexidine or povidone iodine.
- Repeated use of alcohols causes skin irritation and application to open wounds causes necrosis.

Aldehydes

- Formaldehyde is available as formalin (37% solution of formaldehyde and water).
- Kills all bacteria virus and spores.
- Extremely irritating to skin and mucous membrane
- Glutaraldehyde in dilute concentration is less toxic than formaldehyde
- Liquid disinfectant of choice for lenses instruments.

Chlorhexidine

- Available in detergent, tincture and aqueous formulations.
- Because of non-irritating nature to skin. It is used for the preparation of surgical site and for surgical hand scrubs.

- This agent possesses residual activity, and its effectiveness increases after repeated use.
- Chlorhexidine is not effective against some pseudomonas species.
- Chlorhexidine remains effective in the presence of organic material, alcohol and soaps.
- Prolonged use may cause photosensivity.

Iodines

- Good bactericidal, viricidal but poor sporicidal activity (hence not effective against clostridium).
- Iodine acts by binding to bacterial cell wall, forming reactive ions and protein complexes.
- Effectiveness is reduced by the presence of organic materials like blood, necrotic debris etc.
- Concentration greater than 3.5% is toxic to tissue.
- Iodophors are iodine that is complexed with organic molecules such as detergents.
- Free iodine released from the carrier molecules act as disinfectant.
- *Disadvantages*
  i. They corrode instruments.
  ii. Contact dermatitis
  iii. Hyperthyroidism

Phenols

- Oldest known germicidal agent.
- Phenols - cresols (general disinfectants)
- Phenols – bis phenols (Antiseptics)

Quaternary Ammonium Compounds

- Benzalkonium chloride is synthetic cationic detergent.
- Surface-active agents that dissolve lipids in bacterial cell walls and membranes.
- Inactive in the presence of organic material.
- Disadvantage includes neurotoxicity.

Hexachlorophene

- It inhibits bacterial membrane enzyme system.
- Bacteriostatic for gram +ve but inactive against gram –ve and spores.
- Repeated use may promote the growth of gram –ve bacteria.
- Hexachlorophene is inactivated by organic material and alcohols.
- Disadvantage includes skin ulceration.

Antibacterial spectrum of some disinfectants

	Bactericidal	Viricidal	Sporicidal
Aldehyde	+	+	+
Iodine	Kills 99% of bacteria within 30 seconds of application	+	When contact time is greater than 15 minutes.
Alcohol	+	Poor activity	-
Chlorhexidine	Kills 99% of bacteria within 30 seconds of application	Minimal activity	Minimal activity
Phenol	+	-	-
Q.A.C.	+	-	-

Sepsis : rottening or putrefaction is called sepsis.

Asepsis : means a state of being sterile.

Antiseptics : is a chemical agent that either kills pathogenic microorganisms or inhibits their growth as long as there is contact between agent and microbe.

Disinfectant : is a germicidal chemical substance that kills microorganisms on inanimate objects, such as instruments and other equipments that cannot be exposed to heat.

Asepsis and antiseptics : Prevention of wound contamination by bacteria rather than killing of bacteria after they have entered the wound.

On the basis of risk of infection after the use of surgical instruments and equipments, these materials can be classified in to three categories.

i. *Critical items* : The items that are introduced in to the body for therapeutic purposes. The risk of infection is more. Critical items must be sterile. e.g. surgical pack instruments, surgical drains etc.

ii. *Semi critical items* : The item comes in direct contact with mucous mumbrances but the body has barrier to infection. These items should be disinfected routinely to kill all live microorganisms. e.g. thermometers, vaginal speculum, endotracheal tubes, esophageal stethoscope etc.

iii. *Non-critical items* : The items which do not come in direct contact with the patient e.g. face masks, rebreathing bags. Those must be clean and uncontaminated.

Nosocomial Infections : The infections acquired during the course of hospitalization e.g. primary and secondary surgical wound infections.

- The nosocomial pathogens (bacteria, virus, fungi etc.) are transmitted through contact between animals, between hospital staff and animals or through contaminated vehicles.
- Risk of nosocomial infection increases
  - i. Duration of hospital stay increases.
  - ii. Chronic illness in neonates or geriatric animals.
  - iii. If invasive procedures and devices like drains, catheters, tubes etc. are used.
- Nosocomial infection can be controlled by
  - i. Proper cleaning of hands before and after examination/treatment of the animal.
  - ii. Isolation of immune compromised animals and animals that are reservoir of potential nosocomial organisms.
  - iii. A routine surveillance of the hospital should be done to recognize infections in the environment and in hospitalized animals.
  - iv. Hospital equipments should be cleaned and sterilized/disinfected properly.

Chapter 4

Suture Materials and Suture Patterns

Sutures or surgical threads : means a material used to hold the edges of tissue in close approximation.

Objectives

1. To facilitate healing.
2. Haemostatic.
3. To retain drainage tube and implants.
4. To reduce the size of natural opening.

Qualities of An Ideal Suture Material

1. It should be non-antigenic, nontoxic and non-carcinogenic.
2. It should have mono-filamentous texture.
3. It should have no capillary property.
4. It should have adequate tensile strength *in-vitro* and *in-vivo.*
5. It should have good handling property.
6. It should have good knot security.
7. It should be compatible with all kinds of antiseptic disinfectants.

8. It should be easily sterilizable.
9. It should remain intact until union occurs.
10. It should have minimum tissue reaction.
11. It should be cheap and easily available.

Polydioxanoe (monofilament synthetic absorbable) fulfills most of the qualities mentioned above.

Classification : On the basis of absorption in to the body tissue.

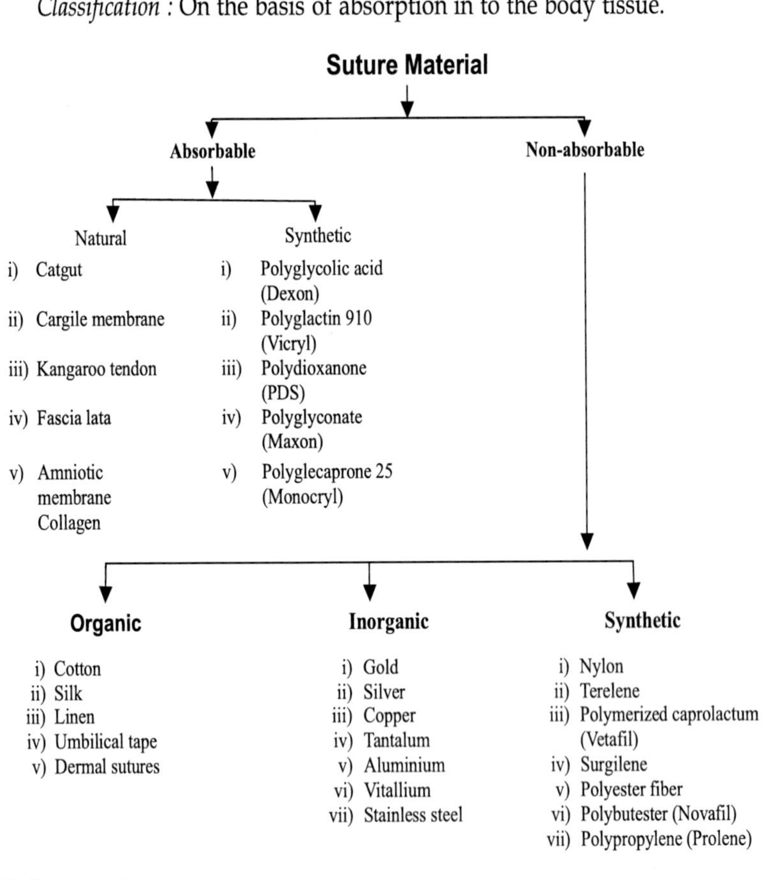

A. Absorbable

Absorbed in the tissue/body.

- Organic in nature.
- Absorbed into the body tissues after a variable period of time.
- Absorption takes places by phagocytosis and enzymatic reaction.
- Mostly used to close the internal organs e.g. (surgical gut).

Natural Absorbable

1. Surgical gut or Catgut [Kit gut – string of a fiddle (violin)]

- Obtained either from sub mucosa of small intestine of ovine (sheep) or the serous layer of bovine small intestine (99% collagen).
- Catgut is composed of formaldehyde treated collagen fibers. Absorption time can also be delayed by treatment with chromic acid, iodine and tannins.
- Sterilized by ionizing radiation or by ethylene oxide. Ethylene oxide prolongs its absorption time. It cannot be autoclaved.
- Catgut is classified by its degree of chromicization or tanning to lengthen absorption time, to increase its tensile strength and to reduce the intensity of soft tissue reaction to the gut.
- Disadvantages of catgut include local antigen-antibody reaction and capillary property.
- Surgical gut is available in USP size 3 (the heaviest) to 7-0 (thinnest).

Type	Chrome treatment	Absorption time
A	Plain or untreated	5 (3-8 days)
B	Mild chromic treatment	10
C	Medium chromic treatment	20
D	Extra chromic treatment	40

Size of catgut	Outer diameter (mm)
4/0	0.203
3/0	0.254
2/0	0.330
1/0	0.406
1	0.483
2	0.559
3	0.635
4	0.711
5	0.813
6	0.914
7	1.016

2. Cargile Membrance

Derived from sub mucosa of bovine caecum and used to cover surfaces from which peritoneum, pleura etc. have been removed. It is rarely used today and is replaced by prolene mesh.

3. Kangaroo Tendon

Obtained from tendon of tail tendon of kangaroo and used for suturing hernial rings, joint capsules. The main advantage was its high tensile strength.

4. Fascia Lata

Obtained from bovine tensor fascia lata and tensor fascia antibrachii (thigh muscles).

5. Amniotic Membrane

Used to repair the gap of body.

6. Collagen

Multifilament suture material procured from the bovine flexor tendon or tendoachilles of beef cattle.

- Absorption is completed within 60 days.
- It is available in plain and chromic form.
- Tissue reaction is less in comparison to catgut and is used in ocular surgery.

Synthetic absorbable : Sterilized by ethylene oxide, since gamma radiation causes loss in tensile strength.

1. Polyglycolic Acid (Dexon)

It is braided multifilament, polymer of glycolide or glycolic acid.

- It lost all tensile strength in 30 days and completely absorbed in 120 days.
- Absorbed by hydrolysis and digestion.

2. Polyglactin 910 (Vicryl)

- It is the braided multifilament polymer of glycolide (glycolic acid) and lactide (lactic acid) (9:1).
- Lost all tensile strength in 32 days and completely absorbed in 70 days.
- Absorbed by hydrolysis (hydrolysis increased in alkaline environment).

- Stable in contaminated wound.
- Used in ocular surgery and closing the muscles.

3. Polydioxanone (PDS)

Homopolymer of p-dioxanone

- It is a monofilament suture material.
- Lost all tensile strength in 56 days and completely absorbed in 180 days.
- It is more flexible than dexon and vicryl.
- It elicits minimal tissue reaction and is absorbed by hydrolysis.
- It can be used in slower healing tissues like tendon and ligaments.

4. Polyglyconate (Maxon)

- It is copolymer of glycolic acid and trimethylene carbonate (32.5%).
- It is an absorbable monofilament suture that has properties similar to polydioxanone (PDS).
- Its strength is superior to that of polyglactin 910 and polydioxanone.
- It has increased tissue drag relative to polypropylene.
- It is stable in the presence of gastric juices and is appropriate for use in gastric surgery.
- Now polyglyconate is investigated for use in the development of absorbable plates and screws alleviating the need for implant removal.
- It has high tensile strength, good knot security and good handling characterstic.
- It is better for tenorrhaphy as compared to other absorbable suturing materials.
- It retains strength up to 4 weeks after implantation.

5. Polyglecaprone 25 (Monocryl)

- It has initial tensile strength superior to that of polyglyconate.
- It is more pliable than polyglyconate, polydioxanone and gut.
- It has less tissue drag than gut.
- It shows strong initial tensile strength but is absorbed faster than polyglactin 910 and polydioxanone.

- It maintains only 20-30% of its initial tensile strength two weeks after implantation.
- Monocryl is mainly used in bladder surgery.
- It is not indicated in gastrointestinal surgery because of rapid loss of tensile strength.

B. Non-Absorbable

They are encysted if buried in the tissues.

a) Organic

1. Cotton

- Its tensile strength and knot security is more when wet.
- Can be sterilized by autoclaving or by chemical means.
- It causes tissue reaction like silk and linen.
- It is weaker as compared to linen
- Disadvantage includes capillarity, tissue reaction and ability to potentiate infection.

2. Silk

- Obtained from cocoon of silk worm.
- Its natural capillarity is decreased by treating it with oil, wax or silicone.
- It has high tensile strength which is lost after 2 years.
- Available as monofilament and braided multifilament.
- Sterilized by autoclaving or by gamma radiation.
- More tissue reaction (silk + gamma globulin (=) acute Inflammation). Encapsulation of the silk with a fibrous capsule usually occurs in 14-21 days
- Should not be used in contaminated wound.
- Degraded by mechanical fragmentation and phagocytosis. Absorption time is >120 days.

3. Linen

- Obtained from flax and composed of cellulose.
- It is available in braided/twisted form.
- Tissue reaction is similar to silk.

- It gains 10% in tensile strength when wet.
- It has excellent knotting property and used for ligatures.
- Pagenstecher's linen – linen thread impregnated with celluloid.

4. Umbilical Tape

It is a cotton tape suture and used to tie the umbilical cord of the new born or as vulvar sutures in cases of prolapsed vagina or uterus.

5. Dermal Sutures

Silk coated with tanned gelatin mostly used in plastic surgery.

b) Inorganic

1. Tantalum

- Inert and is available in monofilament or multifilament forms.

2. Silver

- Ionized in tissues and can cause inflammation.

3. Metal Clip

- To hold the skin in apposition over flat surfaces e.g. Michel wound clips.

4. Stainless Steel

- Introduced in 1934 by Babcock.
- Inert and available as simple or twisted.
- Highest tensile strength and greatest knot security.
- Used to hold slow healing tissues like ligaments, tendons and bones.
- Poor handling quality, tendency to cut through the tissues and broken if kinked and barbs on the end can tear gloves.

c) Synthetic

1. Nylon (Polyamide)

- It is obtained from Hexamethylenediamine and adipic acid.
- Mono or braided multifilament.
- Stimulates minimal tissue reaction.
- Not used within serous or synovial cavity.
- Poor handling and knot security.
- Degrades 15% per year in tissues (chemical degradation).
- Loss of tensile strength occurs after 2 years.

2. Polymerized Caprolactum (Vetafil)

- Polyamide polymer.
- Twisted, non irritant suture.
- Available in 0.3 mm (00), 0.4 mm (0 or heavy), 0.6 mm (extra heavy) and 1.1 mm (special size).

3. Srugilene

- Polypropylene monofilament.

4. Polyester Fiber (Terylene and Dacron)

- Multifilament braided suture and available in plain and coated form.
- Polyester fibers have high tensile strength hence it is the suture of choice in cardiovascular surgery.
- It has a tendency to cut through the tissues. Teflon, silicon, polybutylate or polytetrafluoroethylene (PTFE) coating made the suture material smooth to reduce drag (friction).
- PTFE coating caused flaking in the tissue. However, polypropylene bonds well with the suture. Thus minimizing flaking in the tissues.
- Suitable for skin and cardiovascular surgery.
- High tissue reaction and poor knot security.
- Polyester fiber is available as eyeless needled sutures, prosthesis and mesh.

5. Polybutester (Novafil)

- Copolymer of polybutylene and polytetramethylene. Good for plastic surgery.

6. Polypropylene (Prolene)

- Monofilament polymers of propylene
- It has an extremely high tensile strength and extremely low tissue reaction.
- It has good handling and knotting property.
- It can be sterilized by ethylene oxide.
- It can be used on skin, cardiac muscles and infected wounds.
- It is available as sutures and as mesh for hernia repair, closure of abdominal wall defects.

7. Polyethylene (Ticron)

- Polymerized ethylene.
- It incites minimal tissue reaction.
- It can be autoclaved with least loss of tensile strength.

Sterilization Characteristics of Suture Material

- Autoclaving is safe, if done not more than 3 times, on polyester, nylon, polypropylene and stainless steel. More autoclaving reduces the strength of suture material.
- Steam sterilization is contraindicated for catgut, collagen, fascia lata, polyethylene and polyglycolic acid.
- Gamma-irradiation damages poly glycolic acid, polypropylene, linen and cotton but is acceptable for surgical gut, silk, polyester, nylon and polyethylene, if not repeated more than once.
- Ethylene oxide is safe for all sutures.

Basic Principles of Suturing

- Approximation of cuts edges with least trauma
- Gentle handling of tissues.
- Small size needles and suture material should be used as far as possible.
- The stitches should be little away from incision line.
- The stitches should not be tied tightly.
- Minimal tissue tension and dead space should be obliterated.

Suture Techniques

A. Interrupted Pattern

- Whole suture line is interrupted at many places by multiple sutures.
- Knotting is done for every individual suture.
- Time consuming and requires more suture material.

1. Simple Interrupted Suture

- Commonly used when excessive tension over the entire suture line is not expected.
- A distance of about 1-1.25 cm is usually left between individual stitches in large animals and 0.5 cm in small animals (Fig. 4.1).
- More time consuming and leaves 'rail road track' scar on the skin surface.

2. Interrupted Cruciate or Cross Mattress Suture

- Applied on skin especially on amputated tail stump and digits. Stronger then interrupted (Fig. 4.2).

3. Horizontal Mattress Suture

- Suture line is horizontal to the line of incision (Fig. 4.3).
- Horizontal mattress suture can be applied on skin, muscle, etc.
- Main disadvantages :
  - i. Greater scar formation and delayed healing as a result of eversion
  - ii. During its removal extra cutaneous part of the thread runs subcutaneous which may leads of infection.

4. Vertical Mattress Suture

- Suture line is perpendicular to the line of incision.
- It is an appositional to eversion type of suture (Fig. 4.4).

5. Near and Far Suture

- Far-Far-Near-Near (Fig. 4.5)
- Far-Near-Near-Far (Fig. 4.6)
- No tension on wound edges
- Applied on skin, subcutaneous fascia etc.

6. Quill Sutures

- Modified interrupted vertical mattress sutures causing eversion.
- A plastic or rubber tube is introduced under each loop of vertical mattress sutures on other side external to skin edges (Fig. 4.7).
- Applied on the skin which is under tension to avoided tissue damage.

7. Gambee Sutures

- Gambee sutures are applied for suturing the intestine.
- It is a simple interrupted suture pattern that penetrates the lumen and passes through a small segment of the mucosa submucosa of the same side. The suture then penetrates the submucosa, mucosa toward lumen of the other side and finally comes out through the serosal surface. The knot is fixed outside the lumen (Fig. 4.8).

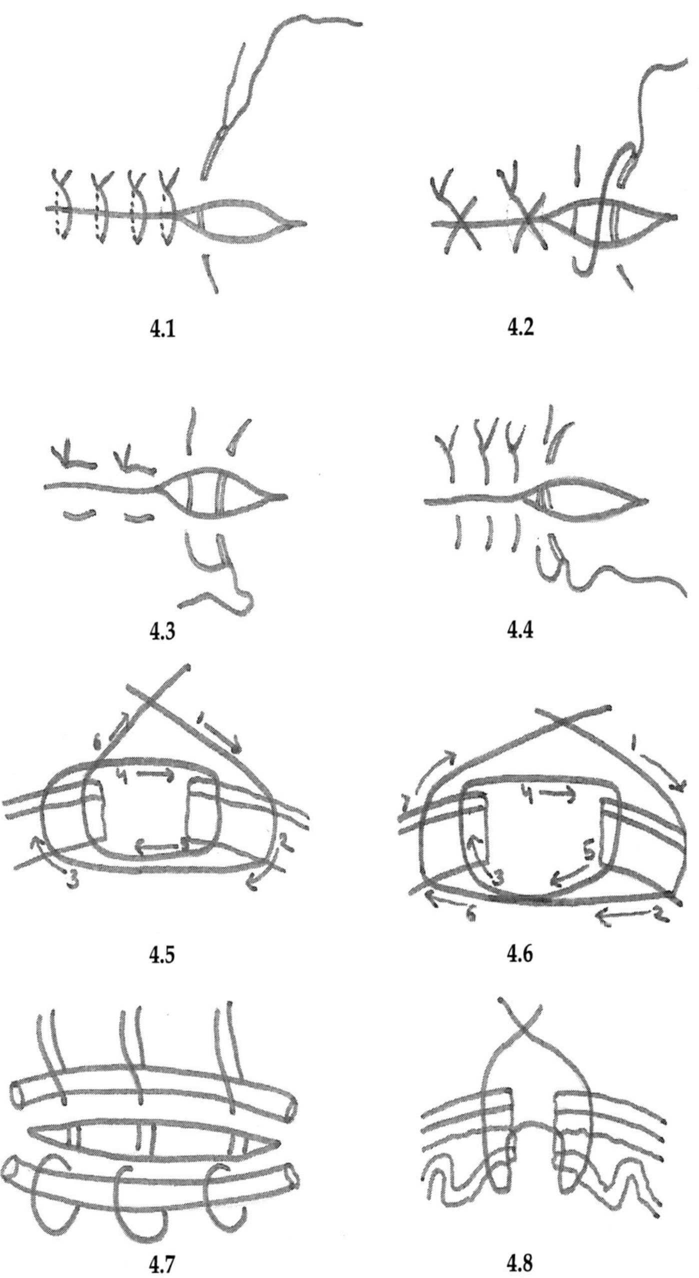

Figures of Interrupted suture pattern : Fig. 4.1: Simple interrupted suture pattern; **4.2:** Interrupted cruciate; **4.3:** Horizontal mattress; **4.4:** Vertical mattress; **4.5:** Far-Far-Near-Near; **4.6:** Far-Near-Near-Far; **4.7:** Quill sutures; **4.8:** Gambee sutures.

B. Continuous Pattern

Requires less suture material, less time consuming and easy to remove. The major disadvantages are:

- A break at any point along the suture line resulting in to total disruption.
- If suture material is of capillary nature and get infected at one place, It will spread to whole suture line. Therefore, It should never be applied for skin closure except in cosmetic ear cropping in dogs.

1. Simple Continuous Suture

- Simple continuous suture pattern is used to suture subcutaneous fascia, muscles etc.
- This suture pattern is started by interrupted suture pattern.
- Subsequent bites are taken perpendicular to the incision line.
- The suture pattern is ended by holding one end of the suture material and then the knot is tied in between the loop and the free end together (Fig. 4.9).

2. Lock Stitch Suture

This suture pattern is also known as Ford interlocking suture or Glover's suture or Blanket sutures.

- Pattern is similar to simple continuous except that the suture material is placed through the loose loop before tightening (Fig. 4.10).
- Disadvantage - more quantity of suture material needed.
- Usually used on skeletal muscles, diaphragm, esophagus.

3. Subcuticular Suture

The suture is placed in subcutaneous tissue only to bring the wound edges in close approximation (Fig. 4.11).

4. Schmieden's Suture

This suture pattern is used for speedy anastomosis of intestine. This method is indicated for quick 1st layer closure of the defect only. It produces inverting effect on wound edges. The bite is made from within outside the lumen of the organ (Fig. 4.12). This technique is not a routine method of closure of hollow visceral organs.

5. Running Suture

This suture pattern is similar to simple continuous suture except that the bites are taken diagonal to the wound edges. This pattern is used for speedy closure of long incision (Fig. 4.13).

(C) Purse String Suture

The suture is used to narrow down the lumen of hollow organs and also to constrict the anal opening after reducing rectal prolapse. For later procedure, the bites are taken at 12, 3, 6 and 9 O' clock position. Both the free ends are tied (Fig. 4.14). This procedure can also be used to secure catheters in position.

Sutures Patterns for Hollow Visceral Organs

Depending on number of tissue layers penetrated by the needles, hollow visceral organ sutures may be classified into two categories:

1. *Seromuscular or intramural* : The needle penetrates only superficial walls i.e. up to submucosa.
2. *Seromucosal* : The needle penetrates all 4 layers (serosa, muscle layer, submucosa and mucosa) and lumen.

1. Seromuscular: (Inverting Suture Pattern)

- Lembert's suture pattern (Fig. 4.15).
- Cushing's suture pattern
- Halsted's inverting suture pattern - modification, lembert and horizontal mattress sutures.
- Czerney suture pattern or Double Lambert's suture pattern

2. Seromucosal

- Jobert's suture pattern (Lembert's suture pattern+ mucosa)
- Connel's suture pattern (Cushing's suture pattern + mucosa)
- Schmieden's suture pattern -end to end anastamosis (Fig. 4.16)

Principles of Hollow Visceral Organ Suturing

1. Preferably three or at least two layer closure should be performed.
2. The first layer may be seromuscular or seromucosal but the second and third layer should always be of seromuscular type.
3. Swaged or eyeless needle should be used for suturing.

4. Inversion should be minimum, to avoid postoperative stricture and stenosis of lumen.
5. Non-reactive absorbable suture material should be preferred.

Classification : The suture pattern can be classified into:

1. Apposition Sutures

a. Simple interrupted suture pattern
b. Simple continuous suture pattern
c. Continuous lockstitch suture pattern
d. Subcuticular suture pattern
e. Pin sutures

2. Inversion Sutures

a. Lembert's suture pattern
b. Czerny's suture pattern
c. Jobert's suture pattern
d. Cushing's suture pattern
e. Connell suture pattern
f. Schmieden's suture pattern

3. Eversion Sutures

a. Horizontal mattress suture pattern
b. Vertical mattress suture pattern

4. Relaxation Sutures

a. Quill sutures
b. Button sutures
c. Near and far sutures

5. Miscellaneous Sutures

a. Purse string suture
b. Buhner's suture
c. Stay sutures etc.

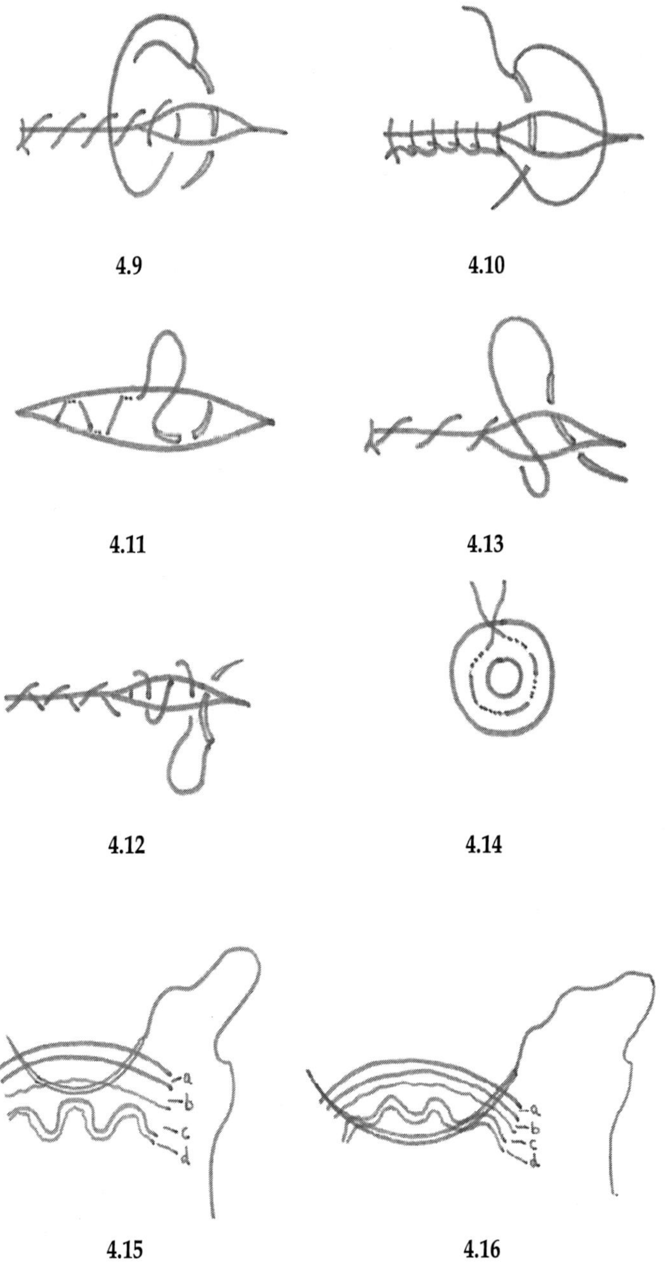

Figures of Continuous suture pattern: Fig. 4.9: Simple continous suture; **4.10:** Lock stitch suture; **4.11:** Subcuticular sutue; **4.12:** Schmieden's suture; **4.13:** Running suture; **4.14 :** Purse string suture; **4.15:** Seromuscular or intramural suture; **4.16 :** Seromucosal suture.

Suture Pattern for Special Purposes

1. Tenorrhaphy or Tenoanastamosis or Tendon Repair

a. *Technique*

- Three loop pulley tendon pattern: Best for round shape ligaments. (Fig. 4.17)
- Locking loop suture pattern or Kessler pattern: Best for flat tendons. (Fig. 4.18a)
- Double locking loop suture pattern (Fig. 4.18b).
- Krackow suture pattern: Best for flat tendons.
- Bunnel's mayer suture pattern (Fig. 4.19)
- Button hole overlapping suture technique (Fig. 4.20, a & b)
- Hoffa method for shortening tendon. (Fig. 4.21)

b. *Suture materials* : Stainless steel wire, nylon, carbon fiber polypropylene and polyglyconate.

2. Herniorrhaphy or Hernial Ring Repair

a. *Technique* : Vest over pant or overlapping sutures or mayo mattress sutures (Fig. 4.22).

b. *Suture material* : Vetafil (1.1 mm), Silk No.2

3. Intestinal Anastomosis

a. *Technique* : Parker Kerr- Ist layer- Lembert suture pattern IInd layer Cushing's suture pattern

b. *Suture material* : Vicryl or catgut.

4. Blood Vessels Repair

a. *Technique* : Simple continuous suture pattern

b. *Suture material* : Polypropylene is least thrombogenic (2-0 to 6-0), Polytetrafluoroethylene (PTFE), polydioxanone with swaged needle.

5. Neuroanastomosis

a. *Technique* : Simple interrupted suture pattern

b. *Suture material* : Nylon and polypropylene

6. Oesophagus Repair

a. *Technique* : Mucosa – simple continuous suture pattern Muscles – Lock stitch suture pattern.

b. *Suture material* : Silk.

7. Urinary Bladder Repair

a. *Technique* : Bell's suture pattern.

b. *Suture material* : Synthetic absorbable (Polyglycolic acid is not used because it may be absorbed prematurely in urine).

8. Vaginal Prolapse

a. *Technique* : Buhner's suture pattern

b. *Suture material* : Umbilical tape

9. Rectal Prolapse or Operation at Perineum for Making Aseptic Condition

a. *Technique* : Purse string suture pattern

b. *Suture material* : Silk or nylon

- *Retention sutures :* to retain gauze packaging inside a wound cavity.
- *Stay sutures :* to retain gauze packaging on the wound surface.

Suture Pattern for Hollow Visceral Organs

1. *Lembert's suture* : May be interrupted or continuous (Fig. 4.23 and Fig. 4.24)
   - The suture is applied from outside the lumen with the needle passing through the serosal and submucosa and returning through muscularis and serosa to the area outside viscera on the same side of the incision. The needle is then passed across the incision to the opposite side and bites are taken in the same manner.
   - The needle penetrates perpendicular to the incision line.
2. *Cushing's suture* : The suture pattern is similar to lembert's suture. The difference is that
   - In this pattern the bite runs parallel to the incision line (Fig. 4.25).
   - Less inversion as compared to Lembert's sutures.

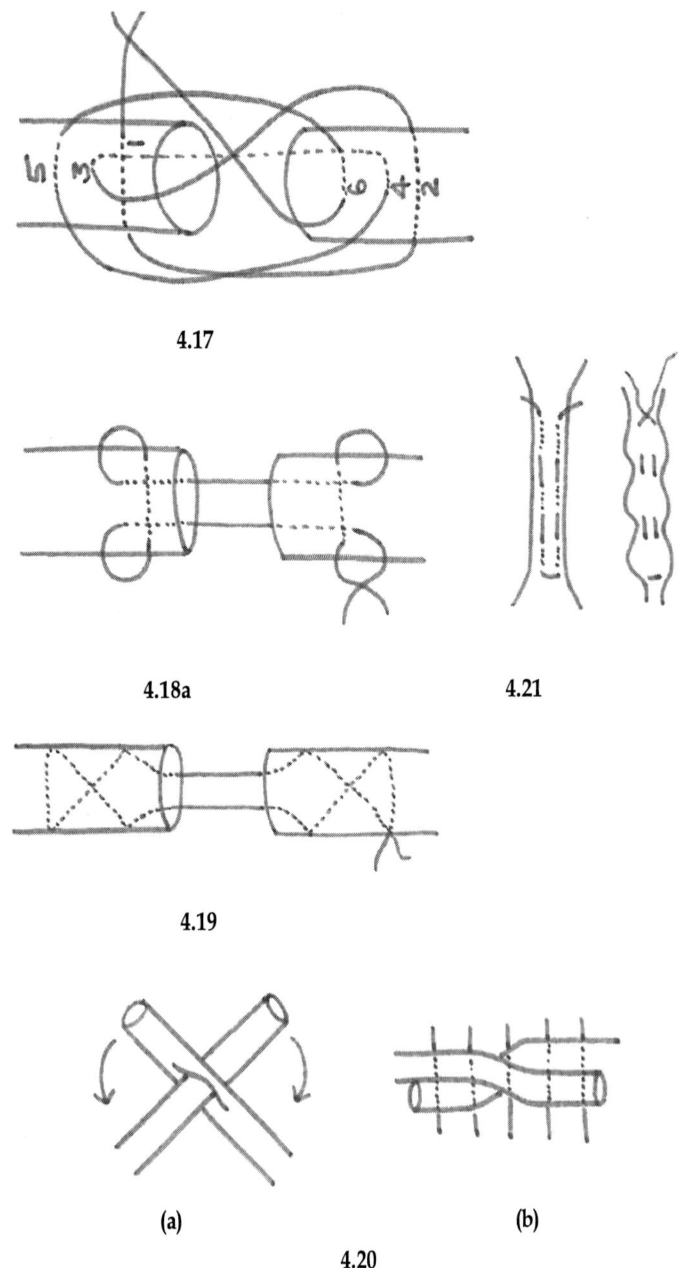

Figures of Suture pattern for special purposes : Fig. 4.17 : Three loop pulley suture; **4.18a:** Locking loop suture; **4.19:** Bunnel's mayer suture; **4.20a&b:** Button hole overlapping suture.

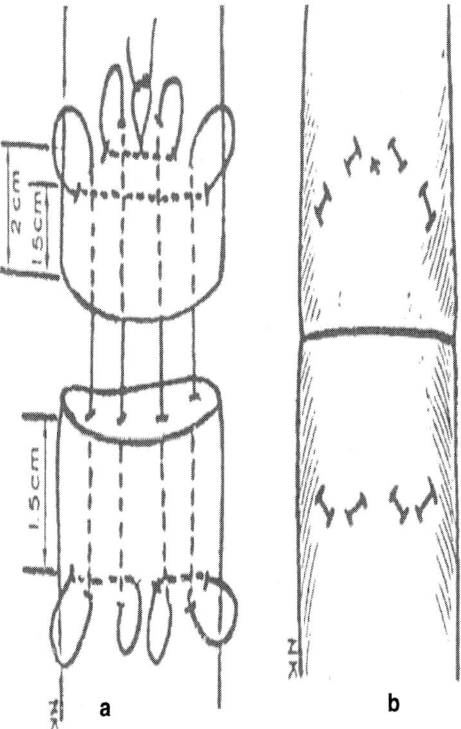

Fig. 4.18b: Double locking loop technique

3. *Halsted inverting suture* : A Lembert's suture with only two parallel but reversing passages through the tissue.
   - Used to reinforce sutures while closing hollow visceral organs (Fig. 4.26).
4. *Jobert's suture :* The suture is very much similar to lembert's suture pattern but the suturing needle penetrates the visceral mucosa. The chances of spread of infection from interior to exterior are more making the suture pattern non preferable (Fig. 4.27).
5. *Connell suture pattern* : The suture is very much similar to Cushing's suture pattern but the suturing needle penetrates the visceral mucosa. The chances of spread of infection from interior to exterior are more making the suture pattern non preferable (Fig. 4.28).
6. *Czerny's suture pattern* : Czerny's suture pattern is the double row of lembert's suture. The first layer closure is followed by second layer closure using Lembert's suture pattern.

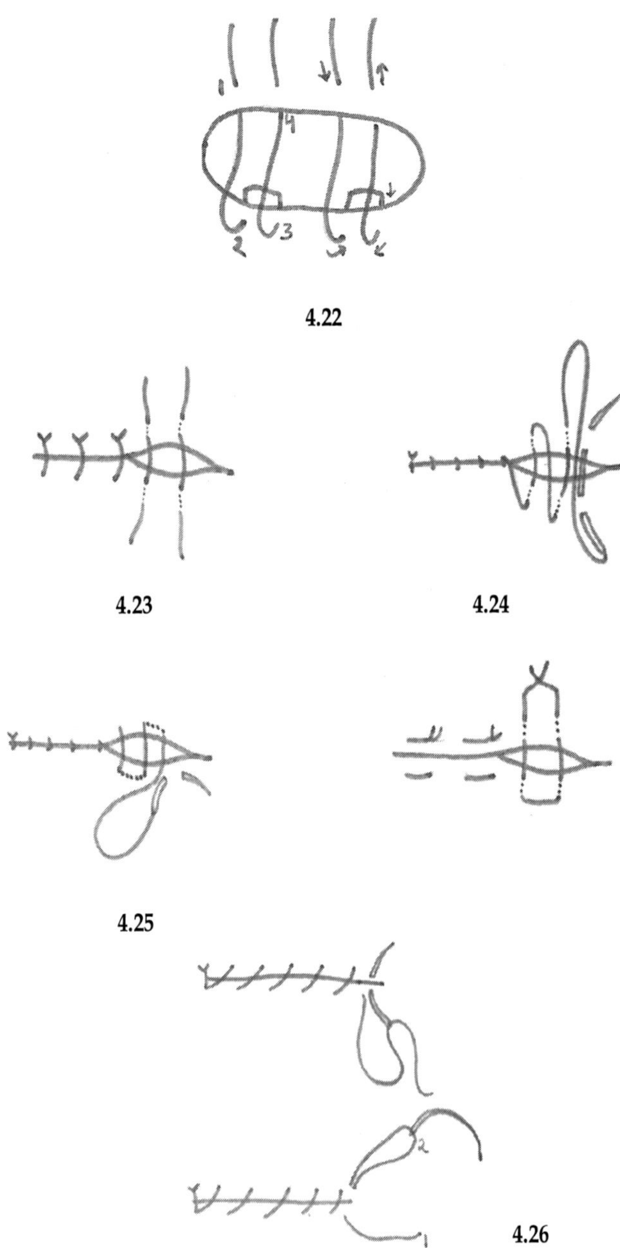

Figures of suture pattern for special purposes : Fig. 4.22 : Vest over pant or overlapping sutute; Figures of suture pattern for hollow visceral organs; **4.23 :** Lembert's interrupted suture; **4.24:** Lembert's continuous suture; **4.25:** Cushing's suture; **4.26:** Halsted inverting suture.

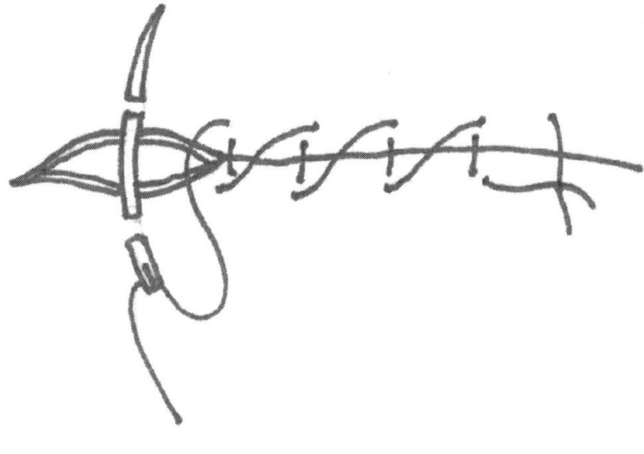

4.27

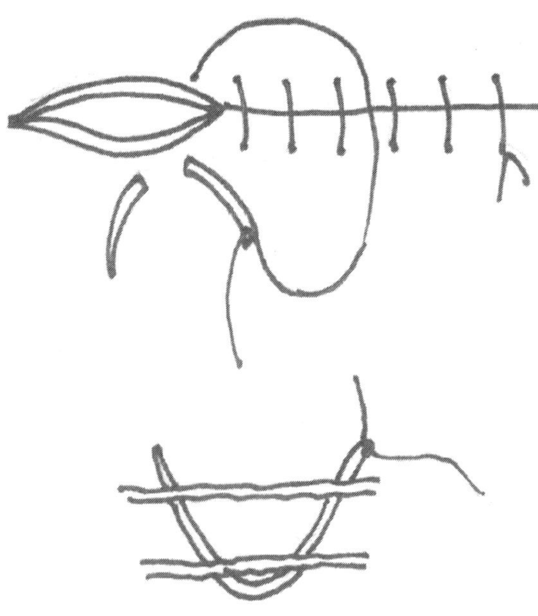

4.28

Figures of suture pattern for hollow organs : Fig. 4.27: Jobert suture ; **4.28:** Connell suture

Alternative Methods of Wound Closure

1. Tissue Adhesives

- Any material which unites tissue is known as tissue adhesives. The tissue adhesives can be classified into two catgories:

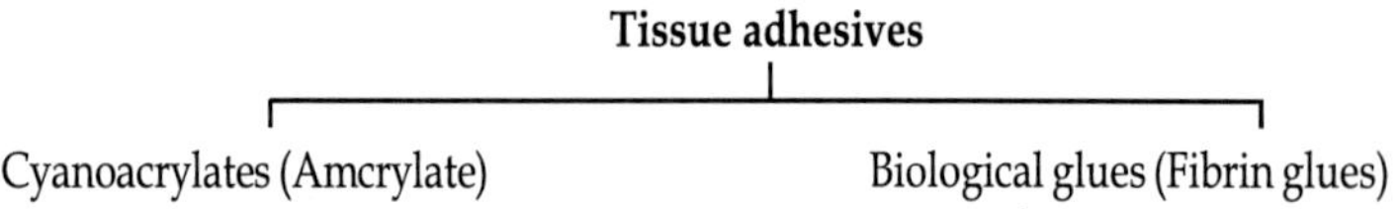

Cyanoacrylates (Amcrylate)

- The first cyanoacrylate, methylcyanoacrylate, was synthesized by Ardis (1949).
- These are the liquid monomer synthesized by formaldehyde and cyanoacetate.
- Polymerization occurs when applied to the tissue. This reaction is catalysed by very small amount of water leading to solid state.
- Properties of cyanoacrylates like tensile strength, flexibility and tissue toxicity depends on the length of alkyl side chain, combination of monomer and polymer and the addition of plasticizer and stabilizers.
- The shorter alkyl chain derivatives (methyl, ethyl and butyl) are more tissue toxic and breakdown quickly.
- Long and branched chain like n-butyl, iso-butyl, isoamyl-2 and N-octyl etc. are almost nontoxic.

Biological Glues (Fibrin glues)

- Due to human blood as one of its component, its use was restricted as a risk of transmitting blood borne diseases.
- Denatured when comes in contact with alcohol or iodine.
- It should be used within 4 hours of manufacturing.
- Snake venom derived fibrin glue is effective in anastomosis, haemostasis, and skin incision closure and for tenorrhaphy.

Uses

- As instant hemostats and for skin incision closure at low tension areas. Tissue adhesives are better than the conventional sutures as regard dehiscence, infection rate, wound healing and cosmetic outcome.
- In internal surgeries like stabilization of osteochondral fragments and aural haematoma in canines, teat lacerations and fistula in bovines and for skin grafting.

Methods of Application

- First of all apply topical anesthetic.
- Prepare the wound aseptically.
- The wound should be dried with sterilized swab and haemostasis should be complete.
- The wound edges should be apposed properly either manually or by applying subcutaneous sutures with no tension on tissue.
- Load the tissue adhesive from vial in to syringe or in a dropper.
- Apply the adhesive over the incision line or wound edges in 2 or 3 thin layers.
- The tissue adhesive should not go in between the wound edges, otherwise it act as a barrier in healing.

Mechanism of Action

- Thin layer of tissue adhesive keep the edges approximated and provides a moist covering under which the epithelium grows faster.

Advantages

- No or very little amount of anesthetic is required.
- No antiseptic wound dressing is required. Only protective covering should be applied to check the self mutilation by the animal.
- No need of suture removal.
- No suture tract infection.
- Very little chance of dehiscence.
- Early wound healing with more cosmetic appearance.

Limitations

- Subcutaneous sutures are required in the tension areas.
- Accidentally it can adhere to surgeon's gloves or other places, but could be cleared using acetone or dimethyl sulfoxide swab.
- In early post-operative days, the tensile strength of healing tissue is less than the sutures.
- Tissue adhesives can not stay in oozing areas.
- If they enter the wound edges, act as a barrier in wound healing.

2. Steri-Strips or Wound Closure Tapes

- These are the reinforced microporous surgical adhesive tape.
- Steri strips are rarely used for primary wound closure and is generally used as an adjunt to sutures or stapler.
- Steristrips are used after application of sucututicular sutures. These strips provide extra support to the suture line.
- *Advantages* :
  - i. Minimal scar formation.
  - ii. Wound closure tape is more resistance to infection than sutured wounds.

3. Surgical Staplers

- Stapling instrument is used in various surgical interventions like skin closure, gastrointestinal anastamosis etc.
- Make sure that the amount of tissue to be stapled is not excessive.
- *Advantages* : Increased efficiency, accurate hemostasis and advantageous in the areas of difficult accessibility.
- Skin staples are made of inert 316 L stainless steel and available in regular (4.8 to 6.1 mm) or wide (6.5 to 7.0 mm) sizes.
- Skin should be apposed by using subcuticular sutures before stapling.
- Staples should not be used in areas under moderate tension because of risk of wound dehiscence.
- Staples should not be placed over the bone or viscera if there is less than 4-6.5 mm between the skin and the underlying tissue.
- A specially designed staple extractor is used for staple removal. Mosquito hemostat can be used to open the staple for removal.

4. Surgical Needles/ Suturing Needles

- The suturing needles are made up of stainless steel.
- The design of the needles varies with size, shape and type of needle point.
- The needles can be classified as: Swaged or eyeless needle/ Eyed, Cutting/ non-cutting and straight/ curved. Curved needles are used in deep cavities.

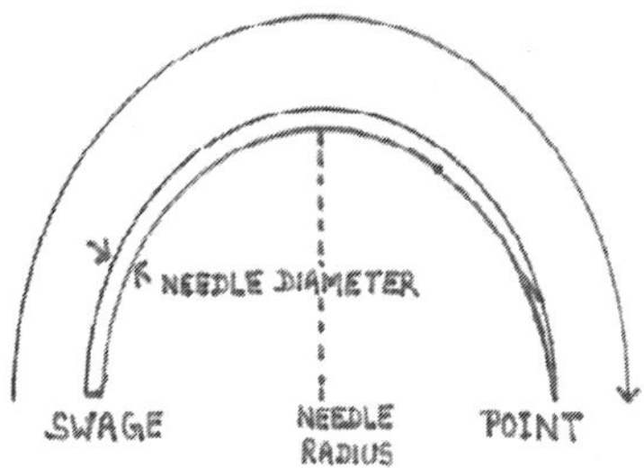

Fig. 4.29 : Parts of a suturing needle

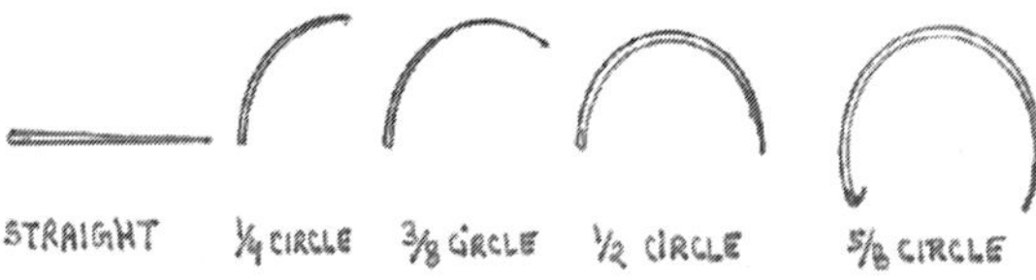

Fig. 4.30 : Shape of the needle

Swaged/ eyeless needle	**Eyed**
• Less traumatic. Tissue disruption minimized by single suture strand swaged to needle (Fig. 4.31). • Presterilized and used once. • Less economical. • No chance of accidental unthreading and loosing during suturing. • Ideal for surgeries of intestine, vessels, nerves, ureters etc.	• More traumatic. Tissue disruption caused by double suture strand with eyed needle. (Fig. 4.32). • These needles are reusable. • More economical but repeated sterilization dull their cutting edges.
Cutting (traumatic)	**Non-cutting (atraumatic)**
• The needle has cutting edges either on convex or on concave surface. The former is called reverse cutting needle. • Used for suturing the dense fibrous tissue and skin.	• The needle point is smooth. • Used for suturing soft tissues, visceral organs, blood vessels, nerves, m uscles etc (Fig. 4.34).

5. Round Bodied Needle

- Designed to separate tissue fibers rather than cut them.
- After the passage of the needle, the tissue closes tightly around the suture material thereby forming a leak proof suture line.
- Blunt point needles are used for suturing extremely friable vascular tissue e.g. liver, spleen and kidney.

6. Round Bodied/Cutting Needle

- *Trocar point needle*: This needle has a strong cutting head which then merges in to a round body.
- *Tapercut needle*: This needle combines the initial penetration of a reverse cutting needle with the minimized trauma of a round bodied needle (Fig. 4.33).
- *Cutting needle* : These needles are required to suture the tough or dense tissue. Cutting needles have a triangular body.
- *Conventional cutting needle:* This needle has a triangular cross sections with the apex cutting edge on the inside of the needle curvature. The effective cutting edges are restricted to the front section of the needle.
- *Reverse cutting needle:* This needle has a triangular cross sections with the apex cutting edge on the outside of the needle curvature. This improves the strength of the needle and particularly increases its resistance to bending (Fig. 4.35).

7. Micropoint Needle

- These needles are used in ophthalmic surgery and microsurgery.

8. Surgical Knots

A proper knot is vital to the better outcome of surgical technique. Failure of knot may lead to wound dehiscence, evisceration, hernia and fatal hemorrhage.

1. *Simple knot*: It is a single half hitch and a primary step of a square knot (Fig. 4.36).
2. *Square knot or reef knot*: It is a simple knot superimposed by another half hitch in the reverse direction (Fig. 4.37).
3. *Granny's knot*: It is a simple knot superimposed by another half hitch but not in reverse direction. Chances of slipping of granny's knot are more (Fig. 4.38).
4. *Surgeon's knot*: Surgeon's knot is a modified square knot in which two primary turns are made instead of one. Second tie is just like square knot. Two primary turns secure the first knot while applying second tie but becomes bulky if a thick thread is used(Fig. 4.39).
5. *Triple knot or reverse knot* : Triple knot is a surgeon's knot superimposed by a third tie similar to second but in reverse direction. Triple knot is recommended for suture materials having poor knot security like nylon (Fig. 4.40).

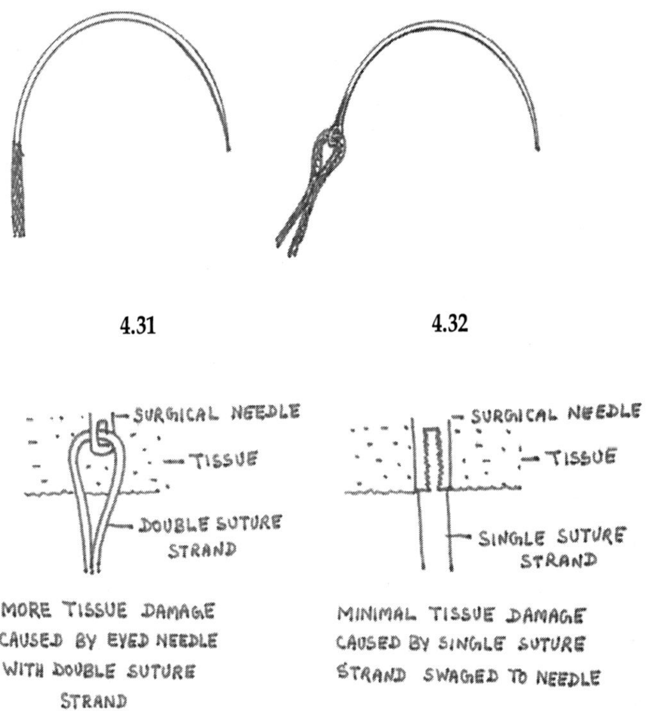

Tissue trauma caused by surgical needles

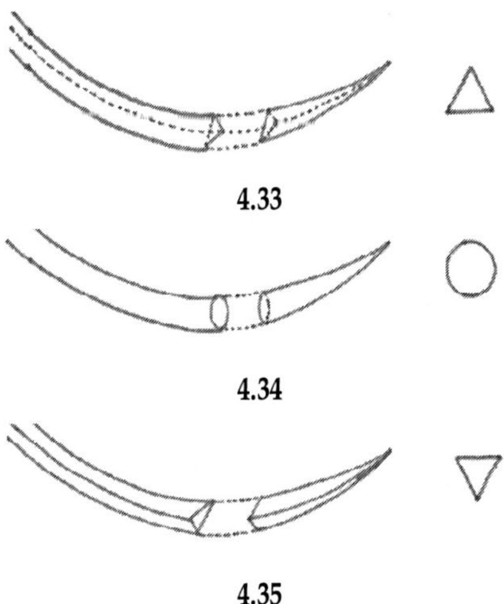

Fig. 4.31 : Eyeless or swaged surgical needle; **4.32:** Eyed surgical needle, **4.33:** Tapercut needle; **4.34 :** Non-cutting or atraumatic needle; **4.35 :** Reverse cutting needle.

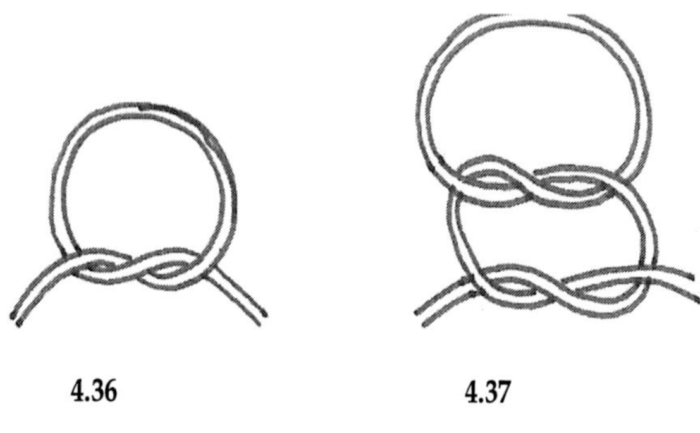

4.36 4.37

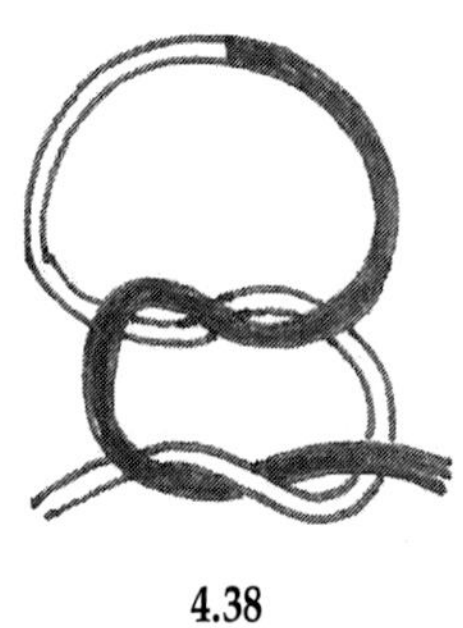

4.38

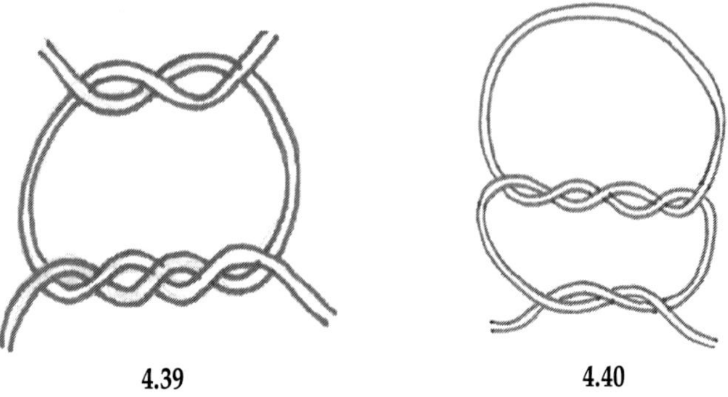

4.39 4.40

Different types of knots : Fig. 4.36 : Simple knot; **4.37 :** Square knot; **4.38 :** Granny's knot; **4.39:** Surgeon's knot; **4.40:** Triple knot or reverse knot.

9. Methods of Tying Knots

1. Single hand knot
2. Double hand knot
3. Needle holder

10. Suture Placement

- Needle holder is used to grasp the needle body (One half to three quarters of the distance from the tip of the needle).
- The needle holder is squeezed to catch the ratchet on the needle holder. Excessive squeezing may damage the needle.
- If the needle is incorrectly placed on the needle holder, it may result in to bent needle and difficulty in penetration of skin.
- The tissue must be stabilized by rat tooth/ thumb forceps before suture placement.
- The needle should always penetrate the skin at 90^0 angle and should be inserted 1-3 mm away from the wound edges.
- The two sides of the suture should become mirror image.
- The tip of the surgical needle should never be grasped by the needle holder. It causes blunting of the needle.

11. Suture Removal

- Sutures should be removed within 1-2 weeks of their placement.
- Early removal of sutures may lead to dehiscence and spread of scar.
- The sutures should be removed after cleaning by an antiseptic like Betadine.
- Suture should be gently elevated with forceps and one side of suture should be cut.
- The cut suture is gently grasped by the knot and gently pulled towards the wound/ suture line until the suture material is completely removed.
- If the suture is pulled away from the suture line, the wound edges may separate.

Chapter 5

Fluid Therapy

There is a delicate balance among electrolyte concentrations, body water and acid base status to maintain body homeostasis. Disturbances in homeostasis results in life threatening abnormalities. The aim of fluid therapy is to replace losses and maintain fluid and electrolyte balance in the body.

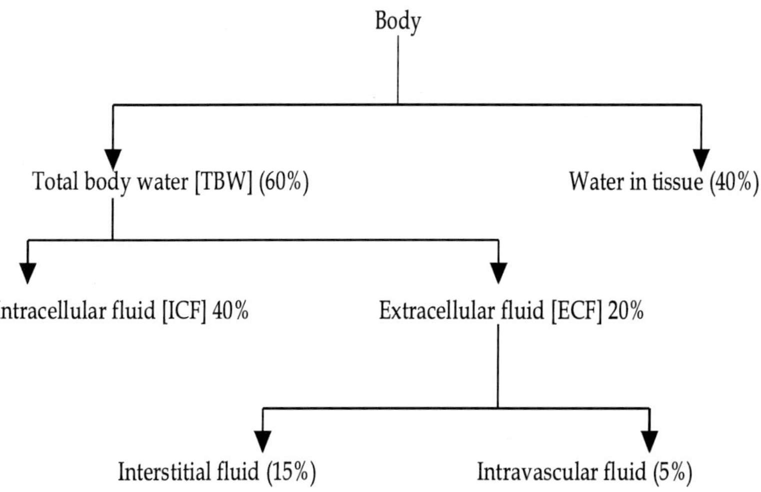

- The water movement between ICF and ECF depends upon their osmotic pressure.
- Main cation of extracellular fluid is Na^+
- Main cation of intracellular fluid is K^+
- Main anion of extracellular fluid is Cl^-
- Main anion of intracellular fluid is PO_4^-
- Other cations of ECF are K^+, Ca^{++}, Mg^{++} and that of ICF are Mg^{++} and Na^+
- Other anions of ECF are HCO_3^-, proteins, organic acids, PO_4^-, SO_4^- and that of ICF are HCO_3^-, proteins, PO_4^- and Cl^-
- Fluid and electrolyte disorders may develop due to inadequate fluid intake or abnormal losses from gastrointestinal, respiratory, urinary tract, exudates from discharging wounds, burn wounds or extensive pleural or peritoneal effusions.

Disorders of Water and Electrolyte Metabolism

Primary Water Depletion

- When the water intake is insufficient and inevitable losses continue e.g. diseases affecting swallowing (esophageal obstruction) and excess renal losses (diabetes and failure of ADH).
- ECF becomes hypertonic and water is drawn in to the ECF from ICF thus the loss is evenly distributed. Tissue catabolism liberates more intracellular water so that ICF contracts. Initially, electrolytes are excreted to maintain ECF tonicity but if the losses continue, to maintain ECF volume, oligourea results with high urine gravity and haemoconcentration. Thirst is marked and mucous membrane is dry. Death occurs when approximately 40% of the water is lost due to medulary failure.
- *Treatment* : Normal saline (0.18%) and 4.3% dextrose.

Mixed Water and Electrolyte Depletion

- This occurs when the body secretions are lost during vomiting and diarrhea. Water and electrolytes are lost but the animal continues to drink, the plasma sodium level will tend to fall so that ECF becomes hypotonic. This provokes diuresis and also causes water movement in to the ICF in an attempt to maintain ECF osmolality. After the initial diuresis, hypovolemia affects renal function so that oligourea occurs.

Thirst is often not marked. Mucous membrane remains moist but the saliva is viscous.

- *Treatment* : Isotonic solutions are used.

Acid Base Disturbances

- Hydrogen ions are generally produced by oxidation of foodstuffs and tissues and immediately buffered by the buffering system. Conventionally the hydrogen ions are measured as pH. Deviation of blood pH below 6.8 and above 7.8 are generally incompatible with life.
- *Osmolality* : Total number of dissolved particles in a solution is called osmolality. Sodium and chloride ions are main contributors of osmolality of serum and increase in their concentration in ECF leads to shifting of water from ICF to ECF.

  Plasma osmolality (P_{osm}) = [1.86(Na^+ and K^+)] + [Glucose (mg/dl) ÷18] + [BUN (mg/dl) ÷ 2.8]
- Normal P_{osm} for canines is about 300 m osm/L.
- *Anion gap*
  - It is the difference between the measured cations (Na^+ and K^+) and the measured anions (Cl^- and HCO_3^-).

    AG= (Na^+ and K^+) - (Cl^- and HCO_3^-).
  - Normal anion gap is 12-14 mEq/L and it represents unmeasured anions, proteins, organic acids, PO_4^-, SO_4^- and is used to determine the cause of acid-base disturbances.
  - AG is generally increased due to increase lactate, salicylates, ketoacids and laboratory errors (underestimation of Cl^- and HCO_3^- or overestimation of Na^+ and K^+)
  - Decreased AG is generally less common and may be due to decrease unmeasured anions (hypoalbuminemia) or lab errors (underestimation of Na^+ and overestimation of Cl^-).

Electrolytes and their imbalances : ECF and ICF compartments exist in a state of equilibrium.

1. Sodium

- The main role of sodium ion is to maintain water distribution due to its osmotic pressure.

- In aldosterone deficiency, sodium ions (Na^+) are excreted and K^+ and H^+ are removed.
- *Hyponatremia* : Sodium concentration is less than 140 mEq/L. Sodium depletion may be due to renal or non-renal causes.

  Etiology
  - Renal causes: Diuretics and hypoadrenocorticism.
  - Non-renal causes: Vomiting, diarrhea, pancreatitis, ascitis, peritonitis, uroabdomen etc.

  Clinical signs
  - Clinical signs appear when sodium concentration reaches < 120 m mol/L and become marked when concentration reaches < 110 m mol/L.
  - Anorexia, lethargy, weakness, vomiting, muscle cramping, seizures and coma.

  Treatment
  - Severe hyponatremia may be corrected with careful administration of 3% saline over 24 hours.
- *Hypernatremia* : It results due to more loss of water as compared to sodium.

  Etiology
  - Gastrointestinal losses (vomiting and diarrhea).
  - Fever and pure water loss (diabetes incipidus).
  - Osmotic diuresis (diabetes mellitus).

  Clinical signs
  - Clinical signs appear when sodium concentration exceeds 170 mEq/L.
  - Clinical signs of CNS are manifested.

  Treatment
  - Hypernatremia can be corrected by administrating 5% dextrose or 0.45% saline with 2.5% dextrose.

2. Potassium

- Kidneys are the main organ of K^+ regulation.
- In presence of metabolic acidosis, K^+ moves out of the cell in to the serum in exchange of H^+.

❒ *Hypokalemia*

Etiology

- Renal losses (hyperaldosteronism, hyperadrenocorticism and polyurea).
- Gastrointestinal losses (vomiting and diarrhea).
- *Drugs*: diuretics, penicillin and $NaHCO_3$.

Clinical signs

- Clinical signs appear when potassium concentration falls below 3 mEq/L.
- Clinical signs includes abnormalities of cardiac muscles, skeletal muscles, kidneys and reduced gastrointestinal motility.

❒ *Hyperkalemia*

Etiology

- Decreased renal excretion: Renal failure, hypoaldosteronism, hypoadrenocorticism, urethral obstruction, rupture of urinary bladder and gastrointestinal diseases.
- Decreased cellular uptake.

Clinical signs

- Clinical signs appear when potassium concentration exceeds 8 mEql/L.
- Clinical signs includes bradycardia.

Treatment

- The animal should be treated immediately with $NaHCO_{3,}$ glucose or 10% calcium gluconate.

3. Chloride

❒ *Hypochloremia*

Etiology

- Pancreatitis, congestive heart failure (CHF) etc.
- Renal losses ($NaHCO_3$, loop/thiazide diuretics, metabolic alkalosis).
- Gastrointestinal losses (vomiting).

Clinical signs

- Clinical sign related to metabolic alkalosis.

Treatment

- 0.9% saline solution if volume expansion is required.
- Chloride containing salts like KCl, $CaCl_2$, $MgCl_2$ and NH_4Cl may be administered orally.

❐ *Hyperchloremia*

Etiology

- Diabetes incipidus, haemoglobinemia and bilirubinemia.

Clinical signs

- Diarrhea.

Treatment

- Therapy with HCO_3^- if metabolic acidosis is present.

Diagnosis of fluid and electrolyte imbalance : This is achieved by a combination of :

1. Accurate history
2. Clinical signs
3. Laboratory examination

1. Accurate History

An accurate history can give valuable information about extent and type of fluid deficit. The owner should be asked about the duration and frequency of gastrointestinal disturbances (vomiting, diarrhea and salivation), polyurea, polydipsia, panting, anorexia and pyrexia.

2. Clinical Signs

❐ *For dehydration* : Dehydration results from either inadequate fluid intake or abnormal losses of body fluids like enteritis, gastritis, vomition, diarrhea, excessive urination in kidney diseases, excessive blood loss, excessive salivation etc. Fluid losses are usually severe in cattle because of milk production which accounts for loss of fluid and electrolyte from the body. Weight loss, altered skin turgor, sunken eye etc.

❐ *For acute Na^+ loss:* Increased pulse rate, decreased pulse pressure and blood pressure, increased capillary refill time (CRT).

❐ *General appearance and body weight:* The dehydrated patient remains dull and depressed. Change in body weight can be a useful guide to the extent of loss if the normal weight is known.

- *Body temperature :* A subnormal body temperature along with cool extremities indicates acute dehydration.
- *Capillary refill time (CRT) :* CRT is an indication of adequacy of perfusion. CRT over 2 seconds indicates hypotension, hypovolemia or peripheral vasoconstriction.
- *Pulse rate :* A rapid weak pulse indicates oligemic shock (due to dehydration) suggests a very large fluid deficit.
- *Mucous membrane :* Dry mucous membrane indicates dehydration. Pale/ white mucous membrane indicates blood loss, anemia and shock.
- *Skin turgor and eye :* Clinical signs express the percentage of dehydration.
  - Loss of skin turgor (skin elasticity and pliability) (5%)
  - Loss of skin turgor + sunken eye ball (5-7%)
  - Loss of skin turgor + sunken eye ball + slow CRT (7-10%)
  - Hypovolemia and shock (12-15%)
- *Urinary output :* Urine output is an indirect measurement of CVP. Normal urine output is 1.5 ml/kg/h. Less than 0.5 ml/kg b.wt/h is considered as oligourea.

3. Laboratory Examination

- *Blood examination*
- *Packed cell volume (PCV):* PCV increases in dehydration. The PCV may be used to calculate fluid requirements. Approximately 10ml/kg should be infused for each 1% raise in PCV over 45.
- *Hemoglobin (Hb):* Hemoglobin increases in dehydration.
- *Plasma proteins:* Plasma protein increases in dehydration.
- *Blood urea:* The blood urea concentration rises with dehydration.
- *Plasma electrolytes:* Measuring the level of electrolytes in the body is very useful.
- *Osmolality:* This is useful to find out hypotonic or hypertonic dehydration.
- *Central venous pressure (CVP):* Normal CVP is 0-6 or 7 cm of H_2O. Serial measurement of CVP should be taken. Low CVP indicates relative or absolute hypovolemia. Increase in CVP occurs in fluid overload or heart failure.
- *Urine analysis*
- pH and specific gravity of urine are very useful particularly when the disturbance is renal in origin. Specific gravity above 1.010 indicate presence of protein, glucose electrolyte etc. in urine.

Dehydration and its evaluation

Body weight loss (%)	Sunken eye	Skin fold test persists for (sec)	PCV (%)	Total serum solids (g/L)	Fluid required to replace volume deficit (ml/kg b. wt)
4-6	Barely detectable	-	40-45	70-80	20-25
6-8	+	2-4	50	80-90	30-50
8-10	++	6-10	55	90-100	50-80
10-12	+++	20-45	60	120	80-120

Methods of Estimating the Size of Volume Deficit

1. *Factorial approach/ calculation of deficiency from history:* A 10 Kg dog inappetant for 3 days, vomiting profusely once daily since the onset of illness and urination decreased in frequency from last 2 days.

   Calculation

   Inevitable water loss 3X10X25 = 750 ml

   Urinary water loss 1X10X25 = 250 ml

   Vomit loss (@ 4 ml/kg) 4X10X3 = 120 ml

   Total deficit 1120 ml

   ECF (33%) = 375ml

   Plasma deficit (25% of ECF deficit) = 95 ml

   The dog therefore needs approximately 95 ml rapidly to support its circulation and a further 1 liter is given slowly to replenish the rest of the deficit.

2. *Clinical approach* : Amount of fluid required is calculated as :

   Amount of fluid required (ml) = % dehydration X body weight (Kg)

   e.g. A 400 kg cow which is 8% dehydrated will require 400 x 8 x 10=32000 ml or 32 liter.

3. *Calculation from PCV*

   Note : Each °C rise in temperature causes 3ml/kg water loss. Insensible loss of moisture from skin and respiratory passage in small animals is about 5 ml/kg/day.

   Fluid needed (ml) = Patient PCV - Normal PCV X 0.66 X body weight (Kg) X

   Treatment : Treatment includes :

1. Correction of the Existing Deficit

- *Restoration of the circulating blood volume :* Plasma or plasma substitutes are preferred. Crystalloid solution can be given @ 90ml/h over 20-30 minutes in order to improve the condition and thereafter infused at a slower rate.
- *Replenishing the rest of the deficit :* This can be done very slowly thus making up the plasma deficit in 24-48 h. 50% of the fluid given in the first 6 hours @ 5-10 ml/kg/h.

2. Meeting the Daily Requirement

Normal daily need vary between 40-50 ml/ kg. However in illness it increases twice the daily requirement depending on the urine output.

3. Replacing Ongoing Losses

The volume of the abnormal losses should be estimated and added to the normal requirement. It may not be possible to measure losses in pleural and peritoneal effusions.

- Vomiting losses - 1ml / kg / vomit
- Diarrheoa - up to 200ml / kg / day

Rate of Infusion

- The fluid requirement may be as fast as possible and several veins can be cannulated simultaneously.
- In moderate deficit, infusion rate may be slower.
- In hypovolemic shock, fluid can be administered @ 3 ml/kg/min. for first 20 minutes.
- In very severe cases fluid can be administered @ 10-15 ml/kg/h.
- Normal maintenance requirement is 5 ml/kg/h.
- The flow rate can be converted to drops/ minute by using the following formula.

$$\text{Drops/min} = \frac{\text{Drops X ml / kg body weight X Body Weight (kg)}}{60}$$

- Fluid therapy should be stopped
  - On hearing moist rales, moist cough and serous nasal discharge indicating pulmonary edema.
  - Increase in CVP.
  - Increase in urine output.

- Route of administration: Intravenous, Subcutaneous, Intraperitoneal, Intraosseous (in young animals), Alimentary, Oral or Rectal.
- *ECF replacement* : e.g. Ringer Lactate and Normal saline.
- *Plasma volume expander* : e.g. Bovine gelatin and Dextran.
- *ECF alkalizers* : e.g. Bicarbonates and its precursors.
- *ECF acidifiers* : e.g. Normal saline.
- *ECF diluents* : e.g. 5% Dextrose.
- *Maintenance solution* : Maintenance solutions are substitute for drinking and for major electrolytes in food. These solutions should not be given subcutaneously.
- *Nutrient solutions* : e.g. Glucose, lipid emulsions and protein hydrolysates.
- *Concentrated derivatives* : e.g. Hypertonic saline.

Choice of fluid in specific conditions

S. No.	Name of fluid	Indication
1.	0.9% NaCl (Isotonic saline)	Plasma volume expander
2.	1.3% $NaHCO_3$ in 5% Dextrose	Acidosis
3.	5% $NaHCO_3$ (Hypertonic)	Severe acidosis
4.	Equal mixture of isotonic saline and isotonic $NaHCO_3$	Acidosis and dehydration and acute intestinal obstruction.
5.	Ringer lactate solution	Acidosis
6.	Mixture of isotonic KCl (1.1%) + Isotonic saline (0.9%) + Isotonic Dextrose (5%)	Metabolic alkalosis (In cattle with abdominal disease)
7.	Isotonic saline + KCl (2.5g/L)	Alkalosis, hypochloremia and hypokalemia
8.	Dextran, balanced electrolyte solution and bicarbonate	Gastric dilatation in canines
9.	Ringer lactate + $NaHCO_3$	Hypovolemic shock

Chapter 6

SHOCK

Shock is a life threatening condition which is usually manifested by serious pathophysiological abnormalities. In most cases it is due to poor tissue perfusion with impaired cellular metabolism.

- It is a clinical state resulting from an inadequate supply of oxygen to the tissues or an ability of the tissues to properly use oxygen.
- Shock can also be defined as imbalance between oxygen supply and oxygen consumption. In other words, the delivery of oxygen does not meet the needs of the tissues.
- Shock is a state in which the vital functions of the body are depressed because of acute reduction in cardiac output and effective circulating blood volume.

Types of Shock

Hypovolemic/Hemorrhagic Shock

Massive losses of intravascular volume lead to hypovolemic shock. Until 10-15% blood volume is lost, the blood pressure is maintained by tachycardia and vasoconstriction. The common causes are :

A. Traumatic Shock

- *Severe injury* : crushing injury to tissues.
- *Severe hemorrhage* : External or internal.
- *Surgical procedures* : If anesthesia is inadequate.

B. Dehydration

- Severe vomiting and diarrhoea.

C. Burn Shock

- Burn shock is caused by rapid plasma loss from the damaged tissues causing hypovolemia.
- More than 25% burn leads to generalized capillary leakage which results in to gross hypovolemia in the first 24 hours.
- Large volumes of colloidal and crystalloid fluids are required to resuscitation.

D. Cardiogenic Shock

- Cardiogenic shock results from impairment of cardiac function resulting in to decrease in stroke volume and cardiac output, peripheral vasoconstriction and venous congestion.
- Impairment in cardiac function may be caused by cardiac tamponade, thrombosis, severe arrhythmias, hypertrophic cardiomyopathies.
- Cardiac pump failure leads to hypotension and compromised tissue perfusion with reduced tissue oxygen delivery.
- Obstructive shock is a form of cardiogenic shock e.g. gastric dilatation and volvulus.

E. Septic/endotoxic Shock

- *Hyperdynamic septic shock (warm septic shock)* : This type of shock develops after severe infection by gram negative microorganisms e.g. peritonitis, leakage at the site of intestinal anastomosis or strangulated intestine.
- *Hypodynamic septic shock (cold)* : Persistant endotoxemia or sepsis leads to cold septic shock.

F. Vasovagal Shock

- Caused by pooling of blood in larger vascular reservoirs (limb muscles) and by dilatation of the splanhnic arteriolar bed.
- It results in to reduced venous return to the heart, low cardiac output and reflex bradycardia.
- The reduced cerebral perfusion causes cerebral hypoxia and unconciousness.

G. Psychogenic Shock

- Psychogenic shock immediately follows a sudden fright or severe pain.

H. Neurogenic Shock

- Neurogenic shock is caused by traumatic or pharmacological blockade of the sympathetic nervous system.
- The end result is dilatation of resistance arterioles and capacitance vessels which leads to relative hypovolemia and hypotension.
- There is low blood pressure, a normal or decreased cardiac output, a normal pulse rate and a warm dry skin.

I. Anaphylactic Shock

- Causes of anaphylactic shock include anesthetics, drugs, serum injections etc.
- Release of histamine and slow release substances-anaphylaxis (SRS-A) causes bronchospasm, laryngeal edema and respiratory distress with hypoxia, vasodilatation, hypotension and shock.

J. Irreversible Shock

Shock may become irreversible due to the severity of vascular impairment and tissue damage.

Sequalae of Shock

1. Recovery
2. Survival with permanent damage to various organs
3. Death

Pathophysiology

Acute hypovolemia

Reduced central venous pressure

Reduced cardiac filling

Reduced cardiac output

Reduced arterial pressure

Peripheral receptors

Central receptors

ADH

Kidney

Angiotensin and renin

Sympathetic nerve stimulation

Norepinephrine release

Increase in heart rate and contractility

Increased intravascular volume and cardiac output

Adrenal medulla stimulation

Release of epinephrine

Vasoconstriction

Deminished secretion from alimentary tract

Skin

Kidney

Oligourea

Maintenance of blood pressure and fluid

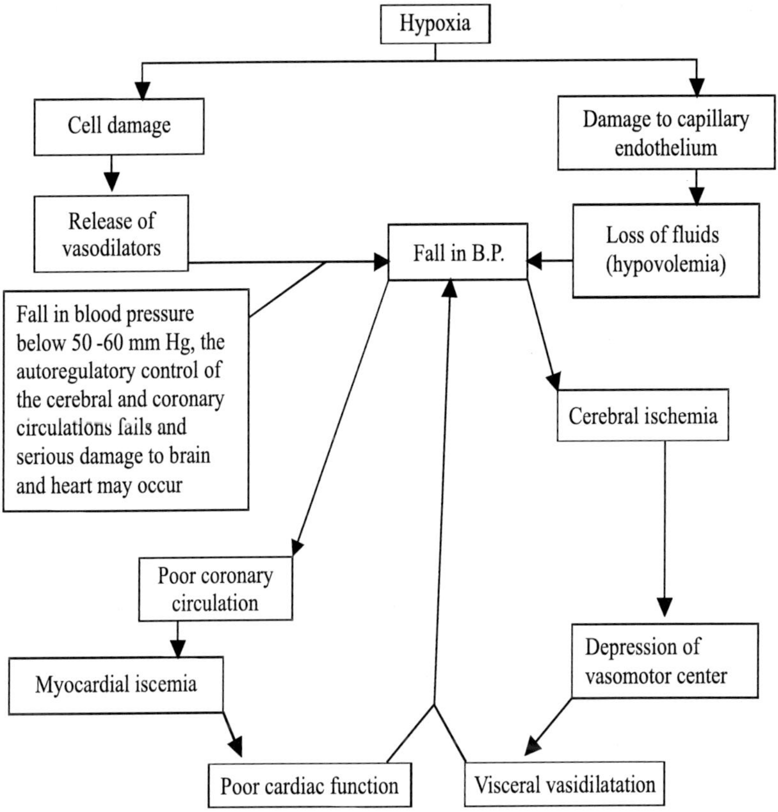

Hypoxia
Cell damage
Damage to capillary endothelium
Release of vasodilators
Fall in B.P.
Loss of fluids (hypovolemia)
Fall in blood pressure below 50 -60 mm Hg, the autoregulatory control of the cerebral and coronary circulations fails and serious damage to brain and heart may occur
Cerebral ischemia
Poor coronary circulation
Depression of vasomotor center
Myocardial iscemia
Poor cardiac function
Visceral vasidilatation

Shock in burns and scald : Severity of shock is proportional to the exuding surface and not to the depth of the burn.

The immediate reaction is nervous (pain and stimulation of afferent nerves)
Inflammatory response evoked by burnt tissue
Excessive exudation and loss of protein rich fluid (sludging of blood in capillaries)
Hypovolemia
Shock

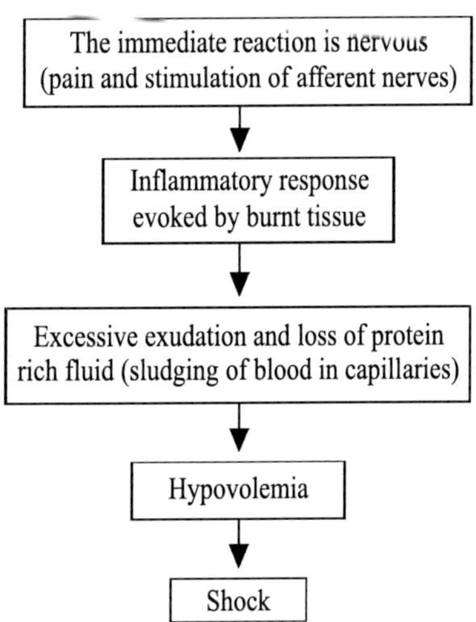

Complications which Aggravate the Burn Shock

1. Burnt tissue is highly susceptible to infections like *Streptococcus sp., Staphylococcus sp.* which causes **septic shock**.
2. Hemolysis of red cells at the burnt site and later severe sludging leads to **anaemia.**

Septic Shock

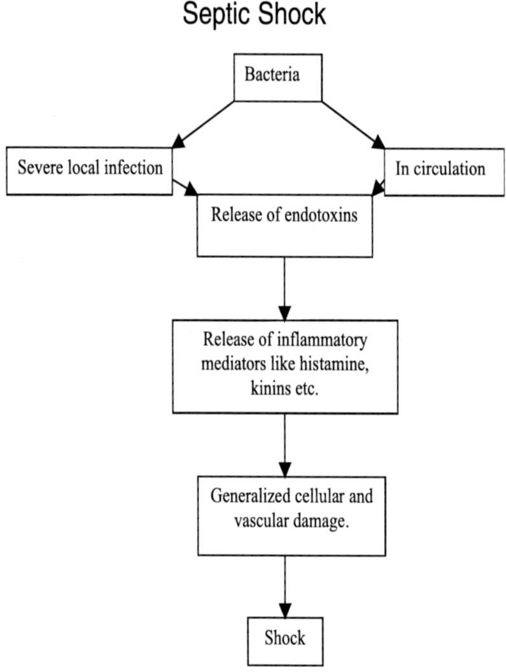

Stages of Shock

1. *Compensatory stage*
   - Slight increase in heart and respiration rate.
   - Blood pressure is normal.
   - Brick red mucous membrane.
   - Capillary refill time is less than 1 second.
2. *Early decompensatory stage*
   - Increase in heart and respiration rate.
   - Weak pulse which is difficult to locate.
   - Pale mucous membrane.
   - Long capillary refill time.
   - Hypothermia and hypotension.

3. *Decompensatory (terminal) stage*
   - Low heart rate.
   - Capillary refill time absent
   - Severe hypotension.
   - Cyanotic mucous membrane.
   - Hypothermia and anuria.
   - Noresponse to fluid therapy.
   - Coma.

S. No.	Parameter	Hypovolemic shock	Septic shock	Cardiogenic
1.	Heart rate	↑	↑	↑
2.	Pulse	Weak	Early stage: strong Late stage: weak	Weak
3.	Mucous membrane	Pale	Brick red	Pale
4.	CRT	↑	↑	↑
5.	Respiration rate	↑	↑	↑
6.	Urine output	Low	Low	Low
7.	Blood pressure	Early stage: high Late stage: low	Low	Low
8.	CVP	Low	Low	Low

Management of Shock

- Early recognition and management are important in the successful treatment of shock.
- The standard ABCD protocol constitutes the basis of initial therapy for animals in shock.

  A - Airway

  B - Breathing

  C - Circulation

  D - Drugs
- 100% oxygen should be administered at a high flow rate.

- In case of extensive trauma, traumatized blood vessels should be ligated.
- Intravenous administration of crystalloid and colloids.
- Whole blood transfer may be indicated as primary fluid replacement during hemorrhagic shock.
- Use of sympathomimetic drugs like dobutamine. These drugs increase the force of contraction of the cardiac muscles.
- Use of vasopressors such as epinephrine (0.1 to o.3 µg/ kg/min.) during life threatening state of hypotension.
- Opioid analgesics are preferred for animals in shock.
- Intravenous administration of antiarrhythmic agents e.g. lidocaine @ 2 mg/kg body weight.
- Patients with septic shock require administration of broad spectrum bactericidal antibiotics.
- Use of glucocorticoids like dexamethasone @ 10 mg/kg body weight and prednisolone @ 30 mg/kg body weight.

Chapter 7

FRACTURE

Dissolution in the continuity of bone/cartilage with or without displacement of fractured fragments is known as fracture.

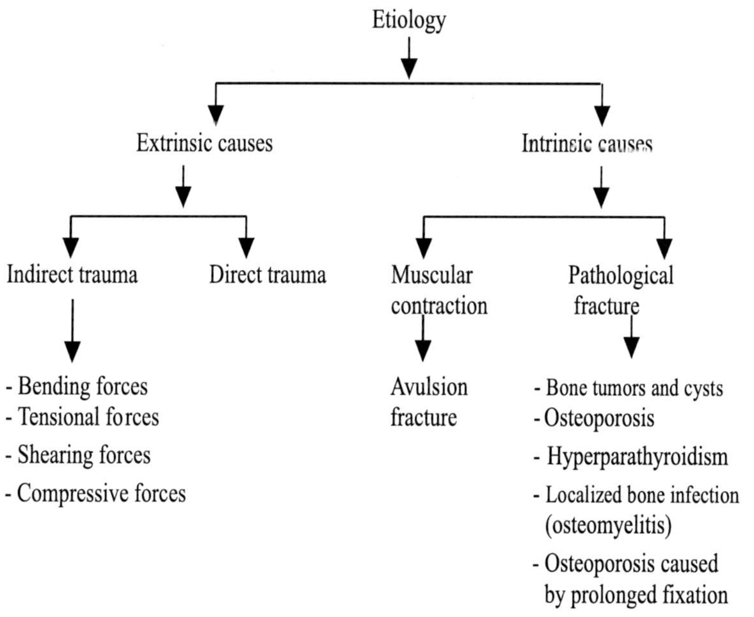

The figure given below shows the general anatomy of the long bone.

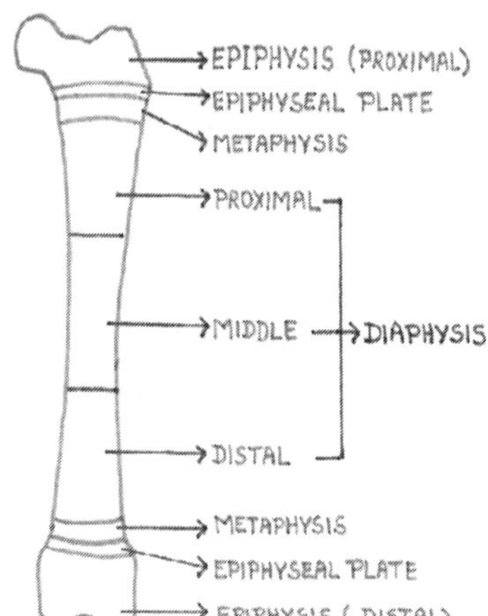

Classification

1. On the Basis of Communication of Fractured Site to the Environment

a. *Simple fracture* : The fracture site does not communicate with the environment.

b. *Compound fracture* : The fracture site communicates with the environment. This type of fractures is more prone to infection.

c. *Complicated fracture* : A closed fracture in which there is considerable injury to important neighboring vessels or nerves or accompanied by the opening of a joint or vascular cavity.

2. On the Basis of Extent of Bone Damage

a. *Complete fracture:* It is a fracture in which there is complete loss of bone continuity and the bone is divided into two or more fragments (Fig. 7.1).

b. *Incomplete fracture:* An incomplete fracture is one where the bone has not completely lost its continuity.

c. *Green stick fracture:* In such fractures, the cortex opposite to the bending force fractures completely, while the cortex under the force remains intact. Commonly seen in immature animals (Fig. 7.2).

d. *Fissure fracture:* When direct trauma applied to a bone is not sufficient to cause a complete fracture, cracks and fissure line will occur. The fissure formed in one cortex of the bone and generally the periosteum remains intact. The fissure line may be longitudinal, transverse or oblique.

e. *Partial or splintered fracture:* When splinters of bone are separated from the main bone i.e. by fire arms.

f. *Sub-periosteal (intra-periosteal) fracture:* A fracture of the cortical bone without rupture of the periosteum.

g. *Deferred fracture:* In which separation of fragments occur only after a varying period after incident due to subsequent violence, strain or concussion e.g. broken back in horses.

3. On the Basis of Number of Fractured Fragments

a. *Single :* When the bone is broken at one place only

b. *Double :* When there are two fracture in same bone

c. *Multiple/comminuted :* When the bone is broken into more than two pieces.

4. On the Basis of Type of Bone Involved

a. *Cortical bone fracture:* Fracture of diaphysis of long bone.

b. *Cancellous bone fracture:* Fracture of skull bone or extremities of long bones.

5. On the Basis of Displacement of the Fractured Fragments

a. *Impacted fracture :* In an impacted fracture, the cortical end of the fracture is forced or impacted into the cancellous bone. Such fractures are seen at the junction of diaphysis and metaphysis of a long bone.

b. *Compression fracture:* Cancellous bone collapses and compresses upon itself. Such fractures are seen in vertebral bodies (Fig. 7.3).

c. *Distracted fracture :* Bone fragments are separated due to sufficient muscle pull. e.g. fracture of olecranon.

d. *Depression fracture:* The fragments are depressed and produce a cavity e.g. fracture of skull bone.

e. *Overriding fracture:* A fracture in which the fragments lie side by side, causing shortening of limb (Fig. 7.4).

6. On the Basis of Direction of Fracture Line

a. *Transverse:* – The fracture line runs transverse to the long axis of bone. Such type of fracture is caused by bending forces (Fig. 7.5).

b. *Oblique:* The fracture line runs oblique to the long axis of the bone. Such type of fracture is caused by bending with axial compression (Fig. 7.6).

c. *Spiral:* The fracture line spirals along the long axis of the bone. Such type of fracture is caused by torsion, twisting or rotational forces e.g. in humerus (Fig. 7.7).

d. *Longitudinal:* A fracture extending in longitudinal direction e.g. split pastern.

e. *Comminuted:* In comminuted fractures, at least three fracture lines inter connect each other at one point (Fig. 7.8).
f. *Multiple:* In multiple fractures, the bone is broken in to three or more segments. The fracture lines do not interconnect each other (Fig. 7.9).
g. *Avulsion:* A fragment of bone at the site of muscle insertion is detached due to its forceful contraction (Fig. 7.10).

7. On the Basis of Stability of Fractured Fragments

a. *Stable fracture:* The fractured fragments more or less interlock after reduction.
b. *Unstable fracture:* The fractured fragments are unstable after reduction.

8. On the Basis of Anatomical Location of Fracture

a. *Diaphyseal fracture:* Fractures that occur in the diaphysis of a long bone. This fracture can further be classified proximal third, middle and distal third.
b. *Metaphyseal fracture (Proximal or Distal):* A fracture within the metaphysis of a long bone is referred as a metaphyseal fracture.
c. *Epiphyseal fracture (Proximal or Distal):* These are fractures of epiphysis.
d. *Condylar fracture:* Fracture of the condyle either medial or lateral or both (Fig. 7.11).
e. *Supracondylar fracture:* Fracture when both the condyles are fractured off the shaft as a unit (Fig. 7.12).
f. *Supracondylar–intercondylar fracture:* The fracture where both the condyles are fractured from the shaft and also from each other ('T' shape and 'Y' shape).
g. *Articular fracture (Intracapsular):* Fracture of subchondral bone and articular cartilage.
h. *Periarticular fracture (Extra capsular fracture):* A fracture near a joint but not entering within the joint capsule.
i. *Trans-cervical fracture:* Fracture through neck of femur.

Fracture dislocation : when a fracture of a bone results into joint instability leading to subluxation or luxation of the joint. It is termed as fracture dislocation. The term *'Monteggia fracture'* is specifically referred to fracture of the olecranon process and dislocation of the elbow joint (Fig. 7.13).

Colle's fracture : Fracture of distal end of radius e.g. abduction of paw is noticed in Colle's fracture.

Down in the hip : Fracture of the external angle of hip.

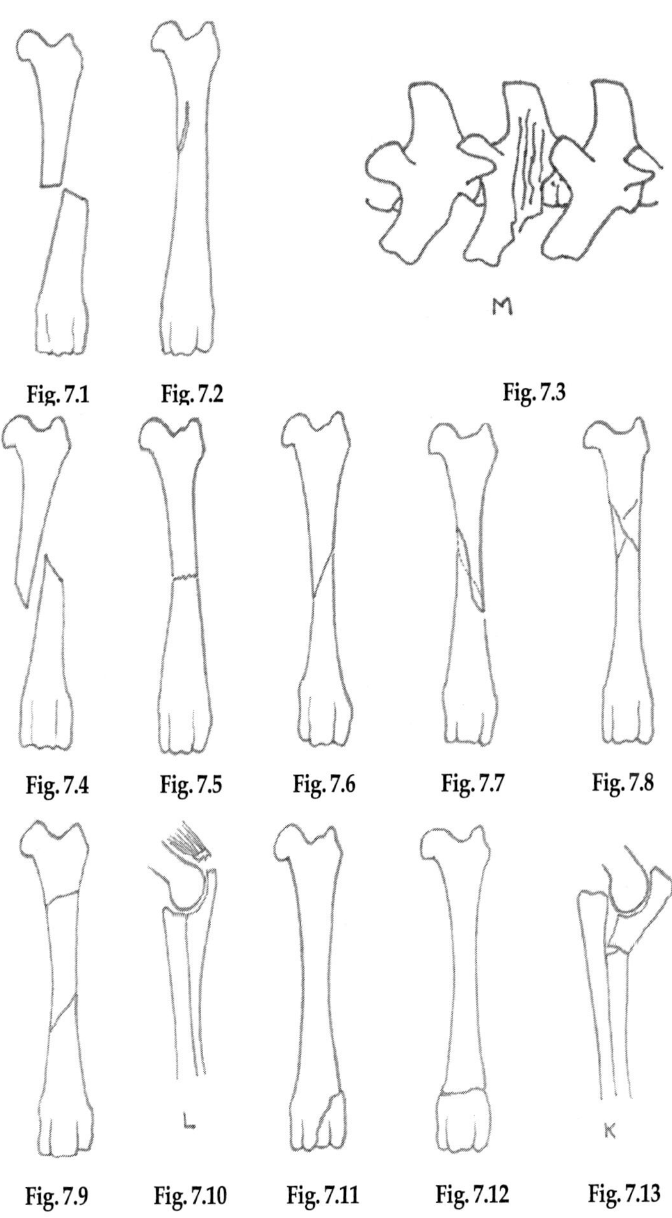

Fig. 7.1 Fig. 7.2 Fig. 7.3

Fig. 7.4 Fig. 7.5 Fig. 7.6 Fig. 7.7 Fig. 7.8

Fig. 7.9 Fig. 7.10 Fig. 7.11 Fig. 7.12 Fig. 7.13

Classification of fractures : Fig. 7.1 : Complete fracture; **7.2:** Green stick fracture; **7.3 :** Comp-ression fracture; **7.4 :** Overriding fracture; **7.5 :** Transverse fracture; **7.6 :** Oblique fracture; **7.7 :** Spiral fracture; **7.8 :** Comminuted fracture; **7.9 :** Maltiple fracture; **7.10 :** Avulsion fracture; **7.11 :** Condylar fracture; **7.12 :** Supracondylar fracture; **7.13 :** Fracture dislocation or Montegsia fracture.

Diagnosis of Fracture

1. *Dysfunction*: Dysfunction is most commonly exemplified by lameness. Dysfunction may also include paralysis with spinal fracture, unconsciousness in cranial fracture, or masticatory dysfunction in mandibular fracture.

2. *Pain*: Pain over the site of fracture is common. In incomplete fractures this may be the only clinical indication.

3. *Local trauma*: Examination of the area around a fracture may demonstrate swelling, hematoma, contusion or laceration if the fracture is open.

4. *Abnormal posture or Limb positioning*: Abnormalities of positioning usually reflects a fracture, deformity, a deviation from the normal anatomical structure, may be caused by displacement of the bony framework as in a fracture or dislocation. The displacement of bone fragments in a fracture may be angular, longitudinal or rotational.

5. *Crepitus*: Crepitus is a sign of fracture that is considered pathognomonic bony crepitus is the gritting sensation transmitted to the palpating fingers by the contact of the broken bone ends on each other. Crepitus may be absent in case of fracture ends are far apart or are interposed by soft tissue or are impacted.

   Pseudocrepitus: e.g. in cases of arthritis, partial luxation of patella.

6. *Radiographic signs*: At least two views including the joints above and below the fracture are needed. The specific radiographic sign of fracture include :

   a. A break in the continuity of a bone.

   b. A line of radiolucency when the fragments are distracted.

   c. A line of radioopacity when the fragments are compressed or superimposed.

7. *Other signs*

   a. Fever

   b. Anemia

   c. Shock – hypovolemic (blood loss)

   d. Nerve injury

   e. Necrosis or gangrene

   f. Fat in synovial fluid.

Fracture Healing

Fracture healing can be divided in to three phases which occur in a sequence but which also overlap to a certain extent.

1. Inflammatory phase (10%)
2. Reparative phase (40%)
3. Remodeling phase (70%)

1. Inflammatory Phase

- When the bone breaks, the soft tissue envelope, including the periosteum and surrounding muscles are torn and numerous blood vessels crossing the fracture line are ruptured.
- The blood vessels are sealed by haemostatic mechanism and accumulated blood in hematoma rapidly clots within the medullar canal, between the fracture ends and beneath the periosteum.
- Since, the haversian blood vessels are torn at the fracture site, blood flow stops within them for a variable distance on each side of the fracture line. Thus, the immediate ends of the bone at fracture site become necrotic.
- The periosteum and marrow bordering the fracture line also become necrotic. Injury to the surrounding tissue and presence of necrotic material at fracture site lead to an immediate and acute inflammatory response.
- Blood and plasma infiltrate the surrounding muscles which, within a few hours, become swollen and edematous. Polymorphs, histiocytes and mast cells soon make their appearance and the process of clearing the debris soon begins.

2. Reparative Phase

- The first evidence of increased cell division is found in about 8 h of the injury, reaching the peak in 24 h. This activity is first seen in the periosteum and tissues immediately around it.
- The hematoma is organized and invaded by fibro-cellular tissue which replaces the clot and lays down collagen fibers and matrix. The hematoma probably plays a role in immobilizing the fracture and serves primarily as fibrin scaffold over which repair cells perform their function.
- The microenvironment around the fracture site is acidic in initial stages which gradually return to neutral and at later stages become slightly

alkaline. This change in pH at fracture site provides an additional stimulus to cell behavior.

- At a short distance from the fracture site and within the deep (osteogenic) layer of the periosteum, the osteogenic cells proliferate and lift the fibrous layer of periosteum within first two days following the fracture. At the same time, osteogenic cells lining the endosteum also proliferate but not to that degree as that of the osteogenic layer of the periosteum.
- The cells within the deep layer of periosteum proliferate so rapidly that within a few days they form a distinct callus around each fragment close to line of the fracture (periosteal or external callus). Simultaneously, capillaries among them also proliferate.
- The osteogenic cells, which are situated deeply within the callus lying within the highly vascular area, become osteoblasts and form bone trabeculae. In some areas, particularly at the periphery of callus, the osteogenic cells that proliferate in the area lacking adequate vascularity (low oxygen tension) differentiates into chondroblasts and consequently cartilage develops in the outer layer of callus. The cartilage thus formed resorbed and replaced with bone by endochondral ossification. The amount of cartilage formation also depends on the degree of fracture fixation. Slight motion at fracture site leads to cartilage formation.
- The periosteal (outer) callus of the two fragments gradually become thicker and fuses forming a bridge (bridging callus). The medullary (internal) and intercortical callus also follow almost the same sequence of events.
- Within a few days, marked vascular proliferation occurs which is accompanied by differentiation of the osteogenic cells in to osteoblasts. The new bone trabeculae of an embryonic type are then laid down.
- The inter-fragmentary gap is invaded by vascular cellular tissue and immature trabeculae of bone with varying amount of cartilage are laid done. At this stage, immobilization of the fragments become more rigid because of callus formation (external, internal and inter fragmentary).
- *Callus* : The cells invade the hematoma and begin rapidly to produce the tissue known as callus, which is made up to fibrous tissue, cartilage or young immature fibers bone.

3. Phase of Remodeling

- It is characterized by slow changes in the shape of the bone to allow function and to restore normal or near normal strength.

- Osteoclastic resorption of poorly placed trabeculae occurs and a new bone is laid down that corresponds to lines of force.
- The callus does not spread indiscriminately in all direction but tends to orient itself towards the opposite fragment.
- The control mechanism that modules this cell behavior is now believed to be electrical.

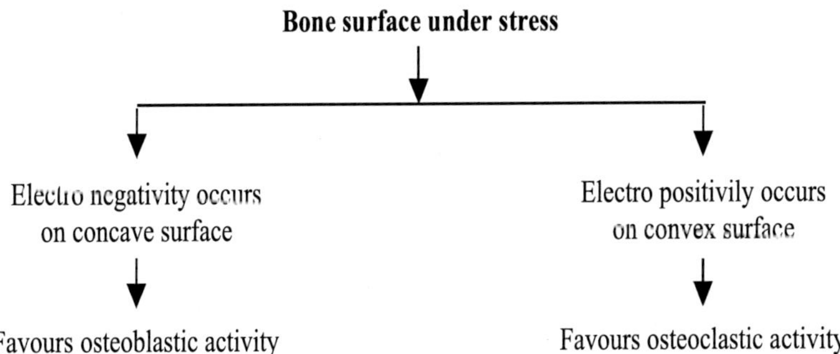

Primary fracture healing : Primary fracture healing occurs where there is absolutely no motion at the fracture site, not even micro movement. Fracture healing with minimum to no external callus is termed as primary healing.

Gap healing : Primary bone formation as it occurs under rigid fixation in areas in which, small gaps are present is called "gap healing".

Contact healing : Primary bone formation as it occurs under rigid fixation in areas in which bone in held tightly in contact is called "contact healing".

Biochemical and Physiological Changes at the Site of Fracture Healing

1. Hyperemia at the site shortly after the fracture.
2. High level of glycosaminoglycans/mucopolysaccharides which gradually decreased.
3. Gradual increase in collagen.
4. Accumulation of calcium hydroxyappatite.
5. An enzyme alkaline phosphatase increases in fracture hematoma about 6-8 times than normal.
6. During 1-2 weeks, fracture hematoma is acidic then neutral and later on alkaline.

Diagnosis of Clinical Union

- Palpable callus.
- Absence of pain on application of angulation stress.
- Absence of movements of fragments at the fracture site.
- Radiographic examination examination.

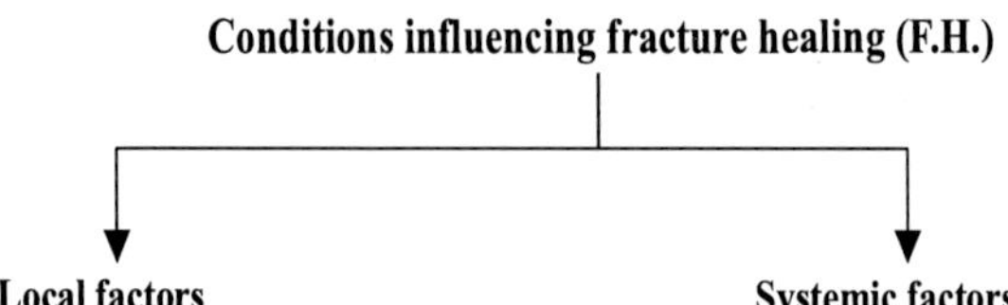

Local factors

1. Degree of local trauma
   ↑ F.H. ↓
2. Degree of bone loss
   ↑ F.H. ↓
3. Distance between fractured fragment
   ↑ F.H. ↓
4. Degree of immobilization
   More motion ↑ F.H. ↓ (non-union)
5. Infection (acidic medium)
   ↑ F.H. ↓
6. Local malignancy F.H. ↓
7. Radiation necrosis of bone F.H. ↓
8. Avascular necrosis F.H. ↓
9. Type of bone involved
   Cancellous F.H. ↑
   Cortical F.H. ↓
10. Type of fracture
    Simple↑
    Compound ↓
11. Type of immobilization
    i) 1. Rigid fixation (DCP): External/periosteal callus: absent or less.
       2. Intercortical callus: Less
       3. Medullary callus: Present
    ii) Pinning / nailing: medullary callus – absent
    iii) External fixation: all type of callus present
12. Site of fracture
    i) Intra articular fracture F.H. ↓
    ii) Extremity F.H. ↑
    iii) Shaft F.H.↓

Systemic factors

1. Age of the patient
   Young F.H. ↑
   Old /adult F.H. ↓
2. Hormones
   GH, T3, T4, Calcitonin, Insulin ↑
   Estrogen ↓
3. Corticosteroids ↓
4. Castration ↓
5. Vitamin A ↑ (high doses) ↓
   Vitamin D ↑ (high doses) ↓
6. Anabolic steroid ↑
   Chondroitin sulfate ↑
   Hyaluronidase ↑
   Anticoagulant (dicoumarol) ↑
7. Anemia, Rickets ↓
8. Hyperbaric O_2 (2h, 2 atm. daily) ↑
9. Physical exercise ↑
10. Denervation ↓
11. Radiation ↓
12. Minerals
    Ca : P ↑
    $ZnSO_4$ ↑

Principles of Treatment: 4 'R'

1. **Removal** of all contaminated and devitalized tissue and restore normal function as near as possible.
2. **Recognition** (clinical history, x-ray and manipulation)
3. **Reduction** of fracture refers to the process of replacing the fractured segments as near to their original position as possible. Complete muscle relaxation facilitates reduction. Reduction may be carried out in three ways.
   - Closed manipulation - by combination of tension and toggling used in areas where bones are easily palpable.
   - Mechanical traction and counter traction - used where muscle exerts a strong displacing force. Gordon's extender can also be used to apply traction.
   - Open approach - the fracture site is surgically exposed under strict aseptic condition. The fragments are manipulated to bring them in apposition.
4. **Retention**/immobilization/fixation - Indicated to prevent displacement of the fragments and to prevent movement and pain.

Points Considered During External Fixation

- Hairs should not be usually clipped.
- Sufficient padding specially at bony prominences.
- Should fit and accurately molded to the configuration of limb.
- In most cases joints above and below the fracture site should be incorporated in the cast.
- After applying the cast, the reduction should be checked by radiography in two planes.

External Fixators

1. *Splints* : e.g. wooden, bamboo, PVC, thermoplastic splints.
2. *Casts* : e.g. plaster cast, fiber glass.
3. Modified Thomas Splint (MTS).
4. *Slings* : Velpau sling and Ehmer sling.

Internal Fixations

1. Steinman Intramedullary Pinning

- The pins may be inserted from within the fracture site *(Retrograde)* or through the extremities of the bone *(Normograde)* (Fig. 7.14).
- Filling the medulary cavity at the fracture site maximizes the resistance to bending and horizontal shear forces. However it can result in damage to the medullary blood supply.
- It is generally recommended to choose an intramedullary pin diameter that fills about 60-70% of the medullary cavity.
- Two or more small diameter pins together can be placed in to the medullary cavity rather than a single larger pin is known as stack pinning (Fig. 7.15).
- Failure is related to mechanical factors such as pin migration, bending and loosening.
- Inadequate seating of the pin in the distal fragment (cancellous bone) will lead to its proximal migration in the postoperative periods.

2. Intramedullary Nailing (K-nail, V-nail)

K-nail should not be used where there are longitudinal or cortical cracks in either proximal or distal fragment of the fractured bone.

3. Interlocking Intramedullary Nail (ILN)

- An ILN is a large diameter pin 6 or 8 mm in diameter with holes to accept screw.
- The nail is placed in to the medullary cavity of a fractured bone and locked to the bone by inserting screws through the holes in the nail and corresponding holes drilled in to cis-cortices and trans-cortices of the bone using a specialized designed zig (Fig. 7.16).
- It provides superior bending stiffness resistance to torsional forces, axial stability and lower implant failure rates than intramedullary pins or bone plates. (Prevent the rotational movements and migration of pins).

4. Rush Pin

It has a hooked end

- A pair of pins is used to immobilize the bone.
- The rush pin is generally inserted from the distal end of the bone (Fig. 7.17).
- Contraindicated in very young animals because of relatively immature and soft cortex and epiphysial region which can easily be damaged by rush pin.

5. Cross Pinning

Useful in compound subarticular fractures of long bones e.g. tibia, metacarpus and metatarsus.

6. Wires

In orthopedic surgery different types of wires are used. They include the rigid Kirschner wire, the flexible orthopedic wire and suture wire.

- *Orthopedic wire*: It is a monofilament soft and flexible wire.
  - *Full circlage*: The wire should be fixed perpendicular to the long axis of the bone and the knot must be twisted down snugly. The full circlage wiring can be used in long oblique fractures, spiral fractures or in fractures that have longitudinal cracks (Fig. 7.18).
  - *Hemicirclage*: Circlage slipping on wedge shaped bones can be avoided by using hemicirclage wire. Hemicirclage wiring is effective in reinforcing longitudinal cracks in the cortex & often in preventing rotation and overriding of oblique fracture fragments (Fig. 7.19).
  - *Tension band wiring or figure of '8' wiring* : It is a form of hemicirclage wiring that is usually used in conjunction with Steinmann pins to achieve stable internal fixation by opposing the pull of muscular attachment on bone. Tension band wiring is used for fixation of patella, fibular tarsal bone, tibial tuberosity, olecranon, greater trochanter of femur, acromian process of scapula, coracoid process of scpula, fractures of the maxilla and mandible (Fig. 7.20).
- *Kirschner wire*: Single pointed Kirschner wires 0.6-1.6 mm in diameter can be used in small animals. They are marketed up to 3 mm diameter and also double pointed. Kirschner wires are used for temporary fixation of fragments, tension band osteosynthesis and intramedullary fixation in small bones. Kirschner wire should be inserted with a hand chuck or low speed drill.

7. Screw

i. Cortical

- These screws are full threaded and used where cortical bone predominates. The screw thread is not as steeply pitched as the cancellous screw.
- The inter-fragmentary compression is accomplished by drilling a long gliding hole (oversized hole) in the near cortex and a smaller threaded hole in the far cortex.

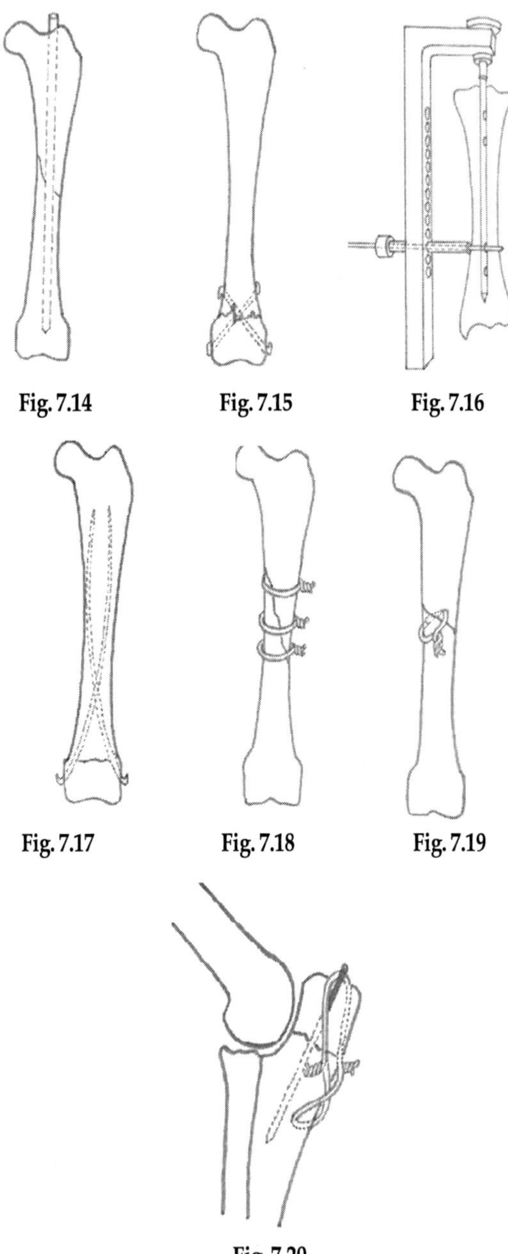

Fig. 7.14 Fig. 7.15 Fig. 7.16

Fig. 7.17 Fig. 7.18 Fig. 7.19

Fig. 7.20

Internal fixations of fracture : Fig. 7.14 : Steinman intramedullary pinning; **7.15 :** Stack pinning; **7.16 :** Interlocking intramedullary nail (ILN); **7.17 :** Ruch pinning; **7.18 :** Full circlage wiring; **7.19 :** Hemicirclage wiring; **7.20 :** Tension band wiring.

ii. Cancellous

- The screws are either partially threaded or fully threaded and used in cancellous bone e.g. fractures of the olecranon, slab fractures of the metacarpus and metatarsus, condylar fractures and longitudinal fractures of the phalanx can be fixed with screw.
- Certain oblique fractures of long bones can also be fixed by application of screw in combination with internal or external support.
- They have a thin core and a deep thread. This large area of thread bone contact in cancellous bone enhances good holding power.
- Removal of partially threaded cancellous screws may be difficult or lead to screw fracture due to deposition of solid bone around the nonthreaded portion of the shaft.

8. Transfixation

- Most useful for treatment of diaphyseal fractures of the radius and tibia.
- A minimum of two intramedullary pins in each fractured fragment are inserted transversely in adult cattle and buffalo. However, one pin in each fragment is considered sufficient in young animals (Fig. 7.21).
- The protruding ends of intramedullary pins are fixed in position by connecting external bars and protected with caps.
- The pins are connected by one or more connecting bars. Depending upon the number of connecting bar they are called as unilateral (having single connecting bar, Fig. 7.22) and bilateral (having two connecting bars, Fig. 7.23).
- The assembly should be removed only after complete union of fractured fragments e.g. 8-10 weeks in adult bovines and 4-6 weeks in young animals.
- Complications: Soft tissue infection, bone necrosis, periosteal reaction around the transverse pins. Pathological fracture may occur at the point of insertion of transverse pins.

9. Hanging Pin Cast

Only one pin is inserted transversely through the proximal fragment.

- This technique has the advantage of preventing rotation of the fractured bone and downward slipping of the plaster cast.

10. Plate Fixation

Most devices approved by ASIF (Association for the Study of Internal Fixation). Plate provide axial compression, counteract rotational forces, do not occlude the intramedullary cavity to compromise intraosseous circulation and can effectively immobilize oblique and comminuted fractures.

Plate classification : Bone plates can be classified according to the function. Each plate type may fulfill one or more different functions, depending on the fracture type and location (Fig. 7.24).

- *Compression plate* : Static compression (a transverse or short oblique fracture can be best treated by compression plate).
- *Neutralization plate* : Splinting of and lag screw fixation (comminuted fracture are anatomically reconstructed).
- *Buttress plate* : Splinting or bridging a fracture area with buttress of the main fragments.
- *Dynamic compression plate (DCP)* : DCP is used for compression and stabilization of a fracture. Compression is achieved by tightening the screws inserted in a specially designed hole in the plate. There are three sizes of DCP used in small animal surgery (2.7 mm, 3.5 mm and 4.5 mm). At least 3 cortical screws on each side of the fractured fragment should be used.

11. Bone Stapling

For correcting valgus and varus deformities of limb bones.

12. Bone Grafts

Cancellous or cortical bone grafts are used to hasten the fracture healing.

- *Autogenous cancellous bone graft*: Harvested aseptically with bone curette from the wing of ilium and proximal part of tibia, femur etc.
- *Cortical allograft*: Harvested from donors of same species. e.g. Freeze dried and freezed grafts or ethylene oxide preserved grafts.

Rehabilitation

- Exercise
- Physiotherapy
- Swimming
- Balanced diet

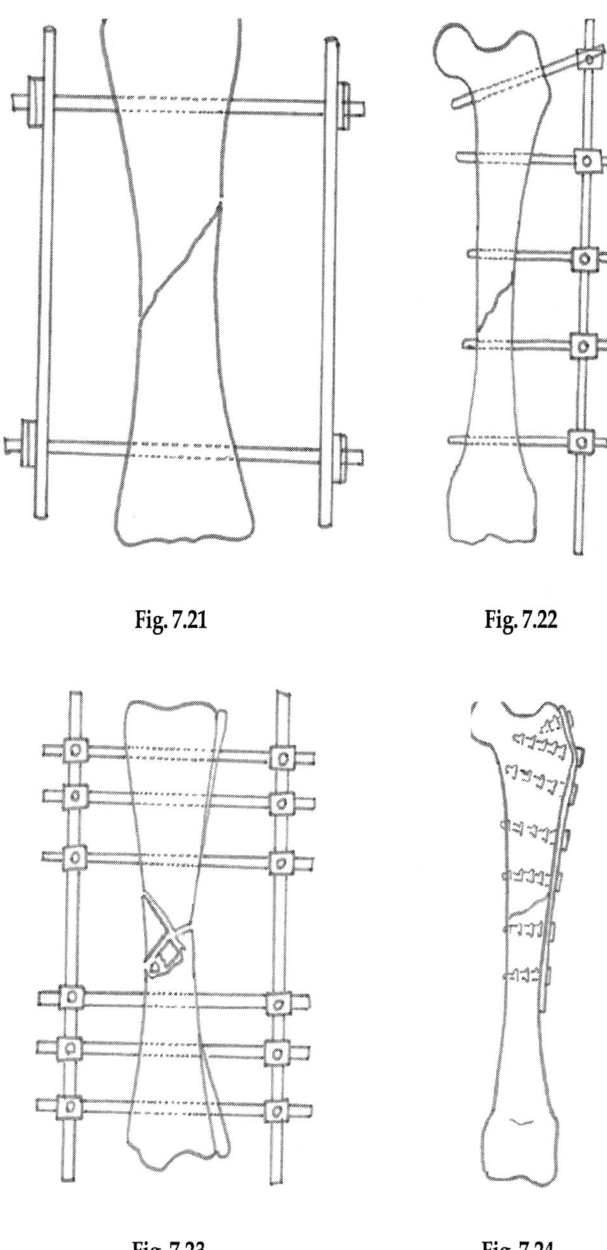

Fig. 7.21

Fig. 7.22

Fig. 7.23

Fig. 7.24

External fixation of fractures : Fig. 7.21 : Transfixation by single pin in each segment; **7.22 :** Unilateral transfixation having single connecting bar; **7.23 :** Bilateral transfixation having two connecting bars; **7.24 :** Bone plate.

Complication of Fracture and Repair

1. *Nerve injury*: Direct trauma and during fracture fixation radial, obturator, peroneal nerve are very prone to injury.

   Sign : Paralysis/recumbent, delayed or non-union.

   Treatment : Spontaneous or anastomosis.

2. *Blood vessel injury*: Direct trauma or at operation time.

   Sign : Diminished pulse, swelling and coldness of distal extremity.

   Treatment : Anti coagulant therapy and anastomosis of blood vessel.

3. *Injury to viscera/ visceral organs*:

   ❒ Rib fracture – Lung, heart, diaphragm, liver etc.

   ❒ Pelvic fracture – Urinary bladder, rectum.

   Treatment : Repair of involved organ before treatment of fracture.

4. *Injures to tendon/ ligament:*

   ❒ Articular fracture, Fracture-dislocation.

   ❒ Affected part should be rigidly immobilized to prevent further damage.

5. *Failure of implant* : Mostly occurs in heavy cattle and buffaloes.

   ❒ Bending of splints.

   ❒ Bending /loosening of plates/ pins.

6. *Infection at the fracture site*:

   ❒ Resulting into delayed union or non-union.

   Treatment – Antibiotic therapy.

   ❒ Removal of died bone (sequestra).

   ❒ Rigid immobilization of fracture site.

7. *Shortening* : may arise from

   ❒ Malunion – overriding.

   ❒ Loss of bone fragments.

   ❒ Injury to epiphysial plate in growing animals.

8. *Joint stiffness* : It occurs mainly due to capsular adhesions and may result from the organization of exudates in the peri-articular tissue.

9. *Post traumatic ossification*: In joint injury → hematoma → ossified.

10. *Avascualr necrosis*: Avascualr necrosis common in fracture of articular cartilage, fracture fragments devoid of soft tissue attachment and excessive periosteal stripping.

    Sign: Nonunion, osteoarthritis.

    Treatment : Rigid fixation, excision arthroplasty – forming a false joint.

11. *Malunion (Angular deformity):* Healing of the bone fragments in an abnormal position. The causes of malunion are:
    - Faulty reduction.
    - Inadequate immobilization.
    - Failure of fixation of the fracture.

    Treatment : Osteotomy is performed and then the case is treated as a fresh case of fracture and managed with appropriate method of immobilization.

12. *Delayed union/Non-union:* Delayed union is prolongation of fracture healing. Nonunion is cessation of fracture healing. The causes are:
    - More gap between the fractured fragments.
    - Loss of blood supply.
    - Damage to the surrounding soft tissues.
    - Compound fracture or Infection.
    - Incomplete fixation.
    - Overstripping of periosteum.
    - If steroids are given.
    - Reaction to orthopaedic implants like plate, intramedullary pins etc.
    - Functional disuse.
    - Early weight bearing.
    - Presence of soft tissue between the fractured ends.
    - Health and age of the animal.

Radiographic Signs of Delayed Union

- Both fractured ends are far apart.
- Presence of very little callus.

Radiographic Signs of Non-union

- No callus formation.
- Sclerosis of bone ends.
- Gap between the bone fragments.
- Medullary canal is completely closed in each fragment.

Clinical Signs of Non-union and Delayed Union

- Abnormal mobility at the fracture site.
- Angular deformity.
- Pain during palpation or during movement.

Treatment of Delayed/ Non-union

- Rigid stabilization.
- Cancellous or cortical bone grafting
- Corrective osteotomy.
- Drilling of multiple holes in the sclerosed fractured ends increases osteogenesis.
- Electrical stimulation at the fracture site.
- Use of Bone Morphogenic Protein (BMP), T_3 and T_4.

Chapter 8

WOUND

A wound is defined as a breach or disruption in the normal continuity of tissue in any body part. The wounds are mainly caused by physical, chemical or biological insult.

Classification of wounds

i) Incised wounds
   - Caused by sharp objects.
   - Minimum loss of tissue.
   - Such wounds heal by primary intention.

ii) Lacerated wounds
   - Caused by tearing of tissues.
   - Inflicted by barbed wires.
   - Such wounds have Jig-Jag borders (Fig. 8.1).

i) Abrasions - are wounds in which the superficial layers of tissue have been destroyed by friction exposing the sensitive tissue.

ii) Contusions or Bruises – There is injury to the skin but without any break or gap in the continuity of tissue surface. Depending upon the extent of the injury and the tissue involved, contusions can further be subdivided in to three categories.

iii) Penetrating wounds
- Caused by long pointed objects and may communicate with body cavities e.g. gored wounds.

iv) Gunshot wounds
- Caused by fire arms.
- The wound may be incised, lacerated or contused, depending upon the velocity of the missile and other related factors

v) Poisoned wounds
- Caused by various types of poisons or toxins.

vi) Bite wounds
- Caused by snake, dog or wild animal bite.

vii) Virulent wounds
- Caused by virus or bacteria leading to the formation of pustules or vesicles e.g. FMD virus, anthrax and tuberculosis causing organisms.

a) **1st degree** - rupture of capillary vessels of the skin and subcutaneous tissue to form ecchymosis.

b) **2nd degree** - larger vessels are ruptured leading to the formation of hematoma.

c) **3rd degree** – tissues are damaged and gangrene may set in.

Seroma: it is a closed collection of serum probably as a result of chronic hematoma in body tissues.

Haematoma: is a collection of blood in an abnormal cavity.

Common sites:

In cow – mammary vein, vaginal mucous membrane

In Bull – penis

Dog – ear flap, vaginal mucous membrane.

viii) Ulcerative – Wound which has no tendency to heal.

ix) Erosive wound – In this type of wound, there is shallow area of necrosis confined only to the epidermis.

x) Punctured wound – These wounds are usually deep and are more prone to anaerobic infection.

xi) Envenomed wound – Inflicted by snakes, ants, wasp, scorpion etc.

xii) Aseptic wound –No infection encountered.

xiii) Septic wound (infected wound) – Micro-organism have invaded the tissues and started multiplying. A contaminated wound may become infected after a lag period of 6-8 hours.

xiv) Contaminated wound – Micro-organisms are present. Strictly speaking all wound other than aseptic wounds are contaminated wounds.

xv) Crush wound – Is one in which severity of trauma is maximum and the status of tissue is completely distorted. Such types of wounds are usually encountered in accidents and very much prone to necrosis/ gangrene.

xvi) Maggot wound- In which the live or dead maggots are visible (Fig. 8.2).

xvii) Avulsion wound – wound in which substantial tissue from the body is lost during injury. It occurs mostly in horn and hoofs.

xviii) Granulated wound – Is one in which excessive granulation tissue is present (Fig. 8.3).

Wound Healing

Wound healing is the restoration of tissue continuity. The biological process of wound healing includes cell regeneration, cell proliferation and production of collagen proteins, proteoglycans to restore both structural and functional integrity of injured area. These events occur in an orderly fashion, beginning with wounding and continue for several months. Higher animals possesses limited regenerative capabilities, therefore, healing in these animals is accompanied by epithelial, endothelial and fibroblastic proliferation with collagen production. Stem cells are being studied in wound healing. The embryonic stem cells are omnipotential cell and one of these cells can develop in to an entire organism. Other stem cells are pleuripotential and can be stimulated to develop in to various specialized tissues.

Process of wound healing : It occurs by two ways:

1. Repair by tissue regeneration i.e. destroyed cells are replaced by cells of their own kind.
2. By the process of substitution where highly specialized cells are replaced by less specialized connective tissue.

1. Repair by Tissue Regeneration

Tissue repair	**Tissue regeneration**
Formation of non-functional scar tissue preceded by an inflammatory reaction.	Is influenced by growth regulating factors that foster the replacement of lost tissue with normal functioning cells. Degree of differentiation $\alpha \dfrac{1}{\text{regenerative capacity of tissue}}$

- On the basis of mitotic capacity, tissues can be divided in to three groups:

  Renewing tissues : Have a continuously active subpopulation of dividing cells from which functioning cells are formed. These cells have a limited life span e.g. hematopoietic cells and epithelial cells.

  Expanding tissue : Cell division is more limited. Cells still retain their mitotic ability but a sub-population of continuously active mitotic cells is absent e.g. liver and bone.

  Static tissue : Do not have the ability to divide e.g. neurons.

- *Difference between hypertrophy and regeneration* : Regeneration begins with tissue loss or damage and is preceded by the classical inflammatory reaction associated with tissue trauma. However, in hypertrophy stimulus it is mechanical in nature.

- *Chalones* : These are tissue specific mitotic inhibitor. It decreases in wounded tissues then cell mitotic rate increases in wounded tissues.
- *Proud flesh* : If irritant, movement or trauma prevents the healing; granulation tissue continues to grow and may be present in abnormally large amounts. This unorganized tissue is called excessive granulation tissue or proud flesh.
- *Keloid* : If collagen tissue deposition enlarges beyond the original size and shape of the wound, it is called keloid.

Regeneration of Selected Tissues

1. Skeletal Muscle

Muscle precursor cell (these cells are derived from satellite cells are structurally undifferentiated cells lies between the basement and plasma membrane of skeletal muscle)

Mitosis and fusion of cells
↓
Myotubes
↓
Muscle fiber

Regenerative healing of transected muscle fibers can be delayed or even prevented if –

i. Any substance is interposed between the cut ends.
ii. Distance between the transected ends is too large.
iii. Loss of large amount of muscle mass.
iv. *Denervation* : In recent cases, denervation atrophy occurs but in long standing cases, loss of regenerative capacities takes place.

2. Smooth Muscle

Smooth muscles have very little regenerating power but heal by fibrous protein reconstitution. Epithelium regenerated rapidly.

3. Liver

In regeneration of liver entire remnant participates in the regenerative process but in other tissues regenerative process confined to the margins of transected tissue. Liver has very high regenerating power.

4. Epithelium and Endothelium

Both have very high regenerative power.

5. Peripheral Nerves

Iinjuries to peripheral nerves are classified according to their severity

i. *Neuropraxia* : Mildest form of injury.

ii. *Axonotmesis* : Physical disruption of one or more axons without injury to the stromal tissue is Axonotmesis. Axoplasm & cell membrane of axon damaged. Schwann cells and supporting connective tissue remain intact.

iii. *Neurotmesis* : Complete severance of all elements of peripheral nerve trunk.

6. Healing by Substitution

In healing by substitution, the destroyed tissue is replaced by granulation tissue. This process can be divided into:

Healing by First Intension or Primary Healing

It occurs in clean incised wound with proper apposition of the incised edges e.g. surgical incisions. Primary healing results in to very little granulation tissue and minimal scarring and contracture.

Healing by Second Intention or Secondary Healing

It occurs if there is considerable destruction or loss of tissue or when the edges of wound are widely separated, necrosis or infection, the healing occurs by second intention. The wound gap is filled by granulation tissue. Secondary healing results in to more scar, more granulation tissue, contracture and more time is taken to heal.

Delayed Primary Closure or Healing by Third Intension

The closure is delayed about 3-5 days to treat local infection or contamination to allow therapy.

Phases of Wound Healing

Wound healing is a complex interrelated process that is divided in to arbitrary phases. These phases are usually known as

1. Inflammatory phase
2. Proliferative phase
    i. Fibroblastic phase
    ii. Epithelialization phase
    iii. Contraction phase
    iv. Remodeling phase

1. Inflammatory Phase (Lag or Preparatory or Substrate Phase)

This phase prolongs up to 6 days and is divided in to:

i. *Stage of inflammation* : The inflammatory response to injury is characterized by a vascular and cellular response which protects the wound against invasion of foreign substances and blood loss. The immediate response to injury is transient vasoconstriction and coagulation followed by active vasodilatation and capillary leak of plasma to the wound area due to release of histamine, serotonin and kinins from mast cell, platelets and a_2-globulin, respectively. The white blood cells, predominate cell is polymorph nuclear cells (PMNs), migrate through vessels specially, venules and eventually concentrates at the site of injury. The wound is filled with an inflammatory exudates in the next few hours. Primary role of PMN is destruction of bacteria. As the PMNs degenerate, their outer membranes rupture and release enzyme containing (collagenase, proteolytic enzymes and PGE_2) granules. These enzymes are released and attack extra cellular debris.

ii. *Destructive stage* : The debridement stage begins 6 h after injury and lasts up to 12 h. Neutrophils and macrophages begin the clean up process by phagocytosis. Macrophages are the most important inflammatory cells for wound healing. These cells precede the onset of fibroplasia during the healing process. Macrophages release a chemotactic substance that not only attracts mesenchymal cells to the area but also influences their differentiation in to fibroblasts and promotes angiogenesis. Monocytes may coalesce to form multinucleated giant cells or become epitheloid cells or histiocytes which are also phagocytic. Monocytes must be present to create normal fibroblast production. Migration of monocytes decreased in the presence of many antiseptics. The destructive phase may prolong in the presence of lot of necrotic debris, wound contamination or large amount of suture material.

2. Proliferative Phase

This phase can be divided into fibroblastic phase, epitheliaization phase, contraction phase and remodeling phase.

i. *Fibroblastic phase* : Just after injury, undifferentiated mesenchymal cells begin to change into migratory fibroblasts. These fibroblasts move into the injured area.

Inflammatory exudates (contains fibrinogen)

Fibrin stabilizing factor (XIII) Ca^{++} 

Fibrin

This fibrin is laid down in the wound and acts as a haemostatic barrier and scaffold. Fibroblasts move by forming a cytoplasmic extension called a *ruffled membrane* which extends from the cell and adheres to a solid substrate (e.g. fiber or capillary). The cell then moves in the direction of ruffled membrane. When the ruffled membrane of two like cells meets, the cells adhere to one another and movement ceases. This process is known as *contact inhibition.* The cell edges free of cellular contact continue to form ruffled membranes and the cells move in the direction of ruffling.

Fibroblasts do not contain fibrinolytic enzymes but when migrating into a wound, are closely followed by new capillaries. The endothelial cells of these new capillaries contain a plasminogen activator. Thus fibrinolysis occurs and the fibrin network is broken down and removed.

Collagen is synthesized by the fibroblasts from hydroxyproline and hydroxylysine beginning on about the 4th or 5th day. The early collagen fibers are called reticulin. Initially collagen fibers are arranged vertical position in the wound. As the wound matures, collagen fibers are arranged parallel to the skin surface. As the collagen content of a wound increases, the glycoprotein and mucopolysaccharide content and synthesizing fibroblast number decreases.

ii. *Epithelialization phase* : Epithelialization is the process where keratinocytes migrates from the lower skin layers and divide. It occurs at about 12 hours following the injury The initial response of cells immediately adjacent to a wound is mobilization. Normally epidermal basal cells adhere to each other and to the underlying layers of the dermis. The proteolytic enzymes released from damaged cells or Leukocytes is responsible for cell mobilization. Following mobilization, epithelial cells enlarge and begin to migrate down and across the wound. These cells usually move across the rest of the basal laminae or along the fibrin deposits. This process is known as *contact guidance.* Migrating epithelial cells stop moving on coming in contract with a like cell and the process is called contact inhibition. Increased mitotic activity of the epidermal cell (around 1-2 mm of the wound) is usually seen after 1-2 day which may be ascribed to the decrease in wound hormone called *chalone*.

    In a sutured incised wound, the epithelial cells begin to migrate immediately after injury and the dermal and subcutaneous tissue of the incision are held together by a cellular fibrin clot. The gap is filled by epithelial cells within 48 hours and epithelial migration ceases within 3-5 days. The epithelial cells also migrate underneath the blood clot, debris or scab and through the suture tract. Keratinization occurs in the uppermost epithelial cells of a wound and the overlying scab is loosened and dislodged by collagenase enzyme.

In open wounds, epithelialization is similar as for incised wound. However, certain differences are observed due to connective tissue regeneration, presence of blood clot and scab formation. Mostly an open wound is initially covered by a blood clot and then by granulation tissue. The migrating epithelium moves under the clot (not through it) and over or into the granulation tissues giving rise to pseudoretepegs. The epithelial cells secrete proteotytic enzymes that dissolve the base of the clot and permits unhindered cell migration. These cells migrate over the wound as a sheet. The process may take weeks to months to epithelialize a large defect completely.

In large open wounds, may epithelialization never be completed or the epithelium in the wounds center may be so delicate that it is continually traumatized, leaving exposed granulation tissue.

iii. *Contraction phase:* In contraction phase, size of the open wound is decreased. Contraction involves the movement of existing tissue at the wound edge. The wound contraction accounts for 40-80% of the wound closure and is best in loose skin regions. The centripetal movement of the skin results from the contractile properties of modified fibroblasts, called myofibroblasts, present in the granulation tissue. Once the contraction begins, it continues until wound edges meet and contact inhibition stops the process. Some wounds fail to contract as they lack contractile myofibroblasts. Different theories of wound contraction has been given by different workers:

- *Picture frame theory* : Fibroblasts within the wound margins migrate towards the center of the wound pulling the skin edges with them.
- *Pull theory* : Mechanism of pull is distributed equally throughout the granulation tissue of a contracting wound.
- *Push theory* : The wound edges are pushed inward by extension of surrounding skin.
- *Sphincter theory* : Contractile material at the wound margin acts as a constricting sphincter.

Disadvantages of contraction

- Contraction of wound near joints may result in the formation of a tight band of scar tissue limiting flexion or extension of the joint.
- Contraction of wound near body openings such as anus, may result in stenosis.

iv. *Remodeling phase/ maturation phase* : Remodeling phase is marked by a decrease in the number of fibroblasts and macrophages. The wound becomes less vascular. The collagen content of the wound begins to stabilize after 21 days. The wound strength continues to increase for months but strength becomes gradually less with time. New collagen fibers are laid down and the old collagen tissue is digested and removed by collagenase enzyme. The increased strength results from intermolecular and intramolecular cross linking of collagen fibers that renders the collagen less accessible to tissue collagenase. Hydroxyproline is the measure of collagen concentration in wound. A scar is never as strong as the tissue it replaces.

Factors Affecting Wound Healing

A. Local Factors

a. *Surgical technique:* Adherence to the Halsted principles is essential for good surgical technique.

b. *Tissue vascularity or oxygen:* Tissue with high vascularity heals more rapidly than poorly vascularized tissue. Any factor which affects blood flow and subsequent O_2 delivery to the tissues will retard the wound healing.

c. *Mechanical stress:* Increase in intra abdominal pressure due to acute tympany may lead to dehiscence of a well apposed abdominal incision.

d. *Movement:* Movement at the site of injury prolongs the healing process and promotes excess scar formation.

e. *Extent of wound surface:* Small clean incised wounds heal more rapidly then the large surface wounds.

f. *Hemorrhage:* Excessive hemorrhage and clot formation at the wound site delays the healing process as the blood acts as a medium for bacterial growth.

g. *Foreign bodies:* Presence of any foreign material in the wound delays wound healing.

h. *Dehydration and edema:* Dehydration delays wound healing, but moderate edema has little or no effect on gain in wound tensile strength. Marked edema has a slight and temporary inhibiting effect on healing.

i. *Radiation and cytotoxic drugs:* Acute radiation and other cytotoxic agents influence the rate of wound healing. Most cytotoxic drugs have their greatest effect on dividing cells. High doses of radiation delays gain in wound strength.

j. *Wound infection:* Infection at the wound site retards wound healing. Wound infection usually results when number of microbes reaches a concentration of 10^5-10^6 organism/gram of tissue or per ml of biological fluid. About 35000 to 60000 bacteria drop into average surgical field each hour. The first 5 hours are safe for primary closure of wound. Bacteria produce collagenase which degrades collagen resulting in to decrease wound strength. The infected wound also had decreased fibroblastic activity. Bacteria changes wound pH, which may also affect local mediators of healing.

k. *Antiseptics*: Antiseptics destroy bacteria but they also injure body cells. Any solution that is not isotonic can injure cells.

l. *Bandaging and biological dressing* : Adherent dressing are detrimental to healing process.

B. Systemic Factors

a. *Age:* Higher rate of wound dehiscence occurs in aged patient which may be associated with nutritional deficiencies, increased susceptibility to infection or decreased rate of fibroplasias.

b. *Obesity:* Incidence of wound dehiscence is relatively more in obese animals.

c. *Malnutrition / hyoproteinaemia:* If serum protein concentration is below 2 g /10 ml, wound healing is inhibited. Decrease in plasma protein decreases fibroplasias.

d. *Vitamin deficiency:*

- *Vitamin A:* It stimulates fibroblasts and the accumulation of collagen. It appears to block the undesirable effects of steroids and radiation on healing wounds. The inhibition of wound healing caused by high doses of cortisone can be completely reversed with high doses of vitamin A. Its deficiency retards epithelialization.

- *Vitamin E*: Vitamin E, like cortisone, stabilizes cellular membranes. High doses of vitamin E retard wound healing and collagen production.
- *Vitamin C:* Its deficiency delays wound healing. Vitamin C is necessary for hydroxylation of proline and lysine for the synthesis of collagen.

e. *Trace elements (zinc):* Normal epithelial and fibroblastic proliferation requires the zinc dependent enzymes DNA polymerase and reverse transcriptase. The deficiency inhibits cell mitosis, fibroplasia and epithelialization. High Zn level can inhibit macrophages, decrease phagocytosis and may also interferes with collagen cross linking.

f. *Anemia and hypoxia:* Anemia associated with hypovolaemia results in increased susceptibility to wound infection and enhanced wound dehiscence.

g. *Systemic disease:* Uremia decreases wound healing by altering enzyme systems, biochemical pathways and cellular metabolism. Poor wound strength in uremia may be due to synthesis of poor quality collagen or increased collagen degradation. Patients with endocrine, hepatic, cardiac disturbances and neoplastic disease show delayed wound healing. In jaundice there is delayed fibroplasia leading to wound dehiscence.

h. *Temperature:* Optimum temperature for wound healing is 30^0C. Decreasing room temperature from 20 to 12^0C wound tensile strength decreases by 20%. It is thought that reflex vasoconstriction is responsible for the decreased healing. There is contraction in heat injured wound.

i. *Anti-inflammatory drugs:*

- *Phenylbutazone, Aspirin and Indomethacin*: In normal doses no effect on wound healing. High doses, delay wound healing by inhibiting biosynthesis of prostaglandins. Oxyphenylbutozne reduces granulation tissue formation.
- *Steroids:* Cortisone and its derivatives decrease the rate of protein synthesis, stabilize lysosomal membranes and inhibit the normal inflammatory reaction. High doses of corticoids limit capillary budding, inhibit fibroblast proliferation and decrease the rate of epithelializaiton. Repeated administration of very large doses of corticosteroids inhibits wound healing. The ill effect of steroids on wound tissue can be reversed by Vitamin A (by stabilizing effect on lysosomal membrane).

Complications of Wound Healing

1. *Hemorrhage* : Severe hemorrhage leads to shock and death. Slight repeated hemorrhage leads to anemia and syncope (cerebral anemia).

   Treatment :

   - Hemostasis by digital pressure.
   - Hemostatic forceps application and ligation of blood vessels.
   - Application of pressure bandage, cautarization with electrocautary or potassium permagnate.
   - Application of Tr. Benzoin.
   - Parentral hemostatics e.g. Styptochrome.

2. *Wound dehiscence* : Predisposing factors include a break in the aseptic technique, obesity, senility, dietary deficiencies and anemia.

3. *Traumatic neuralgia* : It may be primary or secondary in nature. Severe pain along the course of a nerve is known as neuralgia (hyperaesthesia). Primary neuralgia is manifested by pain of prolonged period following the injury. Secondary neuralgia appears during the period of cicatrization.

4. *Traumatic fever and septicemia* : Bacterial toxins produce febrile reaction. Certain pyrogens released form neutrophils and injured body tissues also causes fever by affecting the thermoregulatory center. Massive infection may lead to septic shock.

5. *Traumatic emphysema* : It is a common complication of punctured wounds of the respiratory or gastrointestinal tract.

6. *Tetanus* : It is caused by *Clostridium titani* which releases tetanospasmin resulting in to muscle rigidity. Deep penetrated and punctured wounds are more commonly affected. Protrusion of nictitating membrane is a common sign in equines.

7. *Haematoma and seroma* : Haematoma should not be opened unless it is organized i.e after 5-6 days.

8. *Sinus* : A sinus is a tubular inflammatory tract from a suppurative cavity to the mucous or cutaneous surface along a line of least resistance so as to discharge the purulent exudates to the outside surface. Sinuses may form due to presence of foreign body or dead or necrosed tissue, suture material, parasites etc. Infections like actionmycosis, botryomycosis, inadequate drainage from a suppurative lesion and deep persistent focal infection may lead to sinus formation e.g. Poll evil and Quitter.

Diagnosis

- *Probing*: for depth and direction of the sinus.
- *By dye injection*: Acriflavin solution is injected for assessing the capacity of the sinus.
- By contrast radiography.

Treatment

- Remove the etiological factors.
- Irrigation of sinus tract by irritant solution such as lugols iodine or 10% $ZnCl_2$.
- Making a lower gradient counter opening in the sinus and passing a seton dipped in antiseptic solution. (seton is a bandage strip soaked in an irritant solution which is introduced in to a sinus tract and the end is withdrawn through a fresh opening below the original opening of the sinus).
- Use of antibiotics and anti-inflammatory drugs.

9. *Fistula* : A fistula is an abnormal passage between two internal organs or leading from an internal organ to the exterior or between two cavities. A fistula may be complete (two opening), incomplete or blind (one opening), secretary, excretory, purulent or pathologic.
   - Congenital fistula: e.g. Pervious urachus, anal fistula, rectovaginal fistula
   - Pathological fistula: e.g. Ruminal fistula, reticular fistula, abdominal fistula.
   - Excretory or secretary: e.g. Salivary and teat fistula.

   Treatment : Surgical correction.
10. *Cellulites*: It is a diffuse infective inflammation of the connective tissue and tissue spaces. Multiple incisions to drain out the fluid and antimicrobial therapy are indicated.
11. *Venous thrombosis*: Venous thrombosis may result due to injury to a vein at the wound site. It may be carried to blood stream as emboli.
12. *Adhesions* : An open wound involving the injury to muscles, tendons and other tissues form adhesions during the healing process.

Management of Surgical / Clean / Aseptic Wounds

- The wound should be kept as dry as possible.
- Blood clots and debris should be completely removed.

- The use of mild antiseptic or antibiotic will prevent contamination.
- The sterile dressing should be done on alternate day.
- Suture should be removed after 10 days.

Management of contaminated wound : Traumatic wound of less then 5-6 hours is known as contaminated wound. A contaminated wound can be converted into clean wound.

- The wound should be protected by sterile gauze.
- The area around the wound should be prepared aseptically.
- The wound should be irrigated gently with lukewarm isotonic normal saline or antiseptics.
- All necrosed and dead tissue or foreign material should be removed and irrigation of wound with non irritant antiseptics should be repeated.
- The antiseptic lotion like per chloride of mercury and acriflavin lotion can be used.
- The wound may be closed after providing proper drainage.
- Skin grafting may be attempted in cases when the gap is quite large.

1. *Autograft*: The recipient and donor sites are on the same animal.
2. *Allograft*: The recipient and donor sites are on genetically different animal of same species.
3. *Xenograft*: The recipient and donor sites are on animal of different species.
4. *Isograft*: The recipient and donor sites are between identical twins.
   - Parentral antibiotics for 4-5 days and antiseptic dressing till suture removal are indicated.

Management of Infected Wound

Wound of more than 5-6 h duration is designated as infected wound. Wound infection should be suspected if:

- Signs of inflammation are present.
- Decreased appetite and alertness.
- Increased rectal temperature.
- Increased WBC count.
- Increased serum fibrinogen level.

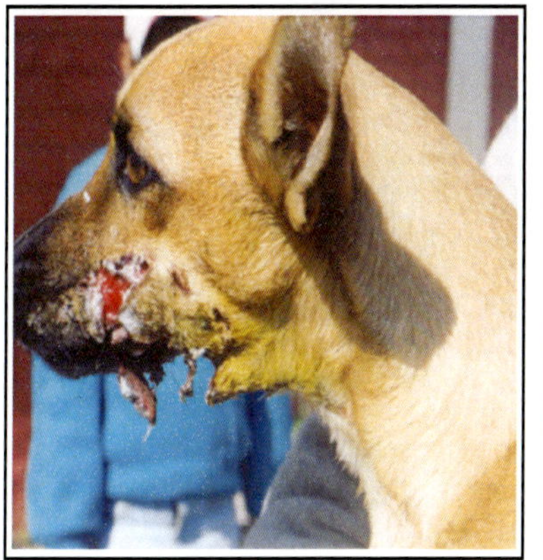

Fig.8.1: Lacerated wound in a dog

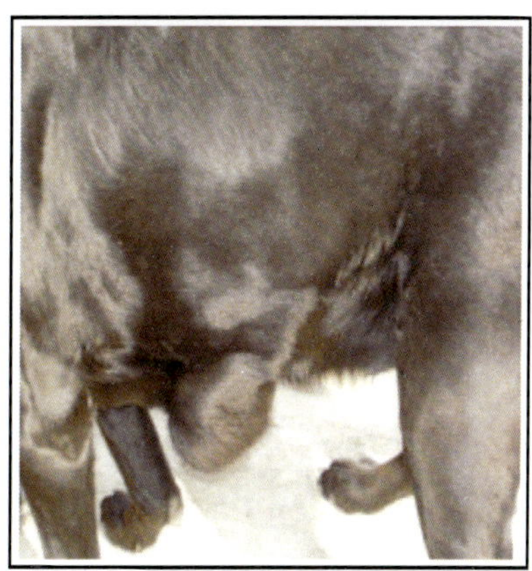

Mammary tumour in a dog

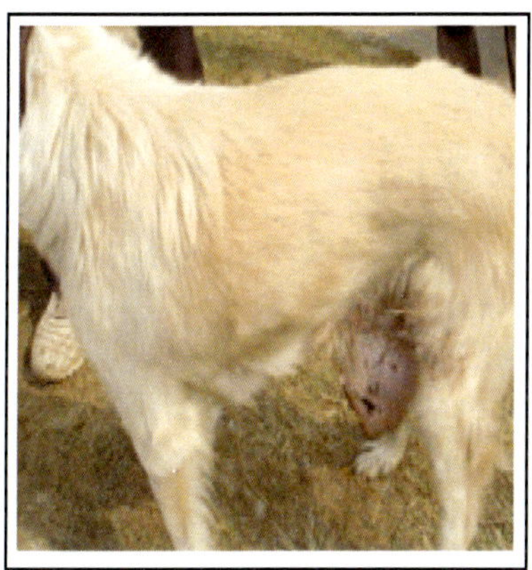

Mammary tumour in a dog

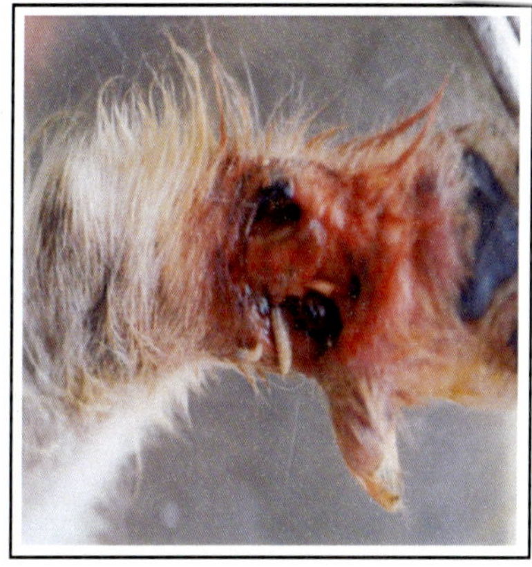

Fig. 8.2: Maggot wound in dog

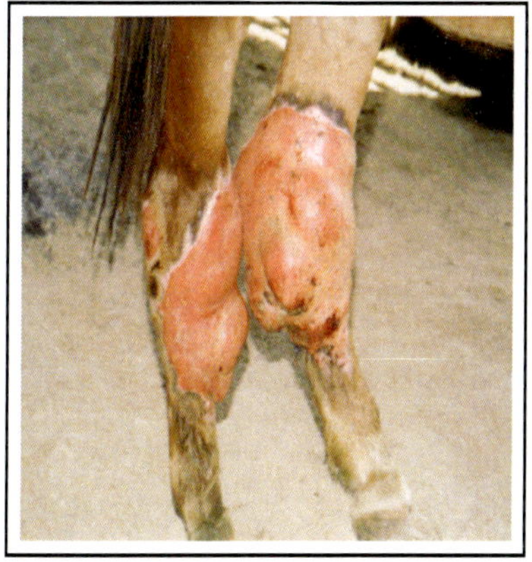

Fig. 8.3: Exuberant granulation in a horse

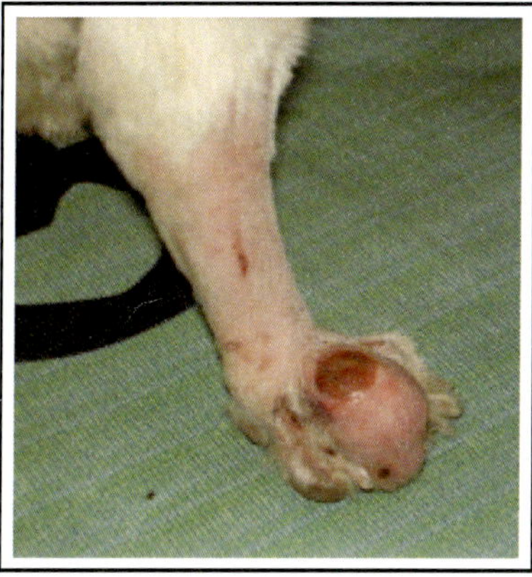

Tummour at paw in a dog

Treatment of Infected Wounds

- *Debridement*: Infected surgical incisions should be opened and all foreign material and necrotic debris should be removed until clean healthy tissue is reached.
- Infected wound should be left open to heal by secondary healing.
- After debridement, the wound should be copiously irrigated with sterile isotonic fluids like normal saline.
- Surgical drains should be placed in the wounds. The drain should be removed when drainage decreases.

Surgical drain : Surgical drain is the device which is used to remove unwanted fluid or gas from a wound or body cavity. It facilitates healing process and used to eliminate dead space.

1. *Passive drains* : Penrose drain. It is used to evacuate a space and should be placed in a dependent position.
2. *Active drain* : Fluid is removed by applying negative pressure to the tube drains.
    - *Antimicrobial therapy*: The antimicrobial agent should be selected only after microbial culture of the wound site.
    - The infected wound should be bandaged until it is completely covered by epithelium.
    - The dressing should be changed daily for 7 days.
    - Generally, infected and deep penetrating wounds are not sutured unless infection is well controlled.

Management of maggot wound – (Traumatic myiasis)

Caused by – *Lucilia cuprina*

Lucilia sericata

Calliphora sp.

Phormia sp.

Treatment

Maggots that are superficial are removed with the help of forceps and gauze dipped in chloroform, turpentine or camphor in oil is allowed to remain in wound for about 24 h.

- Fly repellents like neem oil may be applied on the wound.
- Use of loraxene, himax cream and topicure spray.

Chapter 9

Burn

Burn : Tissue changes due to excessive absorption of heat is known as burns.

Scald : A scald is a burn caused by moist heat and is usually partial thickness.

Etiology

- Dry heat
- Actinic rays (sunburn)
- Irradiation
- Moist heat
- Electricity
- Friction
- Dry heat causes desiccation and charring.
- Moist heat causes boiling or cooking of tissue resulting in coagulation.
- Animal skin, other than pig, do not forms blister.

Classification

1. *1st degree:* Epidermis alone is affected, erythema present.
2. *2nd degree:* Along with erythema, coagulative necrosis of the epidermal cells takes place. Bullae or vesicles are formed.
3. *3rd degree:* Destruction of epidermis, dermis and its components.
4. *4th degree:* The changes are similar to the 3rd degree burn but extend to the subcutaneous fascia and deeper tissues (Fig. 9.1).

   The 1st and 2nd degree burn wounds are more painful than 3rd degree burn.

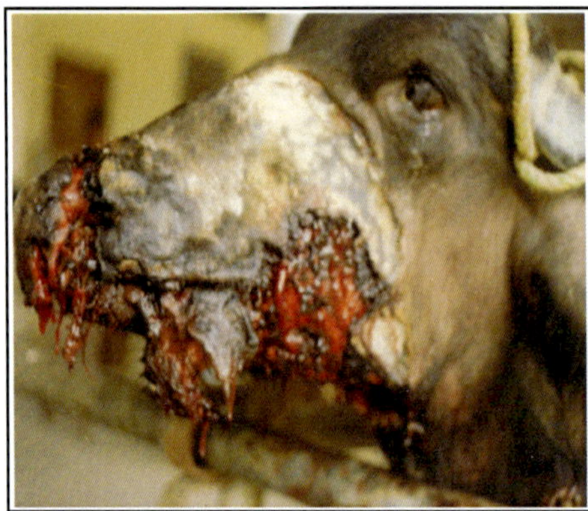

Fig. 9.1: 4th degree burn wound in a buffalo

Patho-Physiology

1. Immunosuppression

- An Immunosuppressive agent is released from severely burned patient which inhibits the migration of peripheral leucocytes and causes the lyses of peripheral lymphocytes from burned patients.

2. Inhalation Injury/Respiratory Tract Burn

- Oral or nasal burn develops stirdor, respiratory distress and laryngeal edema. Endotracheal intubation of such patients should be done before total obstruction.
- Lower respiratory tract burns causes edema with bronchospasm. Treatment included bronchodilators like aminophylline along with steroids. In severe cases mechanical ventilation is indicated.
- Aldehyde (Acrolein) in smoke causes severe pulmonary edema & death.

3. Burn Shock

- Just after burn (first 8 hours), sudden and dramatic changes in circulatory dynamics result in burn shock.
- Causes are fluid loss and fluid shifts, electrolyte imbalances, blood protein losses, myocardial depression, marked increase in peripheral vascular resistance, increased blood viscosity etc.
- Loss of circulatory volume (Hypovolemia) in the first 24 hour through water, electrolyte and plasma protein loss in blister fluid, exudates, edema and by evaporation.
- This is due to vasodilation and increased capillary permeability of the wound, probably mediated by the liberation of histamine, kinins, prostaglandins and fibrin degradation products.
- Considerable heat loss.

4. Burn Toxins

Lipoproteins etc.

5. Burn Wound

In the 1st 24 h after burn, many burn wounds are sterile or have only superficial bacterial colonization.

Severity of Injury

1. *Extent of body surface burnt* : Assessment of burned area in human beings can be estimated on the basis of *rule of nine of Wallace*

   Head and neck-9%

   Hand (each)-9%

   Body (dorsal)-2x9%

   Body (ventral)-2x9%

   Leg (each)-9% (front)

   Leg (each)-9% (back)

   Penile and pubic area-1%

2. *Depth of burn*: Depending on the depth of the skin destruction, the burn can be classified as:

   i. *Partial thickness*: Partial thickness burns heals faster because of remnants of epidermis in hair follicle and sweat glands spread over the wound surface.

ii. *Full thickness*: Healing is slow in full thickness burns and such type of burn is rarely painful due to destruction of most of the nerve endings.

3. *Associated injuries/illness*: Concurrent diseases like renal, cardiovascular or metabolic disorders increases mortality in burn cases.

Treatment

- Immediate care includes application of cold, clean water to the affected part and changes it after every 3 minutes.
- Antitetanus toxoid should be given.
- Partial thickness burns may be relieved by cold water compress and dressings. Cold application retards pain.
- Analgesic or sedative: morphine, ketamine or diazepam in dogs and xylazine or triflupromazine in large animals.
- Hypovolemic shock develops because of losses from burn wound and the formation of inflammatory edema. The lost fluid should be replaced with colloid solution such as synthetic plasma expander e.g. dextran 80.

$$\text{The amount of fluid needed in the first}_t \text{ 4 hours} = \frac{\text{Body wt in Kg x \% burn}}{2}$$

- Fluid requirement can also be monitored by estimating the hematocrit, central venous pressure (CVP) and urine output.
- Urine output should be kept above 1 ml/kg b.wt./h.
- Fluid input will exceed urine output by approximately 3-4 times in the first 48 h. (3-4 ml /kg b.wt/h).
- Mild to moderate degree of acidosis is usually corrected by bicarbonate precursors in electrolyte solutions (lactate, gluconate, acetate etc.). Up to 5 mEq /kg b.wt of Na_2CO_3 can be administered over 30-60 minutes.
- Serum protein should be kept between 3.5–6.5 gm/dl and red blood cells should be given if hematocrit falls below 25%.
- *Treatment of inhalation injury*: Aspiration of fluid from the trachea and bronchi may be needed. Assisted respiration and oxygen is essential. Tracheotomy can be done. Corticosteriods and administration of systemic antibiotics.

- *Local wound therapy/ burn dressing*: Ointments of mafenids and silver sulphadiazine can be applied.
- *Oil based (tulles):* Promotes drying of the wound but tend to adhere and cause pain at dressing changes. The tulles contain Nitrofurazone or Chlorhexidine.
- *Water based cream* : The water based cream should contain antibacterial agents such as Sulphadiazine and 0.5% silver nitrate to reduce the emergence of gram negative organisms in the wet wound environment.
- Systemic antibiotic therapy.
- Skin grafting.
- Physiological dressings include autografts, allografts and xenografts.
- Full thickness burns heal slowly from the wound edges and most of the area requires skin grafting.
- Microbiological monitoring of the wound should be done. Presence of *Streptococcus pyogenes* and other pus forming organisms will destroy skin graft.
- Skin grafts are taken from the areas of normal skin with dermatome.
- The graft thickness should be 15 thousandth of an inch.
- For curing gastric and duodenal ulcers (curling ulcers) H_2 blockers are given.

Complications and Their Treatment

- Acute renal failure and gastro duodenal erosions and ulcerations (curling ulcers) due to stress are the early complications of burn.
- These complications can be treated by restoration of blood volume and maintenance of fluid balance and by administration of H_2 receptor antagonists like Ranitidine, Cimetidine etc.
- Protein losing enteropathy causing hyoproteinaemia (edema and delayed wound healing).
- Chronic scarring.

  Electrical burn : Immediate care of cardiopulmonary resuccitation

Chemical Burns

- The chemicals can be divided into oxidizing agents, reducing agents, corrosives, protoplasmic poisons, desiccants and vesicants.

- Immediate care: Irrigate the burned area with clean water except phenol burns. In case of phenol burns, water increases the absorption of phenol. Polyethylene glycol is of great importance.
- *Treatment* : Neutralization of the injurious agents through irrigation is beneficial.

Frost Bite

- Cold injury to extremities involves either the supporting tissue or primary circulation or both.
- The end results are ischemia, with dry gangrene (mummification).
- *Treatment* : Rapid rewarming of the affected part in warm water at 42°C.

Chapter 10

HERNIA*

A hernia is the protrusion of an organ through a defect in the wall of the abdominal cavity in which it lies.

Classification

1. On the Basis of Anatomical Site

- Abdominal (umbilical and ventral)
- Diaphragmatic

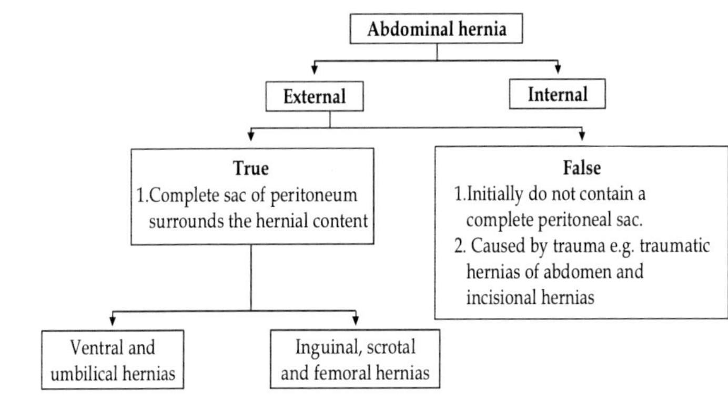

* Dr. A.K. Sharma

- Perineal
- Inguinal (Bubonocele)
- Scrotal (Oscheocele)

2. Congenital/ Acquired

- *Congenital:* Hernia through the anatomical defect at birth (Fig. 10.1 and Fig.10.2).
- *Acquired:* Hernia through the anatomical defect after birth e.g. trauma or incisional.

3. Reducible/Incarcerated and Strangulated

- *Reducible:* When the hernial contents are freely movable and can be pushed back in to the cavity.
- *Irreducible/Incarcerated:* When the hernial contents are fixed in the hernial sac due to adhesion between hernial contents and hernial sac.
- *Strangulated:* Incarceration may cause obstruction of lumen and hamper the blood supply to the herniated mass. Such type of hernia is known as Incarcerated hernia.

4. On the Basis of Hernial Contents

- Intestine, liver, spleen etc.
- Omentum
- Uterus/urinary bladder.

Parts of Hernia

1. *Hernial ring:* Defect in the limiting wall is known as hernial ring.
2. *Hernial sac:* The tissue that covers the hernial contents is known as hernial sac.
3. *Hernial contents:* Organ or a tissue that descends/moved in to the abnormal location is known as hernial contents.

Principles of Herniorrhaphy

1. Reposition of hernial contents in to their normal anatomical position.
2. Closure of the hernial ring either by applying sutures or by mesh/ patients tissue itself (in large hernias).
3. Closure of skin and subcutaneous tissues.

Inguinal Hernia (Bubonocele)

Protrusion of abdominal contents through a defect in the inguinal ring is known as inguinal hernia.

Scrotal Hernia (Oscheocele)

Descendent of abdominal contents (through the defect in the vaginal ring) in to the scrotum named as scrotal hernia (Fig. 10.3).

Femoral Hernia

Protrusion of abdominal contents through the femoral canal is named as femoral hernia.

Diaphragmatic Hernia

Herniation of the abdominal viscera in to the thoracic cavity through thr defect in the diaphragm is named as diaphragmatic hernia.

Hiatal Hernia

Protrusion of abdominal contents in to the thorax through the esophageal heatus of the diaphragm.

Perineal Hernia

Protrusion of abdominal and/or pelvic contents through the defect in the pelvic diaphragm (between the pelvic diaphragm and rectum) (Fig. 10.4).

Umbilical Hernia

Protrussion of the abdominal contents through the defect in the umbilicus (Fig. 10. 5 to Fig. 10.8).

Ventral Hernia

Protrussion of the abdominal contents through the defect in the ventral abdominal wall (Fig. 10.9 and Fig. 10.10).

Ulcer

An ulcer is formed when the surface epithelium of an organ or tissue (skin or mucous membrane) is lost due to necrosis which is replaced by inflammatory tissue.

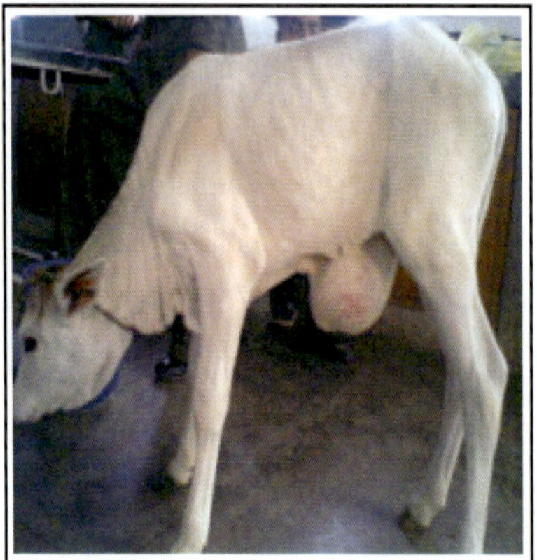

Fig.10.1: Congenital umbilical hernia in a calf

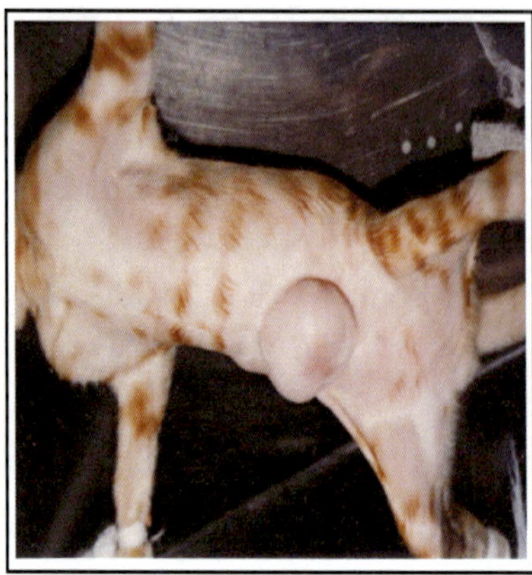

Fig. 10.2: Congenital umbilical hernia in a cat

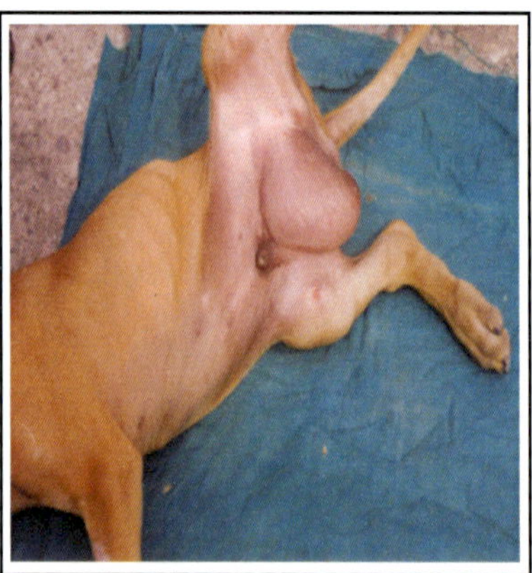

Fig. 10.3: Scrotal hernia in dog

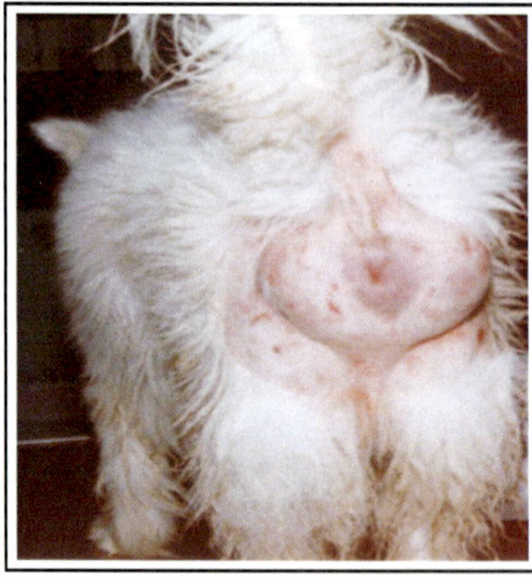

Fig. 10.4: Perineal hernia in dog

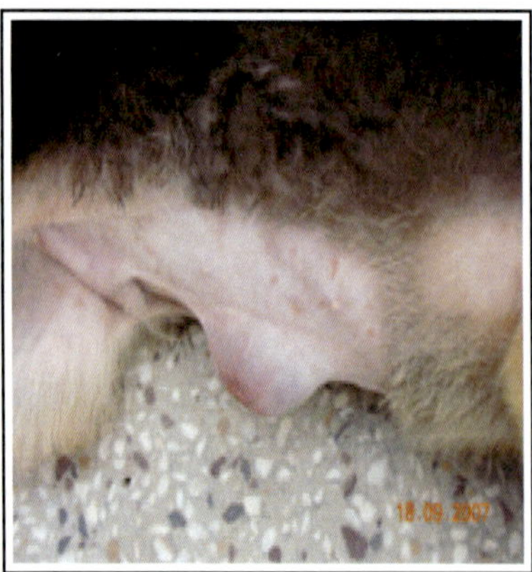

Fig. 10.5: Umbilical hernia in a dog

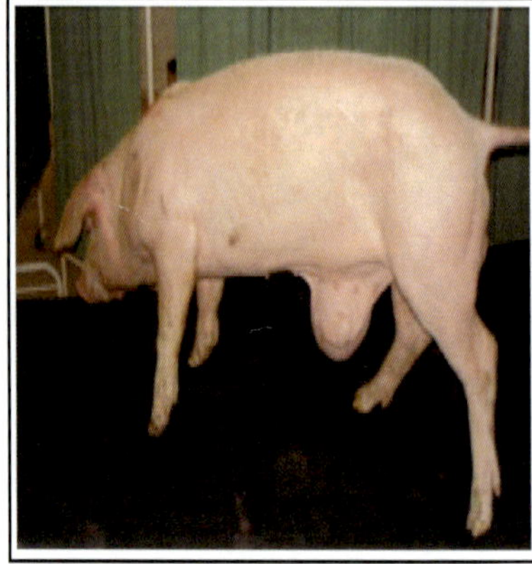

Fig. 10.6: Umbilical hernia in a pig

Classification

1. *Phagedenic ulcer* : An ulcer which is invaded by pathogenic organisms.
2. *Decubital ulcer*: Also known as bed sore, pressure sore or trophic ulcers. Continuous pressure over the bony prominences leads to formation of bed sore.
3. *Indolent ulcer*: Indolent ulcers have no tendency to heal. Such types of ulcers are chronic and painless.
4. *Callous ulcer*: Such types of ulcers have thick callous lining.
5. *Indurated ulcers*: Such types of ulcers have thick indurated edges.
6. *Malignant ulcers*: Such an ulcer is the result of growth of a malignant tumor e.g. rodent ulcer caused by basal cell carcinoma.
7. *Ulcers in different diseases*: e.g. Ulcerative lymphangitis, tuberculosis, glanders etc.
8. *Irradiation ulcers* : Such type of ulcers results from exposure of tissue to radiation like X-rays, UV-rays etc.

Treatment

- Removal of primary cause.
- Antiseptic dressing.
- Application of caustics like carbolic acid and thermocaterization.
- Cryosurgery.
- Excision of ulcer.

Cyst

A cyst is a blind sac lined by a secreting membrane which contains liquid or solid substances.

Classification

Retention Cyst

- *Ranula*: Accumulation of saliva in the salivary gland or its duct.

Congenital Cysts

- *Dermoid cyst* : A dermoid is an abnormal development over the conjunctiva, cornea and eyelid margins which is caused by aberrant migration of ciliated dermal tissue to these sites.
- *Urachal cyst*: The urachal cyst is formed if atrophy of the urachus is incomplete after birth. Urachal cyst exists when secreting urachal epithelium forms an isolated segment from a persistant urachus.

- *Dentigerous cyst*: Development of abnormal tooth in an abnormal position.
- *Branchial cyst*: The cyst arise from remnants of branchial pouch epithelium.
- *Encapsulated cyst:* The cyst develops around the parasites.
- *Degeneration cyst:* Degeneration of new growth leads to degenerative cyst.
- *Exudation cyst:* Accumulation of large amount of fluid in preexisting space e.g. hydrocele.

Treatment

- Destroy the secreting membrane, after evacuating the fluid, by an irritant solution like Tr. Iodine.
- Incise the cyst and debride the cavity.
- Excise the cyst.

Abscess

It is a circumscribed closed cavity containing pus (purulent exudates) surrounded by a limiting membrane 'the pyogenic membrane' (It serves to prevent dissipation of infection). Tissue reactions against the invading organism or foreign body as well as degenerative changes are evident in pyogenic membrane. The pus may consist of dead and living neutrophils, cellular debris, lymph and serum. Various types of pus are sero pus, muco pus, serosanguinous pus, sanguinous pus, sterile pus, dead pus and living or laudable pus (laudable pus is characterized by living leucocytes with substantial activity) (Fig. 10.11).

Classification of Abscess

1. Acute or chronic.
2. Superficial or deep.
3. *Embolic abscess*: Embolic abscess is resulted by an embolus from an abscess to another location.
4. *Hemorrhagic abscess*: In hemorrhagic abscess the contents are blood like or mixed with blood.
5. *Gaseous abscess*: is one in which the content or the pus is cheesy. Very common in udder and yoke gall in working animals.
6. *Dry abscess*: the content are almost desiccated.

7. *Shirt and Stud abscess*: There is an abscess in which two minute abscesses are placed closely and are connected by a narrow channel.
8. *Anorectal abscess*: Abscess in which the continuity between the rectum and anus.
9. *Brodies abscess*: It is a chronic semipurulent lesion over the tibial head. *Mycobacterium tuberculosis* organism is usually associated with such lesions.
10. *Canalicular abscess*: Usually present in udder
11. *Pneumatic abscess (tympanitic abscess)* – when opened, pus mixed with gases is released.
12. *Stitch abscess*: is one which is associated with an infected suture.
13. *Parasitic abscess*: caused by parasites.
14. *Idiopathic abscess*: cause is uncertain.

Etiology: The causative organisms of an abscess are:

- *Staphylococci* sp.
- *Streptococci* sp.
- *E. Coli*
- *Corynibacterium* sp.
- *Pseudomonas* sp.
- *Actinomyces bovis*
- *Actinobacillus lignieresi*

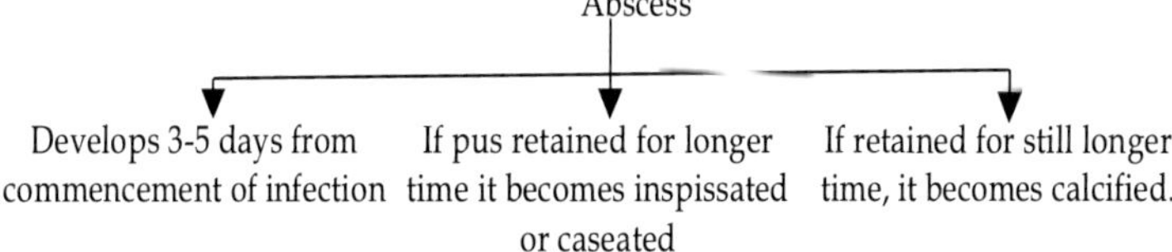

Why Pain is Evident in Acute Abscess?

The rapid formation of exudates in acute abscess develops pressure on the surrounding tissues thereby causing considerable pain.

Pointing of An Abscess

Inflammatory swelling (painful)
↓
Center becomes softer and thin
↓
Finally ruptures leading to escape of pus.

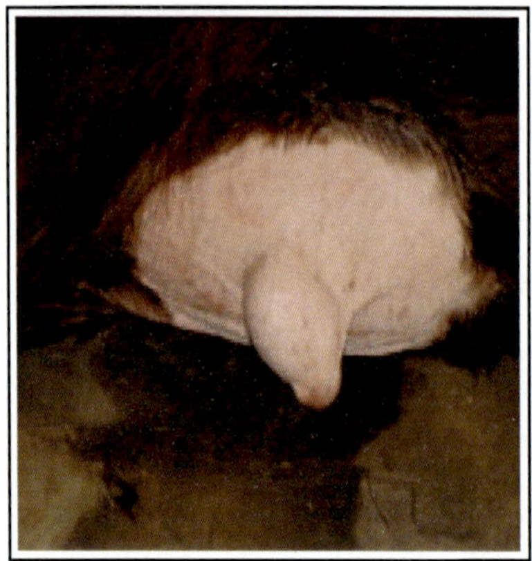

Fig. 10.7: Umbilical hernia in a buffalo calf

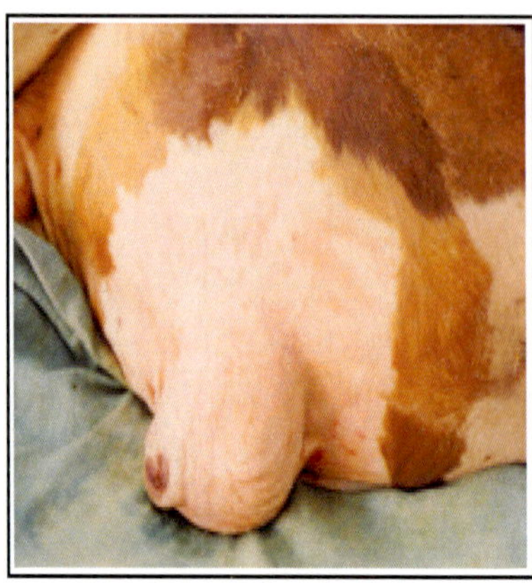

Fig. 10.8: Umbilical hernia in a calf

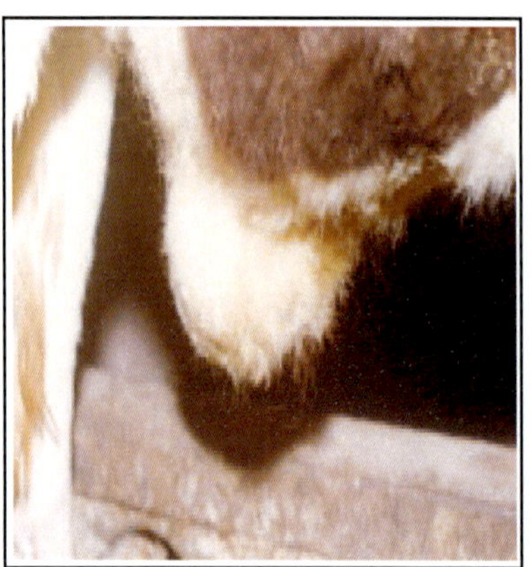

Fig. 10.9: Ventral hernia in a heifer

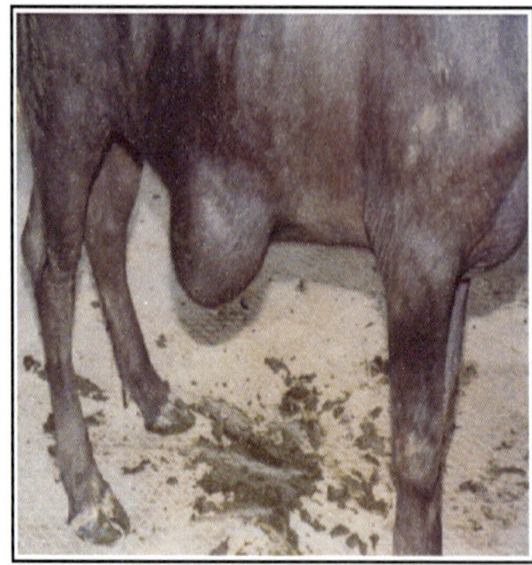

Fig. 10.10: Latero-ventral hernia in a buffalo

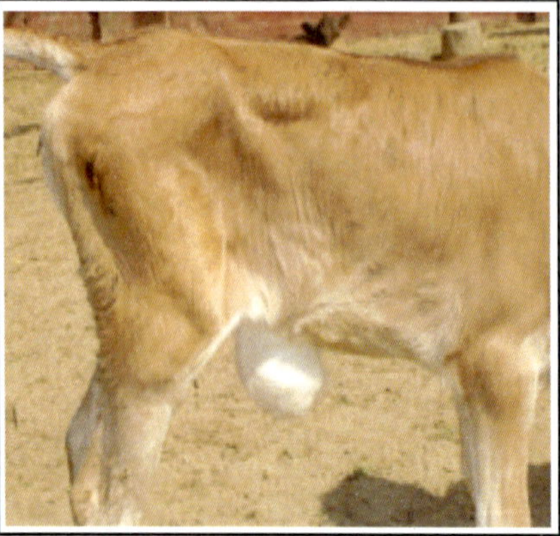

Fig. 10.11: Umbilical abscess in a calf

Treatment : Maturation followed by opening of abscess.

a. Maturation is hastened by use of hot fomentation or by application of mild rubefacient e.g. iodine ointment.

b. The mature abscess should be incised at the most dependent part with a knife (Syme's knife). The incision should be made parallel to the long axis of vessels and nerves running in the area.

c. After opening and evacuation, the abscess should be irrigated with antiseptic lotion.

d. Antiseptic dressing is indicated.

e. Chronic cases should be dressed with irritant antiseptic to promote inflammation and consequent granulation and cicatrisation.

Acne: It is an abscess involving the sebaceous gland.

Furunculosis: It is characterized by group of boils in different part of body. A boil is an abscess involving the hair follicles caused by *staphylococci.*

Antibioma: when an abscess is treated with antibiotics without proper drainage, there will be fibrosis around the abscess cavity and fluid in it may get absorbed making the pus inspissated, such a clinical condition resulting from improper treatment of an abscesses called antibioma.

Sit fast: This condition is common in horses. Sit fast is the dry gangrene of the neck caused by the pressure of the collars

Gall: A gall is a localized acute inflammation of the skin and subcutaneous tissue along with accumulation of inflammatory exudates e.g. Yoke gall in cattle and saddle gall in equines.

Yoke gall: It is the inflammation of skin and subcutaneous tissue on the dorsal surface of neck of bullocks and buffalo bulls.

Etiology: Constant friction/ irritation of the tissue.

Predisposing Factors

- Young bulls/ bullocks are more prone to yoke gall.
- Rough surfaced yoke.
- Unequal size of the bullocks/bulls used in the cart/ plough.
- Heavy load for longer duration.

Clinical Signs

- Warm and painful swelling over the dorsal surface of the neck.
- The swelling may be soft or hard (fibrous). The fibrous swelling is named as tumor neck.
- Yoke gall may change in to an acute or chronic abscess with or without oozing of purulent exudates.

Diagnosis : On the basis of clinical signs and exploratory puncture.

Treatment

- After maturation, the cavity is incised to drain the pus.
- The cavity is irrigated with an antiseptic solution like potassium permagnate (1:1000).
- Daily antiseptic dressing.
- Systemic administration of NSAIDs and Antibiotics.
- Radical surgery is indicated for tumor neck.

Bier's Hyperemia

Bier's hyperemia is used to treat the septic inflammatory lesions of extremities like limbs and tail.

A moderately tight elastic tourniquet is applied just proximal to the lesion to create the passive hyperemia by venous congestion in the affected region. The extravasation of the serum and leucocytes leads to destruction of bacteria and their toxins. The tourniquet is released after 3-4 hours.

The tourniquet should not be very tight.

Differential diagnosis of abscess, hematoma, cyst, tumor and hernia : Exploratory puncture is the most reliable method of differentiating the various lesions. The puncture should be done by sterilized hypodermic needle and the region should be cleaned and shaved. Other methods of differentiation are as follows:

S.N.	Signs	Abscess	Hematoma	Cyst	Tumor	Hernia
1.	Development	Slowly	Quickly	Very slowly	Prolong	Slow
2.	Fluctuation of lesion	Uniformly	Does not fluctuate but may crepitate on feeling with fingers	Very uniformly	Do not fluctuate	Do not fluctuate but it may be reduced by physical pressure in many cases
3.	Pain on palpation	Very painful in acute condition and painless in chronic cases	Painful	Painless	May be painful / painless	Usually painless
4.	Ripening or maturation	Ripes or matures	-	-	-	-
5.	Hernial ring	-	-	-	-	Present

Chapter 11

INFLAMMATION

It is defined as the reaction of living tissue to injury which begins following a sub-lethal injury to tissues and ends with complete healing. The purpose of inflammation is to destroy and remove the irritant and to repair the damaged tissue.

Causes

1. Pathogenic organisms: Bacteria, virus, fungi, protozan and parasites.
2. Chemical poisons: Acid and alkalies.
3. Mechanical or thermal injuries.
4. Immune reaction: Antigen antibody reaction.

Coordinal Signs of Inflammation

1. Rubor (redness) given by cesus
2. Tumor (swelling) given by cesus
3. Calor (heat) given by cesus
4. Dolar (pain) given by cesus
5. Functio – Laesa (loss of function) given by virchow.

Classification of Inflammation

1. On the Basis of Duration of Course and Intensity of Symptoms

a. *Acute*: Caused by severe irritant.
b. *Subacute*: Caused by or repeated attack of irritant.
c. *Chronic:* Characteristic feature is formation of fibrous tissue.

2. On the Basis of Nature of Exudates

a. *Serous inflammation*: inflammation of serous membrane like peritoneum and pleura.
b. *Hemorrhagic inflammation*: blood is present in exudates.
c. *Fibrinous inflammation (croupus):* exudate contains fibrin which cause adhesions e.g. fibrinous pericarditis.
d. *Purulent (suppurative) inflammation*: characterized by the formation of pus.
e. *Phlegmonous inflammation*: caused by pyogenic organism forming a purulent exudate.
f. *Catarrhal inflammation*: mucous surface is affected which is marked by discharge of mucous and epithelial debris.
g. *Membranous or diphtheritic inflammation*: affecting mucous surface, characterized by the formation of false membrane.

3. Based on Sequelae or Tissue Changes

a. *Adhesive*: there is adhesion of opposite surface.
b. *Obliterative inflammation*: inflammation of a lining membrane of a cavity or vessel. Finally there is obliteration of lumen.
c. *Hyperplastic*: formation of new connective tissue in abundance.
d. *Atrophic*: inflammation which leads to atrophy and deformity.
e. *Granulomatous inflammation*: inflammed tissue resembling granulation tissue.
f. *Necrotic inflammation*: death of affected tissue.

4. Based on the Extent of Tissue Involved

a. *Diffuse inflammation*: spread over a large area.
b. *Focal*: confined to a particular spot.
c. *Disseminated inflammation*: there are a number of distinct foci.
d. *Interstitial inflammation*: this primarily affects the stroma of an organ.
e. *Parenchymatous inflammation*: affecting parenchyma of organ.

5. Based on Etiology

a. *Specific*: caused by a particular microorganism.
b. *Traumatic*: caused by injury.
c. *Allergic*: caused by allergic substance.
d. *Toxic*: caused by a toxic substance or inflammation leading to toxaemia.

Termination of Inflammation

Delitescence : disappearance of inflammation in mild cases.

Treatment

1. Removal of etiology.
2. Cold and astringent application.
3. Compression and application of pressure bandage.
4. Fomentation in severe inflammation, in the form of dry or moist heat.
5. For superficial lesion application of local analgesics.
6. Cortisone -as anti-inflammatory agent.
7. For chronic cases - counter irritant.

Gangrene

Gangrene is the invasion and putrefaction of necrotic tissue by saprophytic bacteria.

Causes

1. In Lungs

i. Due to faulty drenching of medicine.
ii. Food may pass into the trachea.
iii. Careless passage of stomach tube into the trachea.

2. In Intestines

Due to the interference with the blood or nerve supply to a part.

(i)

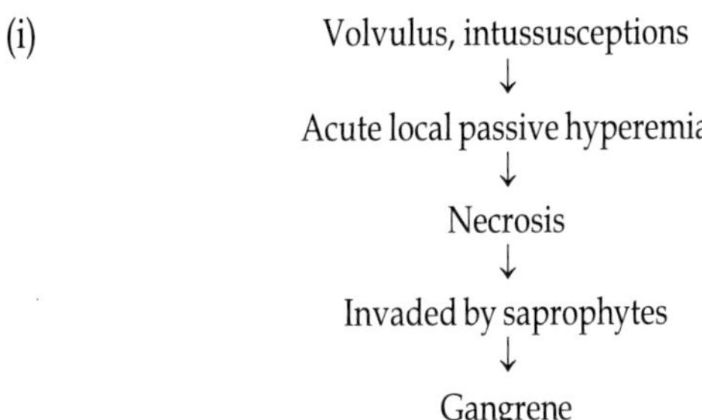

(ii) In horse gangrene of intestine is due to infection by *Strongylus vulgaris.*

Local deficiency of actual blood anurysm and
thrombosis of mesentric artery
↓
Infarction of bowel
↓
Saprophytes invasion
↓
Gangrene

3. Extremities

- Frost -bite (thrombosis of blood vessels), burns and scald.
- Ergot - causes contraction of smooth muscle.

4. Mammary Gland

- Mastitis

5. Traumatic Injuries

- Bed sore (dry gangrene)

Types of Gangrene

1. *Dry gangrene* : Tissue that is poor in moisture and in which evaporation of moisture is possible (e.g. extremities and surface of body). The gangrenous tissue becomes dry and so it is called dry gangrene.
   - Cold, skin has a leathery feel & the tissues are shriveled or mummified.
   - Fe (from Hb) → H_2S (from putrefactive bacteria) → FeS (iron sulphied which is supplied, black or greenish having foul odour)+ H_2
   - The dead tissue is demarcated from the living by a line of inflammatory granulation tissue.
   - Contraction of tissue.
   - Acids which coagulates the fluids cause dry gangrene.
2. *Moist gangrene* : This type of gangrene is seen in internal organs where conditions are conducive for the rapid growth of organisms e.g. abundant moisture (which does not get evaporated) and optimum temperature (part is kept warm by surrounding organs).
   - No demarcation is visible between the dead and living parts.
   - Enlargement of the tissue and severe pain.

- Dead tissue invaded by saprophytes.

  ↓

  Liquefied and production of skatol and indol (foul odour).

3. *Gas gangrene* : Anaerobic spore forming bacteria (*clostridium* group) are pathogenic as well as saprophytic organism.
   - In man caused by *Clostridium welchii.*
   - *Clostridium novyi* - Black disease.
   - *Clostridium septicum* - malignant edema.
   - In animals- *Clostridium chauvoei* (black quarter disease) - causes gas gangrene.
   - Alkalis which liquify the tissues cause moist gangrene.

Termination

- Sloughing of dead tissue
  The process of gangrene is marked by three stages:
  Death of tissue, separation of slough and
  Healing (cicatrisation).

Complications

- Death due to toxaemia or secondary bacterial infection.
- Secondary hemorrhage.

Treatment

- Removal of cause
- Application of an irritant
- Excision of dead tissue

Necrosis

Local death of cells or tissue in a living body due to pathological reasons is known as necrosis.

- The changes that take place gradually in the cells while they are dying is known as Necrobiosis or Apoptosis.
- Necrosis usually preceded by cloudy swelling, fatty change and hyaline degeneration. Severe irritant can cause necrosis directly.

Causes

1. *Poisons*
   - Chemical-Strong acid/alkalis, insecticides, fungicides, lead asrenate, phenol (death by coagulation).

- Poisons of pathogenic microorganisms - toxins produced by bacteria, virus, fungi, rickettsia, protozoa and metazoan parasites.
- Plant poisons - Alkaloids produce necrosis.
  a. Senecio - hepatotoxic
  b. Mushroom-contains toxic glycoside 'Phallin' - renal tubular necrosis.
- Toxins produced within body - e.g. in burn and uremia.
- Animal poisons - cantheridin (from beetles) - cause skin necrosis.

2. *Loss of blood supply* : If O_2 supply and nutrition to the tissue are cut off by blocking blood supply, necrosis results.
   - Passive hyperemia.
   - Ischemia - decreased blood supply
     a. Thrombosis and embolism.
     b. Compression of artery by tumor, ligature, torniquet, abscess, cysts.
     c. Volvulus, intusucception of intestine.
     d. Ergot poisons.
3. *Mechanical injuries* : crushing
4. *Physical agents* :
   - Excessive heat - by denature and coagulation.
   - Excessive cold - by stopping enzymatic activity.
   - Frost bile causes thrombosis of blood vessels.
   - Electric current.
   - X-ray.
   - Ultra Voilet rays.
   - Karyorrhexis - Fragmentation of the nucleus.
   - Karyoschisis - Cracks of the nucleus.
   - Karyolysis - dissolution of nucleus.
   - Chromatolysis - disappearance of nucleolus and chromosomes.

Types of Necrosis

1. *Coagulation necrosis*: cells become necrosed but architectural detail of the tissue is preserved.
2. *Caseation necrosis*: all details of structure are lost.

3. *Colliquative necrosis or Liquefaction necrosis*: liquefaction of tissue may occur in two ways –
   a. by the action of intracellular autolytic enzymes.
   b. by the proteolytic enzymes of leucocytes.
4. *Fat necrosis*: Necrosis of fat in adipose tissue may be of two types.
   - Traumatic – usually in the subcutaneous tissue that is exposed to external trauma – fighting, biting etc.
   - Enzymatic – pancreatic enzymes on the surrounding adipose tissue.
5. Avascular necrosis (bland necrosis; simple necrosis, spontaneous necrosis; anaemic necrosis or aseptic necrosis) where in the necrosis is caused without infection or inflammation.
6. *Ischaemic necrosis*: is due to occlusion of an artery supplying the region.
7. *Embolic necrosis*: caused by embolism.
8. *Diphtheritic necrosis*: is necrosis of a mucous membrance wherein a tough membranous layer called "diphtheritic membrane" formed by coagulated cells and fibrin e.g. Bed sore (this is a local necrosis of the skin and subcutaneous tissue due to constant pressure on bony prominences) and Sit fast (caused by the pressure of the collar on the top of the neck of the horse. Necrosed tissue is cone shaped. Ill fitting saddle may also cause sit fast).

Results of Necrosis

- Liquefaction and removal.
- Liquefaction and formation of cyst.
- Liquefaction and abscess formation.
- Encapsulation without liquefaction.
- Sloughing
- Organization or replacement by scar tissue.
- Calcification
- Gangrene
- Death of individual.
- Regeneration

Chapter 12

SPRAIN, STRAIN AND BURSITIS

Sprain : It is defined as a joint injury in which fibers of supporting ligaments of the joint are ruptured by direct or indirect trauma. Depending upon the degree of ligament rupture, sprain can be classified as follows:

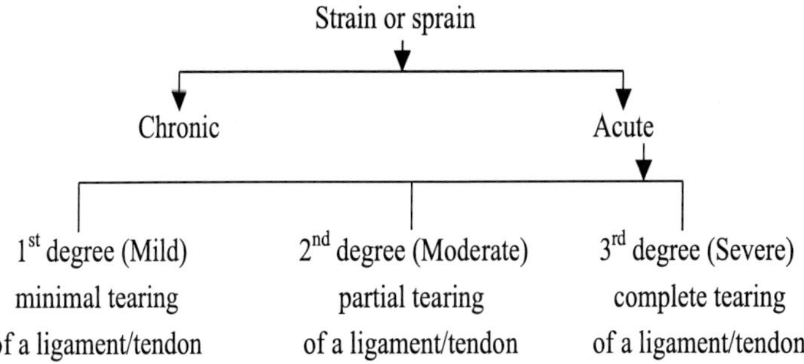

Clinical sign : Characterized by inflammatory symptoms, lameness and persistent instability of the affected joint. Movement of the joint in a direction that puts tension on ligament will produce pain in the area of injury.

Strain : Strain can be defined as injury to a muscle or a tendon due to overstreching or overuse of any part of the muscle tendon unit. Strain may be either chronic, as a result of repeated 'streching' of the involved muscle tendon unit, or acute, as occasioned by single, sudden hyperextensive or hyperflexive action.

Treatment

- Complete rest to the affected area.
- Depending upon the degree of sprain; a support bandage, splints or plaster cast may be applied.
- Most severe forms of sprain may result in luxation of the joint.

Bursitis : A bursa serves to reduce friction between moving parts, such as tendons, ligaments, and muscles or to cushion effects of excess pressure between the movable structures and bony prominences. Inflammation of a bursa is known as bursitis.

Acute bursitis : i. Dry ii. Serous iii. Purulent

Etiology

- Direct trauma.
- An extension of inflammation from local tendonitis.
- Open wounds involving the bursa.
- Bacterial infection.
- Toxaemia of bacterial diseases like influenza and strangles.
- Due to rheumatism.

Symptoms

- In true bursitis, flexion of the affected joint is normal without any pain and lameness. When bursitis extends into the joint causing septic arthritis, pain as well as restricted motion of the joint is evident.
- In dry bursitis, exudation is more or less absent but pain is present.
- In serous bursitis there is pronounced exudation and swelling (carpal hygroma).

Treatment

- Provide proper bedding to the animal.
- Intraarticular injection corticosteroid.
- Application of poultices.
- In cases of purulent bursitis - pus should be drained and infusion of appropriate antibiotics into the cavity.
- In rheumatoid bursitis, use of sodium salicylate is indicated.
- Radical surgery may be required as a last resort.

Chronic Bursitis

- Chronic bursitis results from mild and repeated trauma or it may follow acute bursitis.
- There is swelling, but pain may not be marked
- Chronic bursitis affecting the point of elbow (capped elbow), anterior aspect of knee (capped knee or hygroma of knee) point of hock (capped hock) are frequently encountered.

Common forms of Chronic Bursitis

1. *Cystic from* : The wall of the bursa becomes thickened with fibrous tissue forming a bursal sac which contains a variable quantity of a viscid opalescent fluid. In long standing cases the bursa may contain cartilagenous or calcareous material.
2. *Proliferative from* : The interior of the bursal sac contains vegetative growth.
3. *Fibrous form* : There is extensive fibrous thickening of the bursa.
4. *Hemorrhagic form* : Characterized by the presence of extravasated blood in the bursa.

Symptoms

- Distension of the bursa.
- Skin overlying the inflammed subcutaneous bursa may develop horny or wart like thickenings.

Treatment

- Remove the cause.
- Application of counter irritant e.g. Biniodide of mercury.
- Needle point firing.
- Aspiration of contents followed by injection of an irritant solution like tincture iodine. Afterward a pressure bandage is applied. The irritant destroys the lining of the bursa which is followed by granulation, cicatrisation and obliteration of the cavity.
- Extirpation of the bursa.

Type of Bursitis

Poll evil : is a condition in horses, resulting from the inflammation of atlantal bursa.

Capped elbow (Hygroma of elbow) : It is a condition caused by subcutaneous bursitis at the point of the elbow (Fig. 12.1 and 12.2).

Capped hock (Hygroma of the hock) : It is caused by bursitis of the superficial bursa at the point of the hock.

Deep-capped hock : The distension of small bursa situated between the gastrocremius and superficial flexor tendons at the point of the hock is called deep-capped hock.

Capped knee (Hygroma of the knee) : Distension of the subcutaneous bursa in front of the knee (Fig.12.3).

Capped fetlock : Distension of the subcutaneous bursa in front of the fetlock.

Saddle Gall : Results from continous frictution at neck due to saddle (Fig. 12.4).

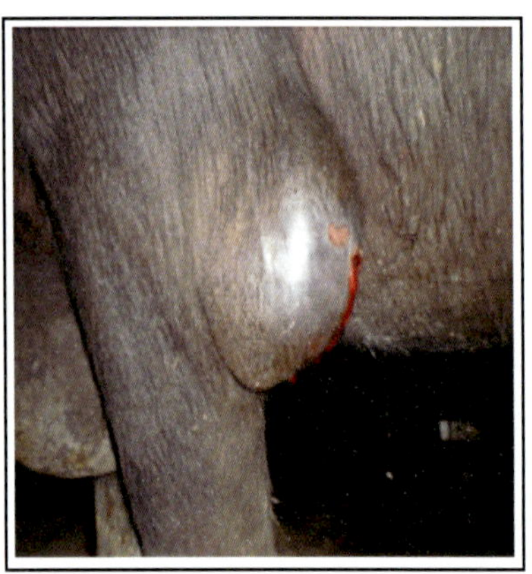

Fig. 12.1: Olecraneon bursitis in a buffalo

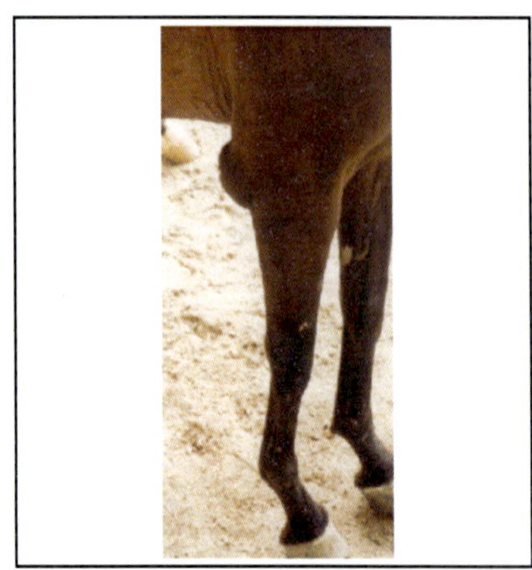

Fig. 12.2: Capped elbow in a horse

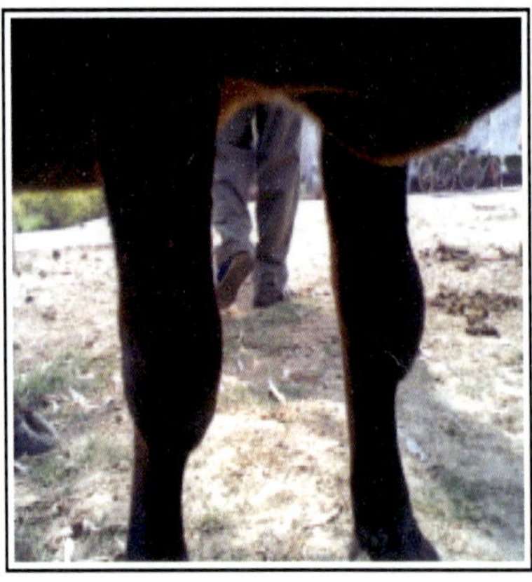

Fig. 12.3: Carpal hygroma in a buffalo

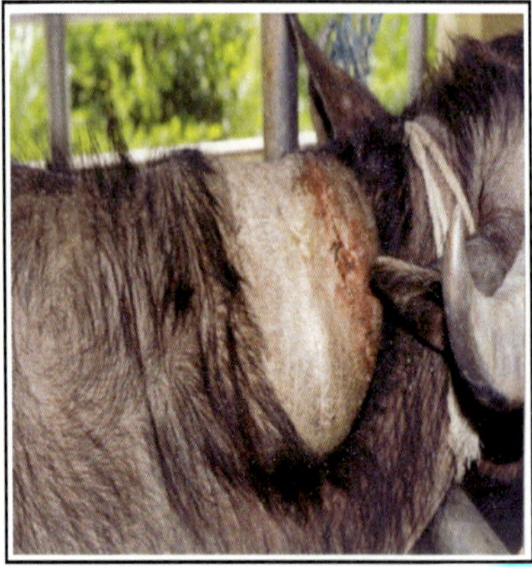

Fig. 12.4: Saddle gall

Fistulous withers (Supraspinous bursitis) : It results from inflammation of the bursa situated over the spines of the 2nd to 5th thoracic vertebrae.

Bursitis intertubercularis (Bicipital bursits) : The bicipital bursa or intertubercular bursa is situated between the bicipital groove of the humerous and the tendon of biceps brachii muscle.

Trochanteric bursitis : Inflammation of bursa situated between the tendon of the middle gluteus muscle and the great trochanter of the femur.

Tarsal cellulites : There is no bursa over the lateral surface of the tarsus the correct term to describe the swelling is tarsal cellulitis.

Chapter 13

ARTHRITIS

Inflammation of the joint is known as arthritis.

Coxitis : Inflammation of hip joint.

Gonitis : Inflammation of stifle joint.

Omarthritis : Inflammation of shoulder joint.

Carpitis : Inflammation of carpal joint.

Types of Arthritis

1. Infectious arthritis/septic arthritis : e.g. joint ill or neonate polyarthritis.
2. Traumatic arthritis.
3. Degenerative arthritis or osteoarthritis on noninfectious arthritis or degenerative joint disease (DJD).

Infectious Arthritis/ Septic Arthritis

- Infectitios arthritis is the inflammation of joint which is caused by microorganisms like bacteria, virus, mycoplasma etc.
- Infectious arthritis with pus in the joint cavity is known as septic arthritis.

Etiology

- Trauma near the joint leads to periarticular infection which may extend to the joint.
- Systemic infection e.g. joint ill caused by omphalophlebitis.
- *Corynebacterium pyogenes, Mycoplasma bovis, Escherichia coli, Staphylococcus sp.* and *Streptococcus sp.* are the common microorganisms responsible for septic arthritis.

Clinical Signs

- Severe lameness with limited motion (due to pain, joint effusions, fibrosis of periarticular tissues and joint ankylosis).
- Swelling of the affected joint (due to effusion of synovial fluid, inflammation, fibrosis of the synovial membrane and joint capsule and bony enlargements).
- Pain during palpation.
- Pyrexia may be present.
- Joint capsule may rupture with oozing of pus.
- Increase in temperature of the overlying skin of the affected joint which can be accurately measured by thermography.

Pathogenesis

- After entrance, the microorganism damages cartilage, synovial membrane and fluid.
- Microorganisms are destroyed by neutrophils and their enzymes (elastage, collagenase etc.). At the same time these enzymes also damages the articular cartilage.
- Articular surface is further damaged by free radicals released by neutrophils and damaged tissue.
- Inflammatory mediators decrease proteoglycan production.
- Decreased production and increased degradation of proteoglycans deteriorates the cartilage.
- The presence of fibrin on cartilage and synovial membrane interferes with nutrient and waste product transportation which makes the joint more susceptible to trauma.

Diagnosis

1. *By radiography* : Radiograph can be taken in anteroposterior and lateral position.
   - *In early stage* : Increase in joint space due to synovial effusion and increased soft tissue density around the joint.
   - *In middle stage* : Narrow joint space due to changes in articular cartilage.
   - *In end stage* : Increase in joint space due to destruction of subchondral bone. Periarticular new bone formation (osteophytes) and calcification of joint capsule and attached sites of the collateral ligaments.
2. *By contrast arthrography* :
   - *Indications* : To evaluate the lesions in the articular cartilage, subchondral bone, synovial membrane, thickness of the articular cartilage, joint capsule tear etc.
   - *Technique* : About 10 cc of 25% solution of triiodinated water soluble contrast media is injected in to the joint.
3. *Arthroscopy* : Arthroscopy is used to make the final diagnosis.
4. *Synovial fluid analysis* :
   - *Synovial fluid culture* : Normal synovia is sterile. Growth of microorganism indicates septic arthritis.
   - *Synovial fluid protein* : >4 gm/dl.
   - *W.B.C. count* : About 50,000 cells/mm^3.
   - Serofibrinous cloudy synovial fluid.
   - Low viscosity of the synovial fluid.
   - Mucin precipitate quality is poor.
   - Increase in neutrophil count : >75%
   - Increased lactate dehydrogenase (LDH) due to damage of articular cartilage.
   - Alkaline phosphatase (ALP), Aspartate aminotransferase (AAT) and LDH increased with severity of disease.
5. *Ultrasonography* : Presence of echogenic (gray) material floating in the joint.
6. *Nuclear scintigraphy* : Technitium 99 is used for nuclear scintigraphy of joints.
7. *CT scan and MRI.*

Treatment : The following steps should be taken :

1. *Treat the primary cause*: treat the systemic infections like omphalophlebitis, metritis, endocarditis, mastitis etc.
2. *Removal of debris and fluids from the joint cavity (Joint lavage)* : After sedation, the animal should be restrained in lateral recumbency. Remove the debris and dilute the fluid in the joint with sterile isotonic fluids.
3. *Antimicrobial therapy* :
   - Antibiotics should be administered after joint lavage because debris in the joint cavity decreases the efficacy of the antibiotics.
   - Specific antibiotic should be used after antimicrobial sensitivity test.
   - Intravenous and intramuscular routes of administration should be preferred.
   - Intraarticular injection and intravenous under tourniquet can be used.
   - Implantation of slow releasing substances (PMMA) with antibiotics.
   - Cephazoline and procaine penicillin are the drug of choice.
4. *Arthrodesis* : Arthrodesis should only be done when all the treatments are ineffective.
5. Use of NSAIDs.
6. In mycoplasmal arthritis, oxytetracycline is the drug of choice.
7. Immobilization of the affected joint.
8. Intraarticular injection of polysulfated glycosaminoglycans (PSGAG), hyaluronic acid (HA) and dimethylsulfoxide (DMSO).

Degenerative Joint Disease

Degenerative joint disease (DJD) is a non inflammatory condition of the articular cartilage resulting from natural ageing, trauma or disease.

Etiology : Etiology of DJD is multifactorial and commonly seen after-

- Hip dysplasia.
- Osteochondritis dissecans.
- Rupture of cranial cruciate ligaments.
- Ligamentous injuries.
- Articular and periarticular fractures.

Clinical Signs

- Severe lameness with abnormality in gait.
- Difficulty in climbing on sloppy areas.
- Severe pain on palpation or manipulation.

- If degenerating articular cartilage and osteophyte formation is evident, crepitation is present.
- Decrease in joint range of motion.
- Joint enlargement.

Diagnosis

1. On the basis of clinical signs.
2. By radiographic examination:
   - Sclerosis of subchondral bone (radiodense area beneath the articular surface).
   - Subchondral bone cysts.
   - Osteophyte formation.
   - Subluxation of joints.
   - Narrowing of the joint space.
   - Intraarticular or periarticular calcification.
3. Laboratory findings : Examination of synovial fluid:
   - *Volume* : Increased.
   - *Colour* : Pale yellow to straw colour.
   - *Viscosity* : Usually normal or decreased.
   - *Mucin precipitate quality* : fair to good.
   - *TLC* : < 5000 cells/mm^3.
   - *Synovial fluid protein* : < 4 gm/dl.
4. Arthrography and arthroscopy.
5. Ultrasonography.

Treatment : The aim of treatment is to restore the affected joint to near normal and to alleviate pain.

- *Rest* : rest plays a major role in the management of DJD.
- Use of NSAIDs e.g. phenylbutazone, flunixin etc.
- Intraarticular injection of hyaluronic acid, corticosteroids and polysulfated glycosaminoglycans.
- *DMSO* : It resolves acute inflammation as well as chronic fibrosis.
- Acupuncture therapy.
- Transfer of synovial fluid.
- Use of counterirritants.

- Physiotherapy like therapeutic ultrasound.
- *Surgical treatment* : Synovectomy, removal of osteophytes and surgical arthrodesis.

Traumatic/ Aseptic Arthritis

Etiology : Direct or indirect trauma to the joint.

- Injury to joint capsule and supporting ligaments.
- Injury to articular cartilage.
- Injury to subchondral bone.
- Intraarticular fracture.
- Injury to menisci.

Clinical Signs

- Pain on palpation.
- Lameness
- Swelling of the joint (Increase in joint girth).
- Warm surface over the joint.
- Reduced joint mobility.

Diagnosis

- On the basis of clinical signs.
- *Synovial fluid analysis* : nearly normal.
- *Radiography* : Distended joint capsule.

Type-I	Type-II	Type-III
• Injury to joint capsule (capsulitis) and synovial membrane (synovitis). • Articular cartilage: normal. • Injury to the supporting ligaments.	• Injury to joint capsule (capsulitis) and synovial membrane (synovitis). • Articular cartilage: disrupted. • Complete rupture of ligaments. Intracapsular fracture.	• Post traumatic DJD.

Treatment

- In acute traumatic arthritis, ice packs should be applied.
- Intraarticular injection of corticosteroids and local anesthetics.
- Use of NSAIDs.
- In chronic cases hot fomentation is recommended.

Chapter 14

Luxation, Subluxation and Dislocation

Luxation/Dislocation : It refers to the displacement of opposing articular surfaces of bone. The direction of displacement is described with reference to the distal bone in relation to the proximal bone.

Subluxation : It refers to partial or incomplete dislocation.

Classification

1. *Acute* : Recent occurrence of luxation.
2. *Chronic* : Luxation existing for a long time.
3. *Recurrent* : Reluxation after correction.
4. *Simple* : No open wound is communicating with the joint.
5. *Compound* : Open wound is communicating with the joint.
6. *Pathological* : Dislocation due to any pathological lesion.

Etiology

1. *Trauma* : During jumping or accidental slipping.
2. *Congenital* : Due to polygenic inheritance.
3. *Pathological* : Due to pathological conditions associated with the joint, ligaments and muscles.

Clinical Signs

- Abnormal mobility of the joint.
- Inability to use the affected part.
- Dislocation of limb joints leads to lameness and no weight bearing by the affected limb.
- Shortening or lengthening of limb with variation in normal angularity of the joint.
- Inflammatory swelling of the joint.

General Principles of Treatment

- Acute dislocations are easy to reduce.
- The animal should be anesthetized or a combination of sedatives and epidural/spinal anesthesia can be used.
- The animal is restrained in lateral recumbency with the affected limb uppermost.
- Traction and countertraction is applied until the articular surfaces of dislocated bone ends come to the same level and then pushed in to their normal anatomical position.
- The reduction may be open or closed.
- After reduction, rest should be given for about 1 month.
- The joint is stabilized by application of sling or cast.

Luxation, Subluxation and Dislocation in Small Animals

1. Coxofemoral Luxation

Luxation of the hip joint is known as coxofemoral luxation (Fig. 14.1).

Classification : Luxation can be classified on the basis of relationship between the acetabulum and femoral head.

i. *Craniodorsal* : Most common in canine and felines (about 80%).
ii. *Caudoventral* : Second most common.

Etiology

- Motor vehicle trauma.
- Sudden fall. Caudoventral luxation develops when the animal falls with the leg abducted and the limb internally rotated.

Clinical Signs

- Mild to severe lameness.
- In bilateral cases, the animal is unable to walk.
- Swelling of the joint.
- Pain and crepitus.
- Abnormally located greater trochanter.

Craniodorsal luxation	Cranioventral luxation
• The limb appears shorter than the contra lateral limb.	• The limb appears longer than the contra lateral limb.
• Adduction and external rotation of the affected limb with outward rotated stifle.	• The affected limb appears slightly abducted and internally rotated.
• The distance between the trochanter and tuber ischii is increased.	• The greater trochanter displaced medially and appears to be absent on palpation.
	• Limb abduction and external rotation are limited due to presence of femoral head in the obturator foramina.

Diagnosis

- On the basis of clinical signs
  i. Leg length changes.
  ii. Change in the distance between the greater trochanter and ischial tuberosity.
- By radiography.

Management / Treatment

- Treatment depends on the type and duration of luxation.
- Delay in reduction causes fibrosis and pelvic muscle contraction.
- Reduction becomes difficult after 4-5 days.
- After reduction (closed or open reduction), exercise should be restricted for 2-3 months.

Craniodorsal Coxofemoral Luxation

Closed Reduction

- The animal should be anesthetized or a combination of sedatives and epidural/spinal anesthesia can be used.

- The animal is restrained in lateral recumbency with the affected limb uppermost.
- Traction and countertraction should be applied.
- The limb is grasped at the hock and mild external rotation and traction are applied.
- The greater trochanter is grasped by the other hand and direct pressure is applied to the trochanter to move it dorsally and caudally towards the acetabulum.
- When the femoral head has moved over the acetabulum rim, the limb is rotated internally to complete the reduction.
- Deep seating of the femoral head in the acetabulum can be done by applying moderate pressure over the greater trochanter and concurrent full range motion of the joint. This process also helps in removal of blood clots from the acetabulum.
- After complete reduction, Ehmer sling should be applied for 7-10 days.

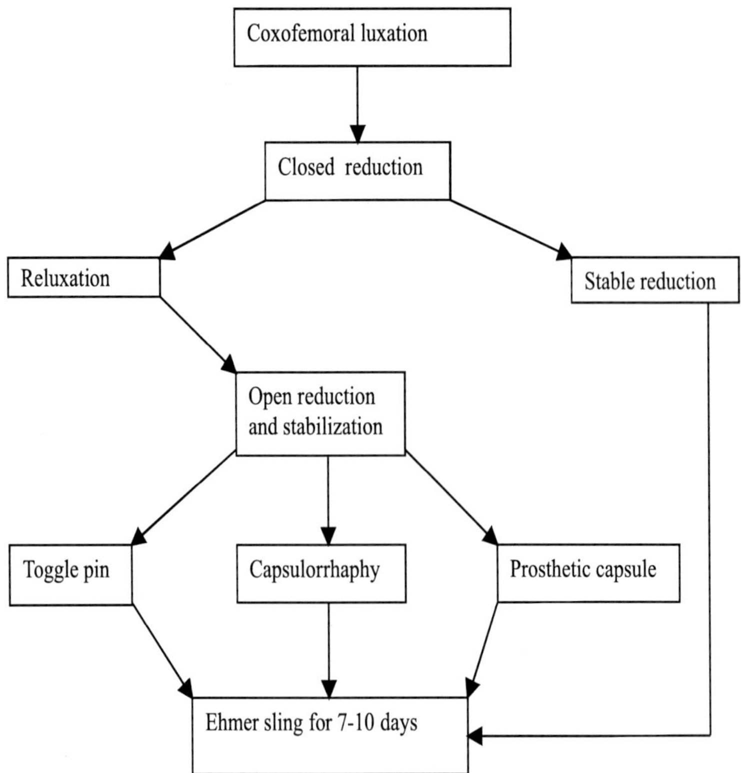

Augmented Closed Reduction

1. Ischial-ilial Pin (Devita Pinning)

- This method is advantageous for stabilizing chronic luxations of hip.
- A Steinman pin is inserted underneath the attachment of the hamstring muscles at the ischium, over the neck of the femur and in to the wing of ilium.
- Pin migration, sciatic nerve injury and septic arthritis are the common complications of this method.

2. External Fixator Pins

- Pins are placed in to the greater trochanter and in to the ilium connected by a rubber band.
- Hemorrhage, sciatic nerve injury, acetabular cartilage damage are the certain complications associated with this process.

Open Reduction and Stabilization

- *Indications*
  - i. Avulsion fracture of acetabulum.
  - ii. If closed reduction failed.
- The femoral head is reduced in to the acetabulum by using the following approaches.
  - i. *Craniolateral approach* : Exposure is not sufficient in craniolateral approach but it can be improved by partial tenotomy of tendon of deep gluteus muscle. This approach is good for capsulorrhaphy.
  - ii. *Dorsal approach* : This approach is recommended in most of the cases because it provides maximum exposure.
- *Stabilization of the joint*
  - i. *Capsulorrhaphy* : Simple circumfential tears of the joint capsule are repaired by suturing.
  - ii. *Modified Knowles toggle technique* : This technique is used to recreate the round ligament or ligament of the head of the femur.

Caudoventral Coxofemoral Luxation

- The animal should be anesthetized or a combination of sedatives and epidural/spinal anesthesia can be used.
- The animal is restrained in lateral recumbency with the affected limb uppermost.

- The affected limb is grasped immediately proximal to the stifle by one hand. The other hand is placed over the tuber ischii with the thumb and palm on the medial aspect of proximal thigh.
- Abduct the limb to relieve the femoral head from the obturator foramen.
- The femoral head is lifted laterally & then cranially in to the acetabulum.

2. Luxation of the Stifle Joint

Etiology : Injury in joint capsule, menisci, cruciate and collateral ligaments leads to luxation of stifle joint.

Clinical Signs

- No weight bearing by the affected limb.
- Pain on palpation.
- Swelling of the joint.

Diagnosis

- Thorough examination of the joint.
- Complete cranial and caudal drawer movement.
- *Joint exploration* : To identify the damaged structures of joint.
- *Radiography* : To identify the avulsion fractures.

Treatment

- *Transarticular pinning* to provide temporary stabilization. The complication associated with this technique is pin migration.
- Application of Schroeder-thomas splint for 1-2 months.
- Reconstruction of the damaged ligaments followed by external splintage.
- Exercise restriction and least walk can be allowed after 3-4 weeks.

3. Luxation of Patella

Luxation of patella is common in canines and it may be lateral, medial or proximal. Lateral luxation is rare and is usually congenital.

Etiology

- Automobile accidents and trauma
- Congenital

Clinical Signs

- In acute traumatic patellar luxation, the animal is unable to bear weight on the affected limb. Pain is evident on palpation or manipulation of the joint. In chronic cases these symptoms are mild.
- In congenital cases, clinical signs vary with the degree or grade of luxation.

Grade 1	• Clinical signs are not present, but lameness may be seen after vigorous exercise.
Grade 2	• Intermittent lameness.
	• Dog carries the leg without pain.
	• The dog flexes and extends the joint several times and bears weight again.
Grade 3	• Bone deformities like lateral bowing and internal rotation of tibia (S shape curve of distal femur and proximal tibia).
	• Luxated patella can be reduced manually.
	• Shallow trochlear groove (coax vara).
	• Mild lameness
Grade 4	• The animal is unable to walk.
	• Marked internal rotation and bowing of tibia.
	• Luxated patella can not be reduced manually.
	• Crab like posture and gait.

Diagnosis

- On the basis of clinical signs.
- Radiography : ***Skyline view*** of distal femur is useful to evaluate the depth and contour of femoral trochlea.

Treatment

- Grade 1 luxations should be treated conservatively.
- Grade 4 luxations are corrected surgically to prevent the permanent bony deformity and disability.

Surgical Methods

1. Trochleoplasty or Sulcoplasty

i. *Abrasion trochleoplasty* : Deepening of femoral trochlea by removing the articular surface and 1-2 mm of subchondral bone is known as abrasion trochleoplasty.

ii. *Recession trochleoplasty* : Deepening of femoral trochlear surface while maintaining the hyaline cartilage is known as recession trochleoplasty. V-shaped wedge is made in the femoral trochlea by a saw. Additional subchondral bone is removed from the wedge. Again the articular wedge is placed over the defect.

2. Tibial Tuberosity Transposition

This technique is used to treat the lateral and medial patellar luxation.

i. The tuberosity is moved to a lateral position to correct the medial patellar luxation.

ii. The tuberosity is moved to a medial position to correct the lateral patellar luxation.

3. Luxation of Scapulohumeral Joint

Lateral and medial scapulohumeral luxations are common in canines. Cranial and caudal luxations are less common.

Etiology

- *Trauma* : Injury to the supporting structures leads to dislocation (mostly lateral luxation).
- *Congenital* : Congenital dislocations are due glenoid dysplasia and capsular laxity (mostly medial luxation).

A. Lateral Scapulohumeral Luxation

Clinical signs

- The animal carries the affected limb in flexion with internal rotation of the foot.
- Pain and crepitus on palpation of the affected joint.
- Lamenes.
- Greater tubercle displaced laterally.

Diagnosis

- On the basis of clinical signs.
- By radiography.

Treatment

i. Closed Reduction and Stabilization

- The animal should be anesthetized or a combination of sedatives and epidural/spinal anesthesia can be used.
- The animal is restrained in lateral recumbency with the affected limb uppermost.

- The limb is held in extension and the humeral head pressed medially while counter pressure is applied over the scapular neck.
- After assessing the range of motion and stability the limb is immobilized by splint/sling for about 1 month.
- Velpeau sling should be avoided in lateral luxation because it promotes lateral translation of the humeral head.

ii. Open Reduction and Stabilization

- Reconstruction of collateral ligaments.
- Transposition of biceps brachii tendon.
- Transarticular pinning.
- Glenoid excisional arthroplasty.
- Arthrodesis.

B. Medial Scapulohumeral Luxation

Clinical Signs

- The animal carries the affected limb in flexion with external rotation of the foot.
- Pain on palpation.
- Medial displacement of greater tubercle of humerus.
- Persistant lameness in traumatic cases and intermittent lameness in congenital cases.

Diagnosis

- On the basis of clinical signs.
- By radiography.

Treatment

i. Closed Reduction and Stabilization

- Contraindicated in glenoid dysplasia.
- The animal should be anesthetized or a combination of sedatives and epidural/spinal anesthesia can be used.
- The animal is restrained in lateral recumbency with the affected limb uppermost.
- After reduction the joint is stabilized by application of velpeau sling (It distracts the humeral head laterally and resists medial luxation) for 1 month.

ii. Open Reduction and Stabilization

- By passing a nylon tape through the bone tunnel in the base of the scapular spine and proximal humerus.

Cranial and caudal scapulohumeral luxation : The transposition of biceps tendon is the method of choice for correction of cranial and caudal scapulohumeral luxations.

6. Luxation of Elbow Joint

Elbow luxation is common in canines.

Etiology : Congenital or acquired (trauma).

Clinical Signs

- The affected limb is abducted, externally rotated and in slight flexion.
- Pain on palpation of the affected joint.

Diagnosis

- On the basis of clinical signs.
- By radiography : Craniolateral view.

Treatment

- The animal should be anesthetized or a combination of sedatives and epidural/spinal anesthesia can be used.
- The animal is restrained in lateral recumbency with the affected limb uppermost.

i. Closed Reduction and Stabilization

- The aim is to hook the anconeus process in to the olecranon fossa and use it as a fulcrum for reduction.
- After reduction, the limb should be stabilized by using cast/slings.
- This technique is depends on the location of anconeal process.

1. If the anconeal process is in the fossa:
   - The limb is extended slightly.
   - The antibrachium is abducted and internally rotated.
   - Pressure is applied to the head of radius medially with concurrent extension of limb.
2. If the anconeal process is lateral to the fossa:
   - The limb is flexed beyond 90 degree.
   - The acetabulum is internally rotated and abducted to push the anconeus in to the fossa.

ii. Open Reduction and Stabilization

- Caudolateral approach should be choosen to open the joint.
- After reduction, the joint should be lavaged.
- Reconstruct the ruptured collateral ligaments and capsule.
- Close the subcutaneous tissue and skin.
- Use of antibiotics and anti-inflammatory drugs.

Hip Dysplasia in Canine

Hip dysplasia is a complex disease of canines. The giant breeds have the highest prevalence of this disorder. It is a disease of young animals (5 months to 12 months).

Etiology

- Combination of nutritional (obesity and rapid weight gain), environmental (excessive exercise) and genetic factors (polygenic) are responsible for hip dysplasia.

Clinical Signs

- The dog is presented with the history of joint instability or joint laxity which is a hallmark sign of hip dysplasia.
- Abnormal hind limb gate.
- Atrophy of the thigh muscles.
- Pain and low exercise tolerance.
- Inability to climb stairs.
- Walking with arched back and a sound 'click' can be audible during walk.
- Untreated hip dysplasia may change in to degenerative joint disease in old animals.

Diagnosis

1. *Clinical signs*
2. *Ortolani sign* : The dog is placed on its back forcing the femur dorsally. The limbs are then slowly abducted. Ortolani signs exists when the femoral head seats in to the acetabulum (popping sound) as the limb abducted.
3. *Bardens sign* : A lateral force is applied on the femur while palpating the femoral head. A palpable lateral movement of the femoral head is considered to be a positive signs.

4. *Radiography :*
   - The dog should be sedated/anesthetized before taking the radiograph.
   - The ventrodorsal position is recommended for taking the radiograph. The dog is placed on its back. The hind legs are extended fully in caudal direction, held parallel and rotated fully in a medial direction.
   - The primary radiographic signs are : shallow acetabulum and small flattened femoral head.
   - The secondary radiographic signs are :

     i. Femoral head subluxation.

     ii. Degenerative joint disease of hip.

     iii. Less concave cranial acetabular border.

     iv. Femoral head becomes less hemispherical than normal.

Mild hip dysplasia	Moderate hip dysplasia	Severe hip dysplasia
• Significant subluxation. • Shallow acetabulum. • No arthritic changes.	• Significant subluxation. • Secondary arthritic changes at the femoral head and neck (remodeling, osteophytes or bone spur formation and sclerosis).	• Significant subluxation and the ball is partly or completely out of a shallow socket. • Secondary arthritic changes like moderate hip dysplasia.

Treatment

Conservative

- Cage rest or exercise restriction.
- Use of analgesics and NSAIDs.
- Reduce the body weight of the animal.

Surgical

1. Pelvic osteotomy : The aim of pelvic osteotomy is to improve joint depth or congruity by placing the femoral head more deeply in to the acetabulum.
2. Total hip replacement : It provides better joint stability and alleviates pain.

3. Pectineal myotomy or myectomy : Myotomy is only pain relieving procedure and does not alter the progression of disease.
4. Femoral head and neck resection : Removal of femoral head and neck is an excellent method of pain relief in dogs with hip dysplasia. In bilateral cases, head and neck resection should be done with a gap of 4-6 weeks between two surgeries.
5. Acetabuloplasty.
6. Derotational femoral osteotomy or varus femoral osteotomy.

Luxation, Subluxation and Dislocation in Ruminants

1. Scapulohumeral Luxation

Luxation/ dislocation of shoulder joint is rare in farm animals. However, cranial and lateral luxations are common in farm animals.

Etiology : Excessive flexion of the shoulder joint during jumping or sudden fall leads to luxation of shoulder joint.

Clinical Signs

- Shoulder lameness but no dropped elbow.
- No weight bearing on the affected limb.
- Shortening of the limb.
- Pain on flexion and extension.
- Prominent swelling on the cranial aspect of the shoulder.
- Depression may be present at the joint site.

Diagnosis

- On the basis of clinical signs.
- By examination of the affected limb : One hand is placed on the point of elbow and the other hand is placed over the humerus and internal and external rotation is applied. Movement of the humeral head confirms the luxation.
- Diagnosis is finally confirmed by radiography.

Treatment

- Reduction of the luxated joint should be performed under heavy sedation or general anesthesia.
- The animal is casted and restrained in lateral recumbency keeping the affected limb uppermost.

- After application of traction and countertraction by ropes, traction is applied caudally with simultaneous manual pressure on the humeral head in a caudal direction.
- After reduction, rest for about three months should be given to the animal.

2. Humeroradial Dislocation

Humeroradial or elbow dislocation is rare in farm animals. Medial and lateral luxations are common.

Etiology

- Traumatic injury.
- Fracture of condyles of the humerus and olecranon process of ulna may lead to dislocation.

Clinical Signs

- No weight bearing on the affected limb.
- The limb is flexed.
- Prominent swelling

Diagnosis

- By clinical signs.
- By plain radiography.

Treatment

- *Lateral dislocation* is reduced by flexion and slight abduction of the limb.
- *Medial dislocation* is reduced by complete flexion with concurrent pressure over the lateral epicondyle of humerus. The anconeal process is used as a fulcrum during reduction.

3. Luxation of Carpal Joint

Carpal joint luxation is common in sheep.

Etiology : Traumatic injury.

Clinical Signs

- Lameness and no weight bearing on the affected limb.
- Prominent swelling of the joint.
- Abnormal mobility of the joint.

Diagnosis : On the basis of clinical signs and plain radiography.

Treatment

- Reduction and immobilization of the joint by plaster cast.

4. Luxation of Fetlock Joint

Luxation of fetlock joint is common in farm animals. The luxation may be open or closed (Fig. 14.2).

Etiology : Severe trauma.

Clinical Signs

- No weight bearing on the affected limb.
- Lameness.
- Pain on palpation.

Diagnosis : On the basis of clinical signs and plain radiography.

Treatment

- By reduction and application of plaster cast/ splints.
- Open luxated joint should be cleaned and irrigated with normal saline.
- After reduction, the skin can be sutured in clean wound. Infected wounds should never be closed and allowed to heal by second intention.
- Daily antiseptic dressing, systemic antibiotics and NSAIDs should be given for few days.
- Plaster cast should be applied for about two months.

5. Coxofemoral Luxation/Subluxation

Coxofemoral or hip joint luxation is common in farm animals.

Etiology

- Trauma
- Dystocia in adult cattle.
- Falling or slipping on concrete floor.
- Metabolic disturbances like Milk fever.
- Indiscriminate use of estrogen hormone.
- Congenital : Shallow acetabulum and small head of the femur.

Classification

Coxofemoral luxation can be classified on the basis of displacement of the femoral head from its normal position relative to coxal tuber and tuber ishii of the os coxae. It may be craniodorsal, caudoventral, cranioventral and caudodorsal. Craniodorsal and caudoventral dislocations are more common in farm animals.

Clinical Signs

A. In Craniodorsal Luxations

- Shortening and outward rotation of the limb.
- While rest, weight bearing on the toe and during walk, swinging limb lameness.
- Cranial displacement of greater trochanter reveals asymmetry as compared to the normal joint.
- Crepitus is absent during palpation of proximal extremity of femur in standing animal.
- Swelling over the hip joint.

B. In Caudoventral Luxation

- The animal remains recumbent and if stands no weight bearing on the affected limb.
- The limb remains extended and the length of the affected limb appears normal or longer as compared to the normal limb.
- Femoral head can be palpated caudoventrally to its normal position.

C. In Cranioventral Luxation

- The animal is usually recumbent.
- No weight bearing on the affected limb.
- The limb remains in extension.
- Concavity at the greater trochanter site.

Diagnosis

- On the basis of clinical signs.
- *Rectal palpation* : Rectal palpation is very much helpful in diagnosing the caudoventral or cranioventral dislocations.

- By radiography.
- The diagnosis should be differentiated from fracture and paralysis.

Treatment

Closed Reduction

- The animal should be deeply sedated or anesthetized and the affected limb should be positioned uppermost.
- Traction is applied by a rope tied at the distal extremity of the affected limb.
- Countertraction is applied by passing a rope under the affected limb in the inguinal region.
- After traction, the femur should be rotated by applying a downward pressure on the stifle and lifting the hock.
- A 'clunk' sound is felt when the femoral head is replaced in the acetabulum.
- The traction is relaxed.
- After correction, the animal should be given rest for 1-2 weeks and kept on the soft floor (to reorganize the periarticular tissues).
- Joint may reluxate if:

    i. Muscular damage is more.

    ii. Joint capsule and supporting ligaments are ruptured.

    iii. Acetabulum is fractured.

    iv. Presence of blood clots and debris in the acetabulum.

Open Reduction

- The animal should be anesthetized and the affected limb should be positioned uppermost.
- After aseptic preparation of the site, a craniolateral incision is made just cranial to the greater trochanter.
- After making an incision, the muscle fascia lata is retracted cranially, muscle biceps femoris caudally and gluteus muscle dorsally to visualize the joint capsule.
- Blood clots and debris are removed.

A. Reduction of Craniodorsal Luxation

- By external rotation and abduction of the limb during traction followed by abduction and internal rotation.
- To minimize the relaxation, the dorsal acetabular joint capsule is reinforced by two screw placed at the craniodorsal rim of the acetabulum.

B. Reduction of Cranioventral Luxation

- Internal rotation is required to correct the luxation.

C. Reduction of Caudoventral Luxation

- External rotation is required to reduce the luxation.
- After reduction the muscles are sutured in different layers.
- Skin is sutured using horizontal mattress or simple interrupted suture pattern
- Daily antiseptic dressing and systemic administration of antibiotics and NSAIDs for 7 days.
- The animal should be kept on soft floor.

6. Femorotibial Luxation

- Femorotibial luxation is rare due to strong collateral ligaments and supporting structures.
- Luxation may be cranial, caudal, lateral and medial.
- Animal is unable to bear weight on the affected limb.
- Joint space is increased.
- Diagnosis can be made by clinical signs, manipulation of affected joint and final diagnosis is made after radiography.

7. Luxation of Tarsal Joint

Tarsal joint luxation occurs at the level of tibiotarsal, intertarsal or tarsometatarsal joint.

Etiology

- Automobile accidents.
- Sudden kicking and falling.

Clinical Signs

- Lamenes and pain on palpation.
- Swelling over the joint.
- No weight bearing on the affected limb.

Treatment

- The animal should be deeply sedated or anesthetized and the affected limb should be positioned uppermost.
- Traction is applied by a rope tied at the distal extremity of the affected limb.
- Countertraction is applied by passing a rope under the affected limb in the inguinal region.
- After reduction, the limb should be immobilized by applying a plaster cast for 2-3 months.

Dorsal Patellar Luxation or Upward Fixation of Patella

- Upward fixation of patella is common in cattle and buffalo.
- Patella gets fixed on the dorsal aspect of the medial trochlea of the femur.
- This affection may be unilateral and bilateral.
- Congenital lateral deviation of patella in calf is also seen (Fig. 14.3).

Predisposing Factors

- Desmitis of the distal part of medial patellar ligament,
- Hyperextension of the limb after slippage over the hard ground.

Clinical Signs

- No clinical sign during rest.
- During movement, the animal has to drag the limb. The limb locks in extended state.
- When the patella returns to its normal position, the release from the extension makes the limb jerk forward.
- In severe cases, the toe becomes worn down.
- Signs aggravates during winter season.

Upward fixation of patella	Spastic paresis
• Mostly occurs in more than 2 years old cattle and buffaloes. • During movement, forwarded movement of the extended limb	• Mostly occurs in less than 2 years of age. • During movement, backward movement of the extended limb.

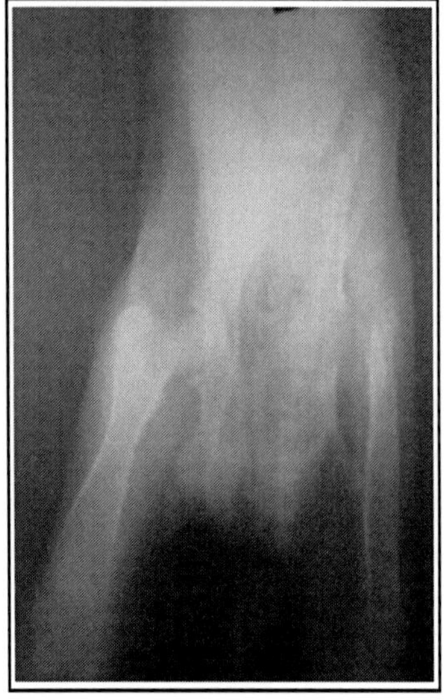

Fig. 14.1: Hip dislocation in a dog

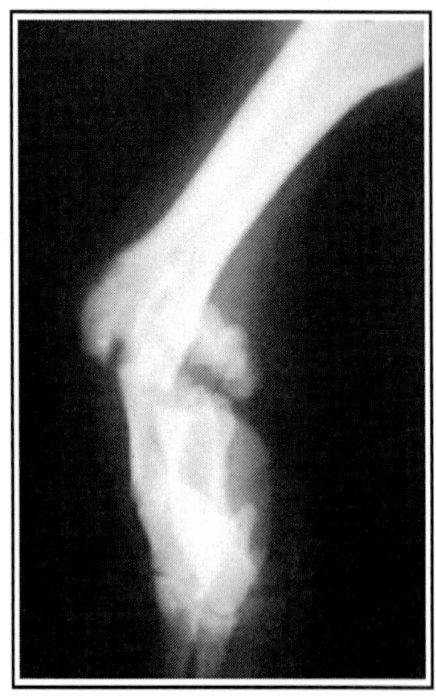

Fig. 14.2: Dislocation of fetlock in a bullock

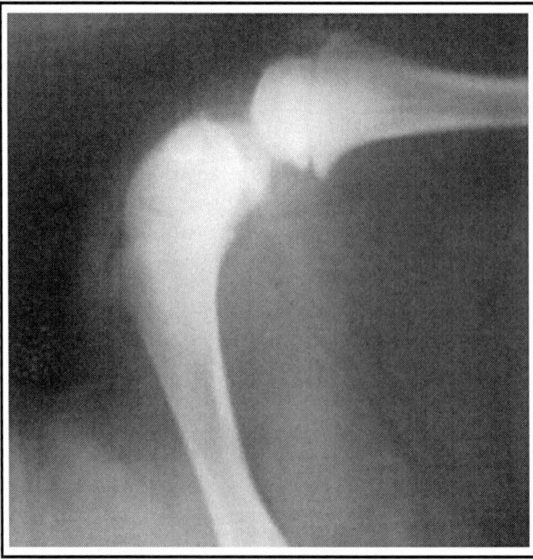

Fig. 14.3: Congenital lateral deviation of patella in a calf

Treatment

- Transection of the distal medial patellar ligament near its attachment on the tibia.
- Operation can be performed in standing or recumbent animal.

The animal is casted and restrained in lateral recumbency facing the affected limb downward. i.e. medial aspect of the affected limb uppermost.

- Both fore limb and the unaffected hind limb is tied together by a rope.
- Slight backward traction is applied on the affected limb by a rope.
- After aseptic preparation of the site, local anesthesia is infiltrated at the insertion of the medial patellar ligament.
- A B.P. blade (No.12) can be used to transect the ligament (Bassi's method).
- Antiseptic like povidone iodine should be applied over the incision site.

Open Method

- After aseptic preparation of the site a one cm incision is made over the cranial aspect of the medial patellar ligament just proximal to tibial crest.
- Fascia is separated to expose the medial patellar ligament.
- A tenaculum or curved hemostat is passed under the ligament to expose the ligament.
- The ligament is transected near the attachment.
- The incised skin is closed using interrupted sutures.
- The sutures are removed after completin of skin healing.
- Bulging of fat through the cut ends of the ligament and immediate relief are the signs of successful treatment.

Closed Method

- A stab incision is made in the groove formed by the middle and medial patellar ligament.
- The sharp edge of the blade should be directed towards the ligament.
- The ligament is transected.
- Any antiseptic like povidone iodine is poured in to the wound which is left unsutured.

Chapter 15

Diseases of Arteries and Veins

Arterial diseases are important because of their serious effect on vital organs like brain, heart and kidney. Thrombosis is the most common complication of arterial diseases but hemorrhage and aneurysm formation may occur.

Arteriosclerosis

- Generalized degeneration of specialized muscle and elastic tissues of media and replaced by inelastic fibrous tissue impregnated with calcium salts.
- It is a disease of tunica media.

Endarteritis Obliterans

- It is a disease of tunica intima.
- Proliferation of fibrous tissue between tunica intima and internal elastic lamina.

Polyarteritis Nodosa

- It is a disease of tunica media.
- Focal necrosis with acute inflammation of tunica media.

Atheroma

- Patchy deposition of yellow lipid in plaques deep in the intima which is covered by fibrous tissue
- It is an intimal disease.
- It is common in dogs due to infection of *Spirocerca lupi* and aorta of adult cattle which is caused by *Onchocerca armillata.*
- The important sites of atheroma and its complications are:

S.No.	Site of atheroma	Complications
1.	Cerebral and carotids	• Generalized chronic ischemia of the brain. • Acute local ischemia i.e. cerebral infarction.
2.	Coronaries	• Chronic ischemia of heart muscles and fibrosis. • Acute infarction.
3.	Abdominal aorta	• Aneurysm and embolism of limbs.
4.	Visceral arteries	• Chronic ischemia of bowel.

Atherosclerosis

- If both diseases (atheroma and arteriosclerosis) occur simultaneously, the disease is named as atherosclerosis.
- Causes of atherosclerosis :
  i. Senility
  ii. High blood cholesterol and lipid.
- In this disease, soft and elastic vessels become harder.
- Lumen of vessel is wider and vessels become tortuous.
- As calcium impregnation increases, the artery becomes very hard (pipe stem).
- Atherosclerosis is common in pig.

Aneurysm : A local enlargement of an artery is known as aneurysm. Aneurysm may be classified as :

1. *True aneurysm* : The sac is formed by the wall of the artery.
2. *False aneurysm* : The sac is formed by the surrounding connective tissue e.g. due to rupture of vessel by trauma.
3. *Cirsoid* : Tortuous complex of dilated arteries and veins.
4. *Berry* : Congenital deficiency of arterial media leads to berry aneurysm.
5. *Parasitic* : Parasitic aneurysm is caused by *Strongylus vulgaris* in the anterior mesenteric artery.

Etiology

1. Hypertension
2. *Weakness of the vessel wall* : It may cause circumferential or localized aneurysm.
   i. *Congenital* : Lack of media and elastic lamina at the site of branching.
   ii. Developmental anomalies of arteries and veins.
3. Traumatic
4. Acquired diseases of aortic wall e.g. Atheroma, arteriosclerosis and polyarteritis nodosa.
5. Parasites e.g. *Strongylus vulgaris.*

Types of Aneurysm

1. *Fusiform* :
   - Long part of the vessel is uniformly dilated around the whole circumference.
   - Local effects are not serious.
   - Fatal retroperitoneal or intraperitoneal hemorrhage.
2. *Saccular* :
   - Pouch is formed on the side of the wall.
   - Local pressure effect on neighboring viscera e.g. esophagus, heart, lungs etc. Pressure on nerve may cause paralysis of the affected nerve.

Sequelae

- Pressure atrophy of the surrounding structures
- Rupture of aneurysm may be fatal.
- Colic in horses.

Arteritis : Inflammation of the wall of the arteries is known as arteritis.

- *Acute* : Caused by microorganisms, parasites and fungi. e.g. equine viral arteritis.
- *Chronic* : e.g. Arteritis of anterior mesenteric artery caused by *Strongylus vulgaris* in equine and polyarteritis nodosa.

Diseases of Veins

Phlebitis

Inflammation of the vein is known as phlebitis which is usually suppurative (pyogenic) or septic in character.

- *Omphalophlebitis* : Infection of umbilicus is known as omphalophlebitis. It is a disease of new born animals.
- *During intravenous injection* : Accidental deposition of irritant chemical/ drugs around the vein causes phlebitis e.g. Accidental accumulation of thiopental (pH 10.5) around the vein.
- In traumatic reticulitis, chronic phlebitis of the involved vein occurs.
- Extension of infection from lungs (pneumonia), udder (mastitis) etc.

Symptoms

- Inflammed vein is enlarged with thickened wall.
- Thrombosis develops after phlebitis (Thyrombophlebitis).
- Sometimes thrombosis may calcified (Phlebolith).
- Sometimes thrombus may form emboli.

Varicose Veins

In this condition, the vein become prominent and tortuous and bulge outward under the skin. (Varix : A localized bulge in the vein, analogous to a saccular aneurysm in an artery). e.g. varicosity of scrotal plexus in the horse and varicosity of supramammary veins in the cow

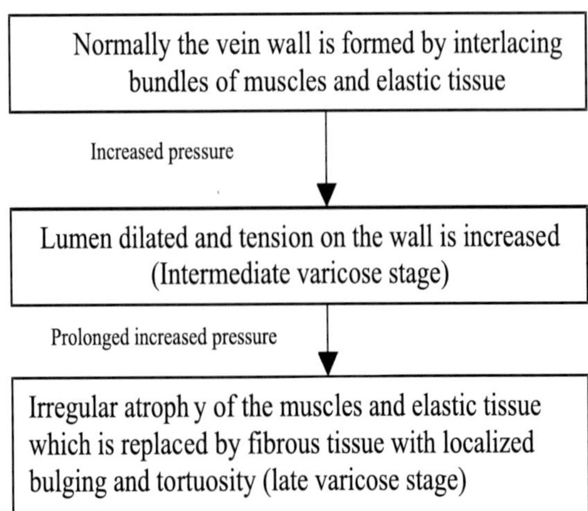

Etiology

- Varicose vein arise when the vein wall is subjected to an increased expanding pressure (tension) over long period (tension) over long periods
- Hindrance to the return of venous blood e.g. mitral stenosis and pulmonary edema.
- External pressure on vein e.g. tumours, gravid uterus etc.
- Ageing
- Post inflammatory weakness of the vessel wall.

Part-B
ANESTHESIOLOGY

Chapter 16

Historical Aspects and General Consideration

- Term anesthesia by Dr Oliver Wendell Holmes (1886).
- Anasthesis (Greece Word) – absence of sensation.

History of Animal Anesthesia

- Paracelsus (1540) produced ether and reported it to have a soporific effect on fowl.
- Sir Humphrey Davy (1800) suggested that N_2O might have anesthetic property.
- Chloroform was discovered by Liebig in 1831.
- Dr. Horace Wells (1844) discovered the general anesthetic properties of nitrous oxide.
- Ore (1875) published the first monograph on intravenous anaesthesia using chloral hydrate. Humbert described its use in horses.
- Rectal anesthesia attempted by Pirogoff (1847).
- In 1884 Kolhler introduced cocaine for local anesthesia of the eye, its use in veterinary practice was popularized by Sir Frederick Hobday.
- Conduction anesthesia by Halstead and Hall (1884).
- G.L. Corning (1885) induced spinal anesthesia in a dog using cocaine.

- Infiltration anesthesia - by Reclus (1890) and Schleich (1892).
- Sendrail (1901) induced subarachnoid anesthesia in horses, cattle and dogs.
- Cathelin (1901) reported epidural anaesthesia is dogs.
- Farquharson and Formston (1940) developed paralumbar anaesthesia technique in cattle.
- Carpentier (1950) introduced phenothiazine derivatives as preanesthetic.
- Dr. C.P. Jackson (1953) a Boston Physician, was first who employ ether extensively in animals.

Anesthesia (Greek word) – insensibility – loss of sensation

1. *Analgesia* – refers of relief from pain.
2. *Tranquilization* – is a state of behavioral change in which the patient is relaxed and unconcerned by his surroundings.
3. *Sedation* – is a mild degree of CNS depression in which the patient is awake but calm.
4. *Hypnosis* – is a condition of artificially induced sleep, or a trance resembling sleep resulting from moderate depression of CNS.
5. *Narcosis* – in man is defined as a drug produced state of deep sleep accompanied by analgesia. In veterinary, the narcotized patient is rarely deeply sleep but is sedated and has decreased sensibility to pain.
6. *Local anesthesia* – loss of sensation in a limited body area.
7. *Regional anesthesia* – insensibility in a larger, though limited, body area.
8. *Basal anesthesia* – is light level of general anesthesia usually produced by preanesthetic agents. It serves as a basis for deeper anesthesia on administration of other agents.
9. *General anesthesia* – is complete unconsciousness produced by controlled reversible intoxication of CNS in which there is lowered sensitivity to environmental stimuli and diminished response to such stimuli.
10. *Surgical anesthesia* – is unconsciousness, accompanied by muscle relaxation to such a degree that surgery can be performed painlessly and without struggling on the part of the patient.
11. *Balanced anesthesia* – is a state produced by combination of drugs, which is characterized by unconsciousness, analgesia and muscle relaxation.

12. *Dissociative anesthesia* – produced by interruption of information flow from the unconscious to conscious parts of the brain.

Reasons for Administration of Anesthetics

i. To alleviate pain
ii. To provide relaxation for surgery
iii. Restraint
iv. Transportation
v. Various diagnostic and therapeutic purposes
vi. Euthanasia

Types of anesthesia : Classified according to method of administration.

i. Inhalation - anesthetic gases or vapors are inhaled.
ii. Intravascular – anesthetic solution is administrated by intravenous, Intraarterial, Intracardiac or Intramedullary (bone marrow) injection.
iii. Other injectable routes – administrated by
    a. Intrathoracic
    b. Intraperitoneal
    c. Intramuscular and
    d. Subcutaneous
iv. Oral or Rectal – by enema (in rectal).
v. Local and conduction anesthesia
    a. Anesthetic is applied topically
    b. Injected locally into or around the surgical site (field block).
    c. Injected around nerves supplying the specific site (conduction).
    d. Injected into epidural or subarachnoid space (spinal).
vi. Electronarcosis – electric current passed through the cerebrum.
vii. Transcutaneous electrical nerve stimulation (TENS, TNS, TES) – local analgesia is produced by low intensity, high frequency electrical stimulation of the skin through surface electrodes.
viii. Hypnosis – anesthesia is inducted by placing the patient in a trance like state.
ix. Acupuncture
x. Hypothermia – body temperature is lowered, either locally or generally, to the level at which anesthesia occurs.

General Considerations in the Choice of Anesthetic Agents

1. History

- The duration and nature of illness determines the duration and type of anesthesia required.
- The patient with the history of epilepsy should not be given agents that reduce the seizure threshold such as Phenothiazines, Methohexital and Enflurane.
- Patient with renal and heart failure require close monitoring during anesthesia.

2. Recent Feeding

It increases the risk of vomiting after induction of anesthesia and in recovery period and thus increases the risk of tracheal aspiration. Fasting of animal is recommended for 24-48 hours in large animals and 6-12 hours in small animals.

3. Relative Size

- Anesthetic doses should be on the basis of mg/kg body weight.
- Small animal → more metabolic rate → larger the dose/ kg body weight.

4. Physical Condition

Fatty animal and animal in poor condition also require reduced doses.

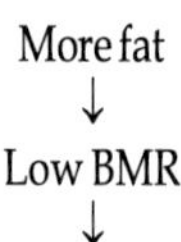

Less doses /kg body weight than
the muscular animals *e.g.* Greyhounds.

5. Species

Each species differ considerably in physiology and pharmacological response to drugs.

6. Breed

- Brachycephalic breeds *e.g.* Bulldog, Pugs etc. are extremely prone to airway obstruction due to long soft palate, redundant pharyngeal-laryngeal tissue and shortened muzzle. They require rapid induction, intubation, oxygen administration and rapid recovery from anesthesia.

- Greyhound exhibit prolonged recovery period following thiobarbiturate anesthesia because of their decreased body fat.
- German shepherds, Boxers, Great Danes have increased sensitivity to CNS depressants and general anesthetics.

7. Age

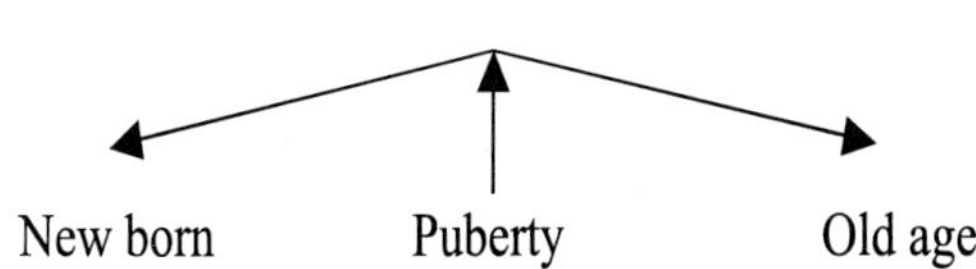

Neonates

- Neonates metabolize and excrete drugs less efficiently than adults.
- Short acting or antagonizable agents with minimal premedication should be used.
- Inhalation anesthetics are preferred over injectable anesthetics.
- Neonates are susceptible to perioperative hypoglycemia, hypothermia and fluid imbalances. Efforts should be made to prevent these complications.

Geriatric Patients

- They have a decreased anesthetic requirement and slowly metabolize and excrete injectable agents e.g. Phenothiazines.
- Fluid therapy should be done because they have significant renal impairment.

8. Sex

- BMR of male (7%) > female. In female BMR rises during pregnancy (due to metabolic activity of fetus).
- Anesthesia should generally be avoided during pregnancy because of teratogenic and abortifacient effect.

9. Genetic Difference

Genetic variation in dose response to anesthetics has been reported

- Rabbits have ability to hydrolyze atropine and cocaine

10. Activity and Biological Rhythms

- Aggressive animals are at greater anesthetic risk because of the lack of evaluation and stress of restraint.
- Active animals (BMR increases) more dose of anesthetic is required.

Preanesthetic physical examination of the surgical patient: It is extremely important to perform a physical examination of the surgical patient before anesthesia.

1. *General body condition*
   - *Obesity* : Obesity increases the anesthetic risk. Venipuncture, catheter placement and monitoring are more difficult in obese animals.
   - *Cachexia* : Cachexia increases the risk of intraoperative hypoglycemia.
   - *Pregnancy* : Pregnancy decreases the MAC of inhalant anesthetics.
   - *Dehydration* : Dehydration increases the risk of anesthetics. Efforts should be made to correct fluid deficits prior to anesthetic induction.
2. *Cardiovascular evaluation*: Heart rate and rhythm, pulse, capillary refill time (CRT) and color of the mucous membrane should be noted at different time intervals during anesthesia.
3. *Pulmonary testing*: Respiratory rate and depth should be noted at different time intervals during anesthesia. Cats are nasal breathers so open mouth breathing in this species indicates dyspnea.
4. *Gastrointestinal diseases*
   - Diarrhea and vomiting causes fluid and electrolyte imbalances.
   - Abdominal distension impairs ventilation and depresses cardiac output.
5. *Metabolism* : Hyperthermia increases the patient's oxygen requirement. Hypothermia will potentiate the effect of anesthesia.

Preanesthetic Laboratory Workup

i. Determination of packed cell volume provides an index of body's oxygen carrying capacity.

ii. Hyperproteinemia can indicate haemoconcentration and dehydration.

iii. Additional tests like BUN, creatinine, glucose, ALT, ALP, calcium and phosphorous may be indicated depending on the disease status.

Patient clasification on the basis of anesthetic risk: American Society of Anesthesiologists (ASA) classify the animals as follows:

Grade	Anesthetic risk	Definition	Example
ASA I	Excellent	Normal healthy patients with no organic disease.	Patients undergoing elective procedures such as ovariohysterectomy, castration etc.
ASA II	Good	Neonatal or geriatric patients or patient with mild systemic disease.	Mild to moderate obesity, simple fractures, complicated cardiac disease.
ASA III	Fair	Patient with moderate systemic disease.	Low to moderate fever, moderate dehydration and hypovolemia, complicated fractures.
ASA IV	Poor	Patient with severe systemic disease that is life threatening.	Patient with shock, high fever, uremia, toxemia, severe dehydration and hypovolemia, diaphragmatic hernia, GDV etc.
ASA V	Guarded	Moribund patient not expected to survive 24 hours.	Patient with advanced multiorgan failure, severe shock and major trauma.

Factors modifying uptake, distribution and elimination of anesthetic agents:

1. *Concentration and rate of injection of the anesthetic agent*: Concentration and rate of injection of a given dose affect anesthetic action, particularly with short acting barbiturates. The more dilute the agent or slower the injection, the less effect produced.

2. *Respiratory function*: Modification of effective ventilation, ventilation - perfusion ratios, and /or alveolar capillary diffusion from any cause will influence both the uptake and elimination of inhalant drug, more specially those of greater solubility e.g. diaphragmatic hernia, pulmonary edema, pulmonary emphysema or atelactasis and recumbency in large animals.

3. *Circulatory function* : Variation in distribution of blood to vessel rich (brain, heart, kidney, hepatoportal system and endocrine glands) and vessel poor group (bone, cartilage, tendon and ligament), to fat (adipose tissue), to muscle (skin and muscles) and to the alveoli themselves will modify the pattern of induction and recovery.

   - Shock → reduction in blood volume → dilution of drug is diminished → induction is rapid → recovery delayed
   - In fear, fever and struggling : induction of anesthesia is delayed and more anesthetic is required.

4. *Recent feeding*: Feeding increases BMR so more anesthetic is required.

5. *Uptake in gas spaces*: With the exception of the GIT, N_2 is the major gas constituent of closed internal body spaces. Due to the high blood/gas partition coefficient of N_2O relative to N_2 and other intestinal gases, administration of N_2O results in transfer of this gas into internal gas spaces of the body. Increased volume or pressure of the gases within these spaces may thus result. Use of nitrous oxide may thus be contraindicated in pneumothorax, pneumoencephalograms, intraocular surgery and in intestinal obstructions requiring prolonged anesthesia.
6. *Solubility of inhalant anesthetic in rebreathing bags*: Due to the solubility of methoxyflurane and halothane in rubber, delayed induction is observed.
7. *Changes in blood constituents*: Drug availability is also modified by the degree of protein binding. Protein binding is diminished by uremia, hypoproteinemia and by administration of drugs competing for the binding sites. Such decreased binding may make more drugs available for specific action.
8. *Preanesthetic medication and previous administration of drugs*: Previous and concurrent administration of certain drugs affects the anesthetic regimen.
   - Opioid analgesics and tranquilizers usually lower the metabolic rate.
   - Atropine causes a slight rise in metabolic rate.
   - Organophosphate toxicity may be potentiated by phenothiazines.
   - Chloremphenicol prolongs barbiturate anesthesia.
   - Hydrogen ion blockers like ranitidine, cimetidine may slow the metabolism of some injectable anesthetics and thus prolongs their effects.
9. *Concurrent disease* :
   - Fever increases the metabolic rate (MR) in accordance with Vanthoff's law, which sates that for each degree Fahrenheit the temperature rises, the metabolic rate is increased by 7%.
   - In toxemia or liver diseases, ability to detoxify anesthetic is depressed.
   - Hepatocellular disease causes reduced protein production with consequent limitation of protein binding.
   - Hyperthyroidism - Increase in metabolic rate and vice versa.
   - Leukemia - Increase in metabolic rate.
10. *Ionizing radiation and anesthetic effects* :
   - X-radiation has been shown to affect:
     i. Potency, onset, duration of action and brain level of barbiturates
     ii. Activity of hepatic microsomal enzyme system.
   - Anesthetic effect of barbiturates (barbital, hexobarbital, thiopental, pentobarbital) is decrease immediately after irradiation (1-3 h).

Selection of the anesthetic agent : The ideal anesthetic agent is one that :

1. Does not depend on detoxifying mechanisms within the body for its destruction and elimination.
2. Permits rapid induction, quick alteration in depth of anesthesia, and rapid recovery.
3. Does not depress respiratory and cardiac centers.
4. Is not irritant to any tissue.
5. Is inexpensive, stable, non-inflammable and non-explosive
6. Requires not special equipment for administration

   No agent available today possesses all these qualities so the agent should be selected according to situation.

Factors to be Considered Include

1. The patient's species, breed and age.
2. Physical status of patient.
3. The time required for the surgical procedure, its type and severity and the surgeon's skill.
4. Familiarity with the proposed anesthetic technique.
5. Equipment and personnel available.

The veterinarian must be used those agent with which he is most familiar.

- Short procedures are done with short lasting agents e.g. thiobarbiturates.
- Long procedures are done with pentobital, inhalation or blanced anesthetic techniques.
- Species difference may prevent the use of some drugs e.g. procaine is lethal to parakeets and morphine is excitatory for cats.
- As a group, the barbiturates are contraindicated for caesarean section because of respiratory depression produced in the newborn.
- In caesarean section - administration of inhalants, use of narcosis and balanced anesthesia or injection of local or regional anesthetics with or without sedation are indicated.

Chapter 17

Preanesthetic Agents

Preanesthetic agents are so named because they are usually given to prepare the patient for administration of an anesthetic agent for one or more of the following reasons:

1. To reduce the amount of general anesthetic needed and increase the margin of safety.
2. To calm the patient so that anesthesia can be administrated without fright or struggling.
3. To reduce secretions of salivary glands (antisialogogue) and mucous glands of the respiratory tract, thus maintaining a free airway.
4. To reduce gastric and intestinal motility and prevent vomiting while the patient is under anesthesia.
5. To block the vagal reflex, thus prevent cardiac slowing or arrest (bradycardia).
6. To reduce pain, struggling and crying during the recovery period.
7. To provide smooth induction and recovery from anesthesia.
8. To be used as an adjunct to local and regional anesthesia to prevent movement of the patient.
9. To provide pre, intra and immediate postoperative analgesia.

Choice of the agent : It depends on:

1. Species/breed/temperament of the patient.
2. Type of major anesthetic agent to be used.
3. Procedure to be performed.
4. Health status of the patient.
5. Facilities and equipment available.

It is Unwise

1. To induce general anesthetics in brachycephalic dogs without administration of a drug to reduce secretions.
2. To induce general anaesthesia in horse without premeditation to ensure a calm induction and to minimize struggling during recovery.

Classification of Preanesthetics

1. Anticholinergics

These agents are used:

- To reduce secretions of the salivary glands and mucous glands of the respiratory tract.
- To reduce gastric and intestinal motility.
- To block the vagal nerve to prevent sinus bradycardia.

Atropine Sulfate

- Obtained from leaves of *Atropa belladona* and also prepared synthetically.
- Atropine blocks acetylcholine at the postganglionic termination of cholinergic fibers in the autonomic nervous system (ANS).
- Causes dilation of pupil (sphincter muscle) but it does not dilate the pupils of birds because their iris is composed of striated muscle.
- Can be given intramuscular, intravenous or subcutaneous routes of administration.
- Duration of action is $1\text{-}1^1/_2$ hours.
- When given intravenously, atropine has
  - i. An initial central vagal stimulation action
  - ii. An intermediate vagotonic action on the conducting mechanism of the heart.
  - iii. Parasympatholytic action.

- Its use should be avoided in cases in which tachycardia already exists.
- Atropine degradation and elimination vary among animal species. The cat, rat and rabbit can destroy large quantities of atropine because they have atropine esterase in the liver.
- It increases the viscosity of the secretions.
- It reduces the tear formation.
- It crosses the blood brain barrier.
- It can prolong thiobarbiturate anesthesia.
- Overdose is characterized by dry mucous membrane, thirst, dilatation of pupils, tachycardia, vomiting and seizures. Overdose can be treated by diazepam.

Glycopyrrolate

- It is a synthetic quaternary ammonium anticholinergic agent and can be given intramuscular, intravenous and subcutaneous route.
- Glycopyrrolate should not be administered to pregnant bitches.
- It produces less tachycardia than atropine.
- Peak effect is obtained 3.0-4.5 minutes after subcutaneous or intramuscular injection and lasts for 2-3 hours. Its antisialogogue effect may persist for 6-8 hours (longer than atropine).
- It does not cross the blood brain barrier.

2. Tranquilizers

Tranquilizers are useful in wide variety of conditions in animals, namely

- As preanesthetic sedative.
- To relieve anxiety.
- To restrain refractory animals during examination or large animals during shipment.
- To prevent animals from licking wounds or chewing bandages and splints.
- As an antiemetic.
  i. Tranquilizers are usually administrated intravenously at least 15 minutes prior to administration of general anesthesia.
  ii. It can be given by intramuscular and oral routes of administration.

iii. *Epinephrine*: It causes ventricular arrhythmias and cardiac fibrillation. Its β-effect may result in further lowering of blood pressure. It is contraindicated in treatment of hypotension caused by tranquilizers. Nor epinephrine or phenylephrine is the drug of choice.

iv. Phenothiazines may potentate the toxicity of organophosphates and the activity of procaine hydrochloride.

v. Their use is contraindicated in cardiovascular and hepatic disease.

Advantages of Preanesthetic Tranquilizers

- The animal is easier to handle during induction of anesthesia.
- The required amount of general anesthetic is reduced.
- Antiemetic action.
- The animal is protected by phenothiazines from ventricular arrhythmias and cardiac fibrillation.
- Smooth recovery.
- No narcotic license is needed.

Disadvantages of Preanesthetic Tranquilizers

- Tranquilizers do not produce true analgesia.
- Cost is many times greater than for combined morphine and atropine.
- Persons handling tranquilizers may become sensitized resulting in urticaria and pruritus.
- When administered to animals in shock or to those with cardiovascular diseases, α-blockade may produce fatal hypotension.
- Permanent penile protrusion may occur in large male animals following administration of phenothiazine type agents.

Phenothiazine Tranquilizers

- Acetylpromazine is most commonly used tranquilizer in small animal practice.
- Phenothiazine tranquilizers can be given orally, subcutaneously, intramuscular or intravenous route.
- The duration of action is 3-6 hours but it may be much longer in patients with hepatic dysfunction.
- All these agents have same effect except potency and duration of action.
- They do not produce analgesia.
- They produce hypotension.

- They have minimal respiratory depressant effects.
- Most phenothiazines are potent antiemetic.
- They depress the thermoregulatory center.
- They lower the threshold to seizures.
- They inhibit myocardium sensitization to catecholamine.
- They have some skeletal muscle relaxant activity.
- No specific antagonist is available.

Chlorpromazine HCl

- It possesses four main pharmacologic properties:
  i. Central depressant action.
  ii. Antiemetic action.
  iii. α-adrenergic blocking effect.
  iv. Enhancing effect on the activity of analgesics, anesthetics and sedatives.
- *Main metabolite*: Chlorpromazine sulfoxide.
- It is not recommended for premedication in ruminants before general anesthesia because of risk of regurgitation due to cardiac relaxation.

Promazine HCl

- It should not be used in animals intended for human consumption.

Triflupromazine HCl

- It is a phenothiazine type tranquilizer containing fluorine.
- Marketed in brown bottles to protect it from decomposition by light.
- Triflupromazine has about 10 times the antiemetic effect of chlorpromazine and 3-5 times the tranquilizing potency.

Acepromazine HCl

- It is a potent neuroleptic agent.
- Most widely used tranquilizer and drug of choice in horses.
- Can be given intramuscular, intravenous, subcutaneous and oral route.
- It possesses antiemetic, anticonvulsant, antispasmodic, hypotensive and hypothermic properties.
- It will reduce or prevent the hypothermic response in susceptible swine exposed to halothane.

- Penile prolapse occurred at intravenous doses of 0.01 mg/kg to 0.4 mg/kg. Persistent paraphimosis may follow use of acepromazine in horses.
- It is effective in preventing cardiac arrhythmias and ventricular fibrillation produced by thiamylal, methohexital and thiopental.

Propiopromazine HCl

- An intravenous dose of 2.2 mg/kg in dogs, cats and monkeys causes ataxia, pupillary constriction, decreased activity and slight prolapse of the nictitating membrane.
- Persistent paraphimosis may occur.

Piperacetazine

- It has tranquilizing and antiemetic effect 35 and 50 times greater than those of chlorpromazine, respectively in dogs. It can be given by intramuscular, intravenous and subcutaneous routes.

Butyrophenone Derivatives

Droperidol

- It is a short acting narcoleptic.
- It has adrenergic - blocking properties, and prevents arrhythmias produced by epinephrine.
- It is a part of innovar-vet (neuroleptanalgesic).
- It has little effect on cardiac output.
- Duration of action is about 2 hours.
- It has antishock and adrenolytic activity.

Azaperone

- It is a narcoleptic and probably the most potent and specific sedative available for swine.
- Used to aggressive sows to allow piglets to be accepted and is used to prevent 'porcine stress syndrome'.
- It may be given as premeditation for cesarean section.
- It has antishock and adrenolytic activity.

Lenperone

- It is used in both dogs and cats.
- Their effects are same as droperidol.

Benzodiazapine Tranquilizers

Diazepam

- Diazepam is insoluble in water and dissolved in propylene glycol.
- Propylene glycol is a cardiopulmonary depressant. Rapid intravenous injection may cause hypotension, bradycardia and apnea.
- Its absorption from intramuscular injection site is unpredictable and erratic due to propylene glycol.
- It has calming, muscle relaxant and anticonvulsant activities in animals.
- It is an excellent preanesthetic agent for animals with a history of CNS disorders.
- The pH of injectable form is 6.4 - 6.9.
- Diazepam appears to act on parts of the limbic system, the thalamus, and the hypothalamus to produce calming effects or taming effect in animals.
- Fear and anxiety are reduced without marked sedation.
- The effect of diazepam occurs at neuronal pathways in which GABA is the transmitter.
- It has broad spectrum anticonvulsant activity.
- Drug passes the placental barrier
- Protein binding is 96%.
- It is useful in patients having CNS disorders like epileptics.
- It can be used as preanesthetic in old and debilitated animals.
- It may cause paradoxic excitement especially when given intravenously in the absence of other CNS depressants.
- Diazepam is metabolized by demethylation and hydroxylation to N-desmethyldiazepam, 3-hydroxydiazepam and oxazepam. These metabolites are all pharmacologically active.
- Diazepam solution should be injected slowly to prevent the possibility of venous thrombosis.
- In healthy animals, it may not produce CNS depression or tranquilization.
- Risk of congenital malformation during early pregnancy.
- It may increase cough reflex and laryngospasm.

- Contraindicated in glaucoma.
- Flumazenil is highly potent antidote for benzodiazepines (0.25-1.50 mg/kg IV or IP). Flumazenil has high affinity for benzodiazepine receptors and will reverse all the CNS effects of benzodiazepines.
- Its duration of action is about 60 minutes.
- Redosing should be done to antagonize large doses of benzodiazepines.

Midazolam

- It is water soluble and may be administered intramuscularly or intravenously.
- It has more predictable effects than diazepam when given intramuscularly.
- It can produce undesirable behavioral changes in dog and cat.
- It is more respiratory depressant than diazepam.
- Its duration of action is shorter than diazepam.
- In ruminants, it is 3-4 times more potent than diazepam.

Narcotic Analgesics

- Mechanism of action: Opioid have three sites of action in the CNS-
  - i. Inhibition of pain transmission in the dorsal horn.
  - ii. Activation of descending inhibitory pathways.
  - iii. Inhibition of somato-sensory afferents at supraspinal level.
- Receptors are mu (μ), kappa (κ), sigma (σ) and delta (δ).
- Mu Opioid receptors are responsible for analgesia and respiratory depression.
- Kappa receptors are responsible for spinal analgesia and sedation.
- Narcotic analgesics may produce CNS depression (most of the species) or excitement (cat) depending on drug and its dose and species of the animal.
- They depress the respiratory and vasomotor center in the medulla.
- They stimulate the vomiting center.
- They may elevate the intracranial pressure.
- They can produce sinus bradycardia.

- The dogs may show panting after administration of non-narcotic analgesics. It may be due to initial stimulation of respiratory center or alteration of thermoregulatory center.

Opioids

Agonists : Produces full range of physiologic response. e.g. morphine, meperidine, oxymorphone, fentanyl, sufentanyil, alfentanil, carfentanil, codein and heroin

Agonist-antagonist : They are agonists/partial agonists at one or more of the opioid receptors and are antagonistic/partial antagonistic at other opioid receptor site. They can partially antagonize the effect of pure opioid agonists. e.g. pentazocine, nalbuphine, nalorphine, butorphanol and buprenorphine.

Antagonists : They reverse the effect of opioid agonists and agonist-antagonists. e.g. naloxone, naltrexone and nalmefene.

Morphine Sulfate

- It depresses respiration.
- It causes vasodilatation and hypotension because of histamine release.
- It may produce significant bradycardia as a result of increased vagal tone.
- It directly stimulates the vomition center.
- Duration of action is 1-4 hours in the dog.
- Chief pharmacological effect is analgesia
- The site of action is nucleus raphe magnus - spinal system
- In the dog it produces marked bradycardia and has significant antidiuretic effects (due to ADI I).
- Morphine is contraindicated in ....
  i. Strychnine poisoning - (It also produce spinal convulsions)
  ii. Uremia (it stimulates secretion of antidiuretic hormone {ADH} - Urine production may reduce as much as 90%).
  iii. Traumatic or hemorrhagic shock (due to severe depression of BP, cardiac out put and lowered O_2 consumption).
- In the cat, morphine in high doses (20 mg/kg) produces mania and tonic convulsions due to dopamine release in the CNS.
- Morphine is inactivated by liver to morphine-3-glucuronide
- It can be used as a sole analgesic and narcotic agent for cesarean section in bitch.

- Morphine is usually injected subcutaneously or intramuscularly but may be given by slow intravenous infusion.

Morphine–Apomorphine narcosis: Apomorphine is a dopamine agonist.

- This combination is used for deep narcosis in the dog.
- Chief use of this mixture is in cesarean section in canine.

Meperidine HCl (Pethidine)

- It is a synthetic narcotic agonist.
- When given IV to dogs, there is a fall in BP due to peripheral vasodilatation.
- At therapeutic doses, it produces less cardiovascular and respiratory depression than morphine.
- Rapid IV, administration must be avoided, since the drug stimulates the central nervous system and causes convulsions.
- Pre-anesthetic dose in dogs is 10-22 mg/kg subcutaneously.
- Duration of action is 1-2 hour.
- 100 mg is equal to the analgesic effect of 10 mg of morphine sulfate.
- Sole agent for cesarean section in dogs.
- Its analgesic and spasmolytic effects make it a suitable preanesthetic for horses having colic.

Methadone HCl

- Synthetic analgesic and narcotic agent.
- Toxicity by the oral, subcutaneous and intravenous routes is in the ratio of 3:2:1 respectively.
- Barbiturate dose is reduced by one half in dogs @ 1 mg/kg IV or SC.

Oxymorphone HCl

- Semi synthetic narcotic analgesic with a potency approximately 10 times that of morphine.
- Duration of action is 1-3 hours.
- It produces less respiratory depression than morphine.
- It can be used in dog and cat.
- It produces more sedation and less hypnosis than morphine.

- The anesthetic dose of barbiturates is reduced 1/3 to 2/3rd.
- It can be antagonized by levallorphan, nalorphine or nalxone.

Fentanyl citrate and carfentanil

- Fentanyl is synthetic narcotic agonist that is 500 times more potent than meperidine and 250 times more potent than morphine.
- It is not recommended for use in the cat
- It has short duration of action (less than 30 minutes)
- Action can be reversed by the narcotic antagonists.
- It produces bradycardia due to increase in vagal tone
- Fentanyl is a basic drug. This makes fentanyl more lipid soluble and increases penetration through the blood brain barrier.
- Fentanyl, unlike morphine, usually does not produce vomiting in dogs. However, the anal sphincter is relaxed.

Carfentanyl

- Carfentanyl is a congener of fentanyl which is 12000 to 18000 times more potent than morphine and has been termed *super fentanyl.*
- It is administrated by swabbing or spraying over the buccal or nasal mucosa.
- Used almost exclusively for capture of exotic species of animals.
- Action reversed by morphine antagonists, e.g. cyprenorphine or deprenorphine.
- Its potency compared to etorphine and fentanyl is 20:15:1.

Sufentanyl

- The analgesic potency of sufentanyl is 5-10 times that of fentanyl.

Alfentanyl

- Alfentanyl is 1/5th to 1/10th as potent as fentanyl and its duration of action is 1/3rd that of fentanyl.

Thiambutene HCl

- White powder, aqueous solutions may be boiled but do not withstand autoclaving.
- It crosses the placenta and depresses fetal respiration.

- When given subcutaneous, it is about 1/5th as active as morphine sulfate and 3-4 times more active than meperidine on a weight basis.

Etorphine HCl (M-99)

- It is an oripavine derivative and used extensively for restraint of wild animals.
- Etorphine is 80-1000 times more potent than morphine
- The effect of etorphine can be antagonized with
  i. Nalorphine (etorphine/nalorphine ratio 1:10 to 1:20)
  ii. Diprenorphine (etorphine/diprenorphine ratio 1:1 to 1:2).

Butorphanol Tartarate

- It is a synthetic analgesic with both narcotic agonist and antagonist properties.
- Its analgesic potency is 3-5 times more than morphine.
- Antagonistic potency of butorphanol and nalorphine is 50 times less than naloxone.
- It can produce bradycardia.
- Respiratory depressant effect is similar to morphine.
- Duration of action is 1-4 hours.
- It is a good analgesic and fair sedative.
- When it is combined with acepromazine, benzodiazepine or $á_2$ agonist, a very good neuroleptanalgesia is produced.

Pentazocine Lactate

- It is an analgesic having agonist antagonist properties.
- It produces minimal CNS and cardiovascular depression and mild respiratory depression.
- Duration of action is about 2 hours.
- Naloxone hydrochloride- specific antagonist.

Buprenorphine

- It may cause slightly more respiratory depression than butorphanol.
- Duration of action is 6-8 hours.

Uses

- To sedate and calm the patient prior to local or general anesthesia.
- To provide pre and postoperative analgesia.

Disadvantages

- It causes marked respiratory depression and should be used with caution in patients with respiratory diseases.
- It can cause hypotension.
- It produces sinus bradycardia which can be treated by anticholinergics.
- It can cause an increase in intracranial pressure and should be used with caution in patients with head trauma.
- It can cause excitement in some patients.

Non opiate analgesics: (α_2-agonist) : e.g. Xylazine, Detomidine, Medetomidine, Romifidine, Oxymetazoline, Dexmedetomidine, Azepexole etc.

1. Clonidine is the prototype compound of α_2-agonist.
2. They can produce analgesia, sedation, anticonvulsant and calming effect.
3. Analgesia and sedation is produced by stimulation in the CNS.

Xylazine HCl (Rompum)

- It is a thiazine derivative.
- It is a potent non-narcotic sedative and analgesic as well as muscle relaxant.
- Sedative and analgesic activities are related to CNS depression mediated by stimulation of α_2-receptors.
- Its sedative effect lasts for 1-2 hours and analgesic effect lasts for 15-30 minutes.
- Muscle relaxant effect is based on inhibition of intraneural transmission of impulses in the CNS.
- Thiopental dose reduced to $1/3^{rd}$ –1/2 of the estimated dose.
- Xylazine induces hyperglycemia in cats and dogs, resulting from inhibition of insulin secretion.
- It produces mydriasis in cats due to CNS inhibition of parasymphethetic tone to iris by postsynaptic α_2-adrenergic receptors.
- Swine are resistant to xylazine, requiring 20-30 times the ruminant dose.

- Xylazine induced second degree A-V block which can be abolished by prior IV, administration of 0.011 mg/kg atropine sulphate
- Emesis (in normal doses) and acute abdominal distension (in large doses) occurs (Parasympatholytic effect → gastrointestinal atony → accumulation of gases. This feature makes radiograph interpretations of upper GI tact less certain.
- It decreases the gastrointestinal sphincter pressure.
- It has a wide margin of safety. Increasing dosages do not in general increase the degree of sedation but rather the duration of effect.
- Xylazine induced bradycardia may occasionally lead to heart block and death in dogs.
- It can cause marked vasoconstriction.
- It also induces hypotension, hypoventilation and excessive salivation.
- It sensitizes the myocardium to catecholamine thus making dysrrhythmias more likely.
- If xylazine is used in dogs as a preanesthetic prior to halothane, it causes an increased probability of cardiac arrhythmias and lowers the threshold to ventricular fibrillation. This reaction may be due to its ability to potentate cardiac sensitization to epinephrine.
- Ruminants regurgitate and become tympanitic under its effect.
- It decreases respiratory rate and depth.
- Large doses of xylazine or used with CNS depressants, significant respiratory depression may occur.
- It causes relaxation of the larynx and suppresses the cough reflex.
- It can cause hypothermia by depressing the thermoregulatory center.
- Administration to very excited animals may result in to paradoxic increase in excitement.

Uses

- As preanesthetic sedative prior to local, regional or epidural anesthesia.
- It can also be used before injectable or inhalant general anesthesia.
- It is used for minor diagnostic or manipulative procedures.
- Xylazine along with opioid produces profound sedation and analgesia.

Precautions

- Xylazine should never be used with tranquilizers.
- Bloat is common in Great Danes and Irish setter. So xylazine should be used with caution in these breeds.
- It should be used with caution in animals with cardiovascular, respiratory, hepatic or renal diseases and in debilitated animals.
- Xylazine should be used with anticholinergics because of its vagotonic effect.
- It can be absorbed through break in the skin and mucous membrane. So the persons administrating xylazine should be careful.
- Xylazine is contraindicated in the last trimester of pregnancy in cattle, since abortion may occur.

Medetomidine

- It is 10 times more potent than xylazine and 6 times more potent than detomidine.
- Cardiopulmonary and respiratory effects are similar to xylazine.
- Atropine is more effective than glycopyrrolate in preventing bradycardia caused by medetomidine.
- Antagonist: Same as xylazine. Atipamizole is the most effective because of its α_1 and α_2 selective ratio.
- It is recommended for young and healthy dogs.

Romifidine

- It provides less ataxia than xylazine in horses.
- Effects are longer lasting than xylazine.
- Dose: 1 mg/kg of xylazine is equal to 100 µg/kg romifidine.

α_2-antagonists : α_2-antagonists should be given slow intravenously or intramuscularly because of risk of hypotension and tachycardia caused by rapid intravenous injection.

- A combination of 4-aminopyridine (0.3 mg/kg) and yohimbine (0.125 mg/kg) intravenously will antagonize a dose of 2.2 mg/kg of xylazine in dogs.
- Yohimbine: Cattle @ 0.125 mg/kg b. wt. intravenously.

Horse @ 0.075 mg/kg b. wt. intravenously.

Dog @ 0.1 mg/kg b. wt. intravenously.

Cat @ 0.5 mg/kg b. wt. intravenously.

- Atipamizole is a specific antagonist for medetomidine.
- Idazolxan @ 0.05-0.1 mg/kg body weight in all species.
- Doxapram: It is a general CNS stimulant. Doxapram @ 2 mg /kg IM reverses xylazine atropine sedation in dogs. It is not a true antagonist.
- Tolazoline works better than yohimbine in cattle (0.44 mg/kg intravenously) It is also effective in sheep dog and cat @ 2.0 mg/kg b. wt.

Neuroleptanalgesics : These are the combination of neuroleptic (tranquilizer) and analgesic (narcotic) to enhance the CNS depressant effects of each drug.

Fentanyl Citrate – Droperidol: (Innovar –Vet)

- Used to produce neuroleptanalgesia (it is a state of CNS depression and analgesia produced without the use of barbiturates and volatile anesthetics).
- Fentanyl citrate (0.4 mg) + Droperidol (20 mg).
- Dose in Dog - 1 ml/10-15 kg b. wt. IV.
- This combination is sufficient for minor surgery.
- The mixture produces sedation, analgesia, immobilization, respiratory depression, panting and bradycardia.
- *Advantage* : Easy to administer, wide margin of safety, quite recovery and partial reversibility with Opioid antagonists.
- A mixture of 4-aminopyridine (0.5 mg/kg) and naloxone hydrochloride (0.04 mg/kg) IV, antagonize the CNS effects of droperdol-fentanyl.

Lytic Cocktail

- Consists of

  40 mg Atropine sulfate (32 mg/ml of solution) +

  200 mg Methadone hydrochloride (10 mg/ml) +

  Promazine hydrochloride (250 mg/ 5 ml)
- *Dose in horses:* One ml / 50 kg body weight.

Etorphine - Acepromazine (Immobilon, L.A.) For large animals.

- Used in horses, wild and zoo animals.
- It has been used to immobilize horses for minor surgery e.g. castration.

Etorphine - Methotrimeprazine (Immobilon, S.A.) For small animal

Etorphine antagonist - Deprenorphine (0.272 mg/kg IV).

Neuroleptanalgesic combinations for dog and cats

S.No.	Neuroleptic (Tranquilizer)	Analgesic (Narcotic)
1.	Acetylpromazine @ 0.1mg/kg i.m. or i.v. Maximum total dose 1 mg	Oxymorphone@ 0.2 mg/kg i.m. or i.v. Maximum total dose 3 mg
2.	Diazepam @ 0.2-0.4 mg/kg i.m. or i.v. Maximum total dose 10 mg	Oxymorphone @ 0.2 mg/kg i.m. or i.v. Maximum total dose 3 mg
3.	Acetylpromazine @ 0.1mg/kg i.m. or i.v. Maximum total dose 1 mg	Meperidine @ 2-4 mg/kg i.m. or i.v.
4.	Acetylpromazine @ 0.1mg/kg i.m. or i.v. Maximum total dose 1 mg	Butorphanol @ 0.2-0.4 mg/kg i.m. or i.v. Maximum total dose 20mg
5.	Diazepam @ 0.2-0.4 mg/kg i.m. or i.v. Maximum total dose 10 mg	Butorphanol @ 0.2-0.4 mg/kg i.m. or i.v. Maximum total dose 20mg

Note : Diazepam should not be mixed in the same syringe with the opioid as it will cause precipitation. So while administering the opioid and diazepam, give the opioid first and then give diazepam 2-3 minutes later to prevent diazepam induced behavioral changes.

Chapter 18

GENERAL ANESTHESIA

General anesthesia : reversible complete loss of consciousness along with analgesia.

- Unconsciousness occurs due to depressant action or functional disruption by stimulation in brain by anesthetic agents.
- Analgesia is probably due to blockade of synaptic transmission in the dorsal horn of the spinal cord.

Qualities of An Ideal Anesthetic

- Not dependent on the body for detoxification and excretion.
- Rapid induction, quick alteration in the depth and rapid recovery.
- Wide margin of safety, minimal depression of vital centers and low toxicity.
- Non irritant to tissues.
- Nonflammable, nonexplosive and chemically stable.
- Inexpensive and not requiring expensive equipment for administration.
- Produces good muscle relaxation and analgesia.

Theory of anesthetic effect : The theory given by Mayer (1989) and Overton (1901) is most accepted. According this theory the anesthetic effect is proportionate to the coefficient of solubility in water and fat.

Stages of anesthesia : Given by Guedel and there are four stages depending upon neuromuscular signs.

Stage–I (stage of voluntary excitement) : Characterized by in-coordination and analgesia. Dilatation of pupils, voiding of urine or faeces are other signs of excitement. In ultra short acting anesthetics like thiopentone, this stage passes off unnoticed.

Stage–II (stage of involuntary excitement) : It is characterized by unconsciousness.

Stage–III (stage of surgical anesthesia) : Characterized by unconsciousness abolition of sensation and neuromuscular reflexes, slow and regular breathing and loss of swallowing reflex. The cerebral cortex is affected first and is always last to recover from the effects of anesthesia.

Stage–IV (stage of medullary paralysis or over doses) : The animal is in anesthetic shock. If corrective measures are not adopted, the animal is likely to die.

	Drugs			**Anesthetic stage**	
1.	Diethyl ether	I	II	III	IV
2.	Nitrous oxide	I	II		
3.	Trichloroethyline				
4.	Ketamine				
5.	Phencyclidine				
6.	α-Chloralose	I	-	III	IV
7.	Enflurane				
8.	Barbiturates				
9.	Halothane				
10.	Methoxyflurane				

Inhalation anaesthesia : This is a technique of administrating anesthetic agents via the lungs. Now a days this usually consists of a volatile agent being vaporized in a vaporizer by oxygen and then being administered to the patient through an anesthetic breathing circuit of which there are several designs. Nitrous oxide is the only anesthetic gas now used in anesthesia which is administered through flow meter and then passes in to breathing circuit. Inhalation anesthesia can be grouped into 3 phases :

1. Pulmonary phase
2. Circulatory phase
3. Tissue phase

Vessel rich group (brain, heart, intestines, kidney, liver and spleen) and muscle group (skeletal muscles) are the tissues which are primarily involved in uptake of inhalation anesthetics. An alveolar concentration is a readily measured index of brain anesthetic tension. Once induction is achieved vaporizer concentration should be adjusted to proper level to maintain anesthesia. Recovery from anesthesia can be hastened by assisted ventilation, increased O_2 flow and stimulation of anesthetic patient. The clinical signs of general anesthesia results from the action of anesthetics on the CNS.

Vaporization of volatile anesthetic agents : A vapor may be thought of as a gas below its critical temperature. Both liquid and gaseous phases exist simultaneously and in a closed container, a state of equilibrium is attained when the number of molecules leaving the liquid phase equals the number of molecules reentering it.

Anesthetic agent uptake : The depth of anesthesia is related to the partial pressure of anesthetic agents in the brain. For anesthetic action to occur the anesthetic agent must be capable of crossing the blood brain barrier to the CNS. Therefore, it must be lipid soluble. The mechanism for a gas to dissolve in the patient's blood and other tissues relies on pressure and pressure gradients between the tissues or phases. The following are definitions or terms which may be used when describing the uptake and distribution of anesthetic gases.

i. *Dalton's law of partial pressure* : The constituent gases in a gas mixture acts independently of each other and the pressure exerted by a mixture of gases is the sum of the individual pressures exerted by each gas. The component of total pressure that each gas exerts is termed its partial pressure.

ii. *Graham's law* : The rate of diffusion of gases through certain membranes is inversely proportional to the square root of their molecular weight.

iii. *Fick's law of diffusion* : The rate of diffusion of gas is directly proportional to the concentration gradient.

iv. *Partition coefficient* : It is the ratio between anesthetic concentrations each of two phases when equilibrium exists between these phases e.g. blood/gas, tissue/gas, and tissue/blood. Blood/gas partition coefficient of certain anesthetics are as follows

Nitrous oxide	-	0.47
Enflurane	-	1.78
Halothane	-	2.3
Chloroform	-	8.4
Diethyl either	-	12.1
Methoxyflurane	-	12.0

- Agents with high tissue/blood coefficients require longer induction periods.
- Anesthesia can be induced most rapidly with those gases having a low blood/ gas partition coefficient.

Methods of Administration or Breathing Circuits

1. *Open method* : Cones, cotton and jars are used in open method of administration e.g. ether and chloroform.
2. *Semi open method (non-rebreathing)* : This method is less economical. Non-rebreathing circuits with Stephen valve, Ayres T piece and magill apparatus are used. There is minimum resistance to breathing.
3. *Closed method rebreathing* :
   i. *To and fro system* : No valve are necessary methoxyflurane can not be efficiently administer with this system.
   ii. The circle system.
   iii. *Circle system with vaporizer inside circle (VIC)* : An increase in ventilation will increase the inspired concentration.
   iv. *Circle system with vaporizer outside circle (VOC)* : Assisted or controlled ventilation can be used safely in VOC.
4. *Semi closed or partial rebreathing* : A part of expired gases escape usually through pop-off value. It is a safe system and can be divided in to :
   - Semi closed method with CO_2 absorption.
   - Semi closed method without CO_2 absorption.

Anesthetic equipment : Anesthesia machine and breathing systems are required for administration of liquid or gaseous inhalant anesthetics to the patient for general anesthesia. The breathing system supplies oxygen and anesthetic to the patient and eliminates carbon dioxide from exhaled gases.

Basic Components of the Anesthetic Machine

i. Cylinders for oxygen and nitrous oxide or sources of these gases from a bank of large compressed gas cylinders.

ii. Pressure gauges

iii. A regulator

iv. Flowmeter

v. Vaporizer :

   a. VIC- *e.g.* Ohio# 8 glass bottle vaporizer and Stephen vaporizer.

   b. VOC- *e.g.* Tec vaporizers, Fluotec Mark 2 and Tec mark 3 vaporizer.

Pressure of gases in an anesthetic machine : It varies at different locations in an anesthesia machine.

- *High pressure areas (about 2200 psi)* : Cylinder to a regulator.
- *Intermediate pressure areas (37-50 psi)* : Just after regulator to flowmeter.
- *Low pressure areas (0-30 cm of H_2O)* : From flowmeter to common gas outlet.

Knowledge of these pressures at different locations of an anesthesia machine facilitates safe operation of an anesthesia machine.

1. *Cylinder for O_2 and N_2O* : These cylinders are supplied with color code.

Kind of gas	Cylinder color
Oxygen	Green
CO_2	Gray
N_2O	Light blue
Cyclopropane	Orange
Helium	Brown
Ethylene	Red
CO_2+O_2	Gray and green

2. *Pressure gauges* : The gauge indicates pressure on the cylinder side and attached to the regulator.

3. *Regulator* : A regulator reduces the high and variable storage pressure to a lower and more constant pressure which maintains constant flow to the Flowmeter.

Flowmeters : A flowmeter measures and indicates the rate of flow of gases to the vaporizer. The scale in the glass tube indicates rate of gas flow in ml/min. or L/min. Flowmeters are calibrated at 760 mmHg and 20°C. A flowmeter's indicator should be read at the top except for a ball type float, which is read at the center. The indicator should move freely in the glass tube.

- The flow control knobs are labeled with the gas symbol and are colour coded.
- The size of the float may be >1 cm.

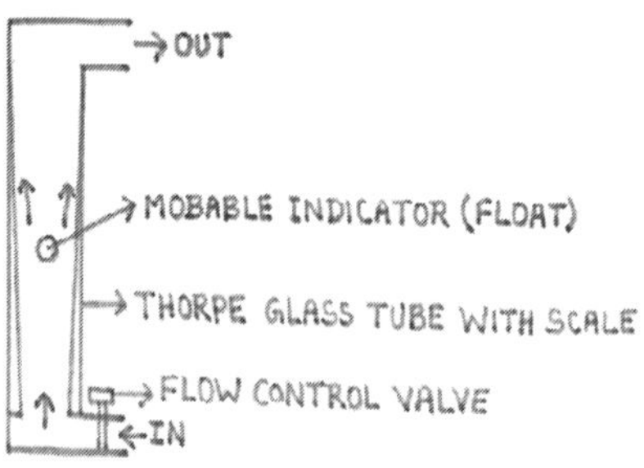

1. *Safety devices for pressure and flow of oxygen* : These devices alert the operator to a dangerously low pressure or flow of oxygen by an alarm. The machine may be designed to cut off the supply of al other gases (N_2O) to prevent the delivery of hypoxic mixture.
2. *Flush valves* : Oxygen is supplied to the flush valves of an anesthesia machine at about 50 psi. It delivers a high flow (35-75 liter/ min.) of oxygen to the breathing system which can quickly fill a breathing system. Pediatric breathing system like Bain circuit and Mapleson system should not be filled via the flush valve due to danger of over pressurization of the patient's respiratory system.
3. *Vaporizers* : A vaporizer is designed to change a liquid anesthetic in to its vapor. The specific amount of vapor adds to carrier gas, oxygen alone or with nitrous oxide, which is delivered to the patient. There are many different designs depending on which type of agent is to be vaporized and where in the circuit the vaporizer is positioned. There are two positions in the circuit in which the vaporizer can be placed : Either vaporizer in circuit (VIC) or vaporizer out of circuit (VOC). Vaporizers are also classified on the basis of resistance to flow.

- VOC- High resistance vaporizers are used in VOC unit *e.g.* Plenum type vaporizers.
- VIC- Low resistance vaporizers are used in VIC unit *e.g.* Ohio # 8 and Stephen vaporizers.

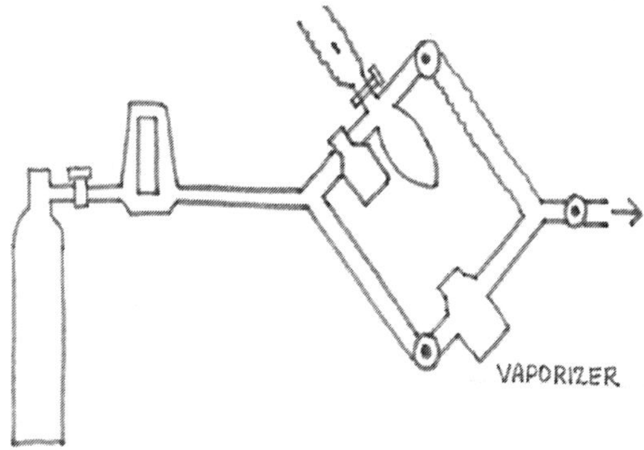

Vaporizer Out of Circuit (VOC)

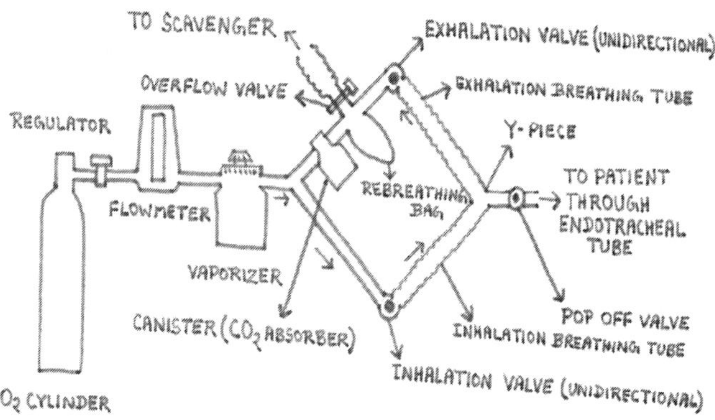

Vaporizer In Circuit (VIC)

Breathing systems : Anesthetic breathing systems supplies anesthetic gases and oxygen to the patient and remove CO_2 from exhaled gases and provide a means to support ventilation.

- Doubling the radius of conduits decrease the resistance 16 times.
- If the circuit length is halved, resistance is also decrease to half.
- Endotracheal tube has the smallest diameter of the breathing circuits.

Rebreathing System / Circle Breathing System

- After excretion of CO_2 (chemical absorbent soda lime) all the exhaled gases are return to the patient.

- In rebreathing system, anesthetic agent, oxygen, heat and moisture are conserved. However, it imparts more resistance e.g. circle system and to and fro system.
- Breathing system that induces least resistance to gas flow should be chosen for spontaneously breathing patients.

Components of the Circle System

- *Y piece* : It is made of plastic and contributes to the mechanical dead space.
- *Breathing tubes/ hoses*

  i. Breathing tubes are made up of rubber or plastic.

  ii. These tubes are corrugated to reduce the chance of kinking and subsequent obstruction.

  iii. Rubber tube may bulge during intermittent positive pressure ventilation. This means that some of the energy used to ventilate the patient is wasted in expanding the hoses. Modern plastic tubes/ hoses are free of this problem.

  iv. *Size of the breathing tubes/ hoses*

    i. 15 mm i d (internal diameter)- for animals> 7 kg.

    ii. 22 mm i d (internal diameter)- for smaller patients.

    iii. 50 mm i d (internal diameter)- for large animals.

- *Unidirectional valves* : (Inhalation or exhalation valves)

  i. These valves directs the flow of anesthetic gases

    a. Toward the patient on inspiration.

    b. Away from the patient from expiration.

  ii. These valves allow rebreathing of exhaled gases only after the absorption of the carbon dioxide.

  iii. Valves should be checked time to time because they contribute to the resistance of breathing.

- *Fresh gas inlet*

  i. Fresh gas inlet is the location from which the gas enters the circle system.

  ii. It is located on the absorbent canister near the inspiratory one way valve or on the inspiratory one way valve.

- *Pop off valve (overflow valve)*

  i. Pop off valve vents gases to the scavenger system to prevent the build up of pressure and allows rapid elimination of anesthetics from the circle when 100% oxygen is indicated.

  ii. The exhaust port of the valve diverts gases to the scavenger system.

  iii. Pop off valves are safety features of the closed or semi closed circle system.

  iv. The valve should remain open except during positive pressure ventilation.

- *Reservoir bag*

  i. It is made up of rubber or neoprene.

  ii. The reservoir bag allows controlled ventilation i.e. respiratory rate and tidal volume can be assessed.

  iii. If the pop off valve is closed, the bag provides compliance to slow the build up of pressure.

  iv. The size of the reservoir bag should be at least 6 times the patient's tidal volume.

  v. Spontaneous deep breath should not empty the bag.

  vi. Common bag sizes are 1, 2, 3 and 5 liter.

  vii. A large bag impairs monitoring and slow changes in anesthetic concentration when setting on a VOC machine are altered

  viii. The bag should be about ¾ full of anesthetic gases for optimum condition.

  ix. *Functions*

  a. It allows visual observation of patient ventilation.

  b. It protects the patient from excessive pressure in the breathing system.

  c. It provides a means of assisting or controlling the ventilation of the patient.

  d. It allows accumulation of the gas during exhalation so that a reservoir of anesthetic gas is available and it prevents dilution with room air in non-rebreathing system.

- *Manometer* : Manometer is attached at the top of the absorber for assessment of inspiratory pressure (in cm of water) during controlled ventilation.
- *Vaporizers* : Refer parts of the anesthetic machine.
- *Absorber assembly* : It includes absorbent for CO_2.
  - i. The absorbing canister may be single or two stacked containers.
  - ii. Air space between the absorbent granules should be equal to or more than the tidal volume.
  - iii. Absorption of the CO_2 is the fundamental in a rebreathing system.
  - iv. Calcium hydroxide is the major component of soda lime and barium hydroxide lime.
  - v. Granular size of absorbents is typically 4-8 mesh.
  - vi. Soda lime changes from white to violet with use. The absorbent should be changed when the color reaction appears in 2/3rd of the absorbent.
  - vii. Absorption of the CO_2 is exothermic reaction which can be detected on the canister.
  - viii. Amount of absorption is about 26 liter/ 100 gram.

Rebreathing Circuits / Circle Breathing System

- Closed circle system
- Low flow circle system
- Semi closed circle system
- To and Fro system
  - i. In To and Fro system CO_2 absorbent canister is located between the endotracheal tube connector and a reservoir bag.
  - ii. This system is suitable for both small and large animals, if proper canister is available.
  - iii. The gases pass back and forth through the absorbent during ventilation.
- *Advantage* : The system is portable and easy to disassemble for cleaning.
- *Disadvantage* : Heat produced during CO_2 absorption may be transferred to the patient during inspiration and inhalation of alkaline dust.

S. No.	Properties	Closed circle system	Low flow circle system	Semi closed circle system
1.	Flow of gases	The fresh gas flow equals uptake of anesthetic gases and O_2 by the patient and system	Oxygen flow is greater than the patient's O_2 consumption	Fresh gas inflow is greater than the patient's uptake of O_2 and anesthetic
2.	Rate of gas flow	4-11 ml/kg/min.	10-15 ml/kg/min. but less than 22 ml/kg/min.	22-44 ml/kg/min.
3.	Use of N_2O	Generally not used in closed system because hypoxic gas mixture may develop. Denitrogenation (empty the reservoir bag via the pop off valve and refill the system with fresh gas) should be done 2-4 times during the first 15 minutes and every 30 minutes thereafter to prevent exhaled N_2 from diluting the O_2	–	N_2O can be safely used. Nitrogen accumulation is not significant because nitrogen is eliminated through the pop off valve.
4.	Economy	Relatively economic, retain heat and humidity and relatively safe for the environment.	Same as closed system	Semi closed system retains less heat and humidity and is less economical compared to closed and low flow system.
5.	Dependency of CO_2 absorption	Depends on CO_2 absorption	Depends on CO_2 absorption	Dependency is less because CO_2 is partially eliminated through the pop off valve
6.	Disadvantage	Inadequate delivery of anesthetic from a concentration calibrated (VOC) vaporizer during induction. This problem can be solved by higher flow for first 15-30 minute followed by a low flow technique.	Same as closed system	–

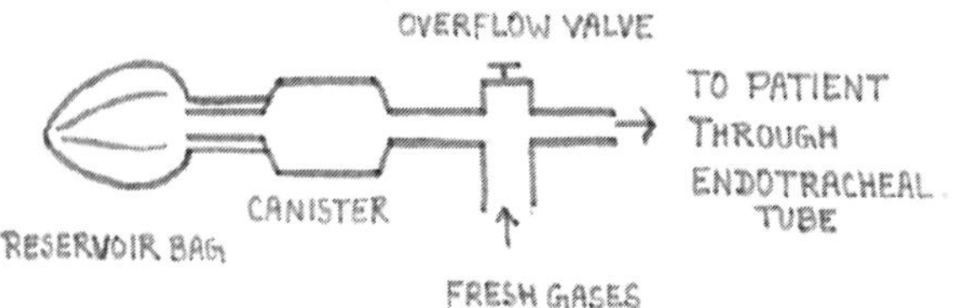

To and Fro System

Non Rebreathing Circuits

In non rebreathing circuits, fresh gases from the anesthetic machine (with anesthetic vapor) pass in to a reservoir and the patient breaths from that reservoir.

- Exhaled gases pass in to atmosphere, either directly or through an exhaust valve.
- There is no need of CO_2 absorbent in Mapleson system. This system depends on high fresh gas flow to flush the exhaled CO_2 from the system.
- The Mapleson systems are simple and easy to use, inexpensive, impart little resistance and allow the inspired concentration of anesthetic to be changed rapidly.
- Development of excessive airway pressure may lead to barotraumas to the lungs (pneumothorax).
- Classification of Mapleson system :
  - i. Mapleson A : The Magill circuit and lack Co-axial circuit.
  - ii. Mapleson B and C : Not used in veterinary practice.
  - iii. Mapleson D and E : Bain circuit
  - iv. Mapleson F : Ayer's T- piece circuit.
- *Disadvantage of Mapleson system :* Mapleson system require higher flow rates of fresh gas which decreases economy and promotes hypothermia and drying of respiratory tract.

1. Magill System

- The Magill system contains
  - i. Fresh gas inlet
  - ii. An overflow valve near the patient

iii. Corrugated tube connecting the patient end of the system to a reservoir bag.

- The system is good for patients under spontaneous ventilation.
- In controlled ventilated patients, some rebreathing of expired gases occurs.
- The volume of the reservoir bag and corrugated tube should be = the patient's tidal volume.

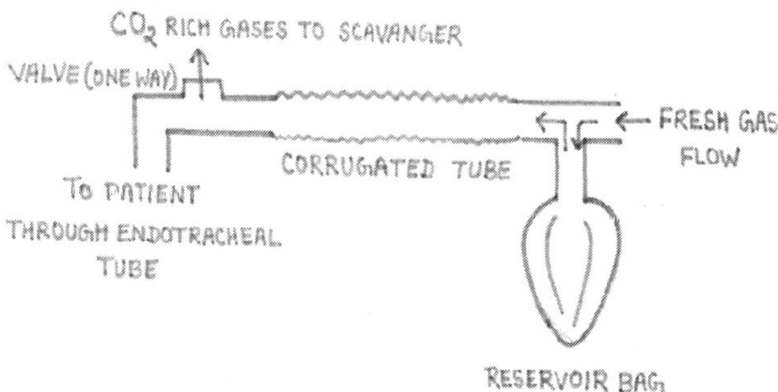

Magill System

2. Bain Coaxial System

- Bain coaxial system is designed as a tube within a tube.
- Internal tube

  i. Diameter-0.7 mm i. d. (internal diameter).

  ii. Supplies fresh gases to the patient through endotracheal connector (15 mm) or a mask (22 mm).

- External corrugated tube : It exhaled gases from the animal to a reservoir bag and finally passes out through scavenger.
- Recommendation for total fresh gas flow in to a bain coaxial system depends on minute volume, body weight and body surface area.
- During spontaneous ventilation recommended flow rates are variable.
- Recent studies suggests fresh gas flow of 1.5-3.0 times minute volume. Less than 2-3 times the minute volume will result in small amount of rebreathing of CO_2
- Bain system is effective in reducing loss of heat and humidity.

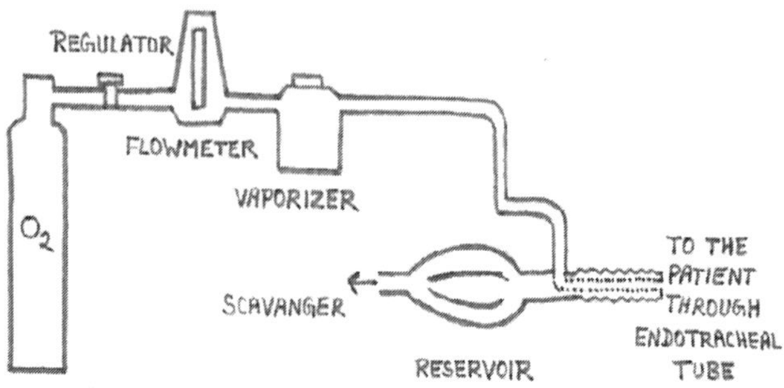

Bain Coaxial System

3. Ayer's T- Piece

- It consists of expiratory limb (corrugated tube), reservoir bag and T piece.
- The T piece is a T shaped tube with an internal diameter of 1 cm.
- During spontaneous ventilation:
  - i. Fresh gas flows towards the patient during inspiration.
  - ii. Gas flows towards the reservoir during expiration and to the next inspiration.
- 2-3 times the patient's minute volume is recommended to prevent dilution of inspired anesthetic concentration and rebreathing of CO_2.

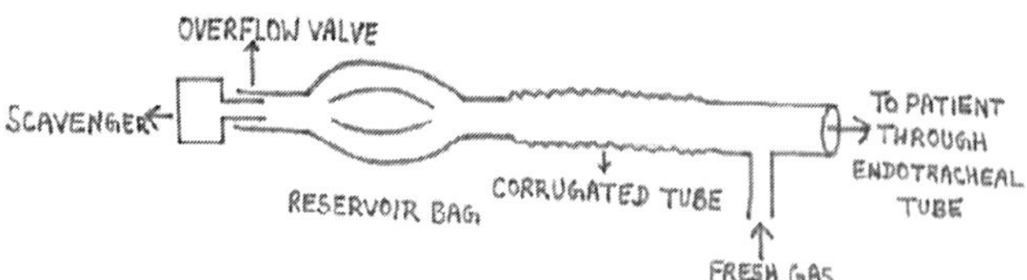

Ayre's T piece System

4. Stephen Slater System

Not used (obsolete) in veterinary practice.

- The system contains 2 one way valve.
  - i. Direct the gases from reservoir to the patient.
  - ii. Direct the exhaled gases away from the system.
- The recommended total fresh gas flow is equal to the patient's minute volume.

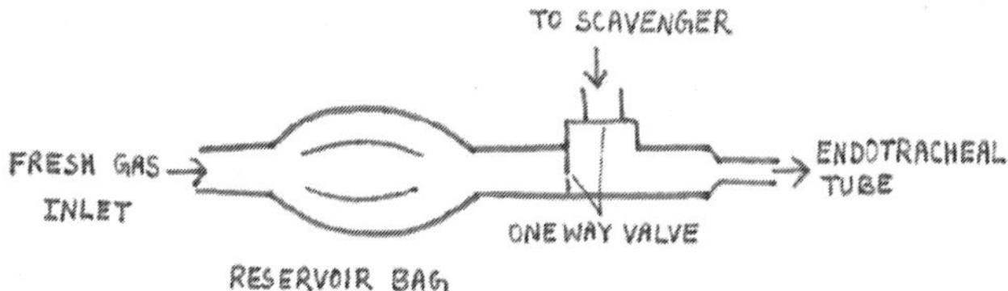

Stephen Slater System

Resuscitation Bag (AMBU Bag- Assisted Manual Breathing Unit):

- Resuscitation bag facilitates resuscitation.
- Resuscitation bag also have non rebreathing valve.
- During compression of the bag, gases enter the patient's respiratory system.
- During decompression of bag, gas flows from the patient's respiratory system through the exhalation port.
- Ambu valve allows the patient to inhale room air only.

Chapter 19

Injectable Anesthetics and their Combinations used for General Anesthesia*

Injectable Anesthesia

Injectable anesthetics are the agents which are administered to the patient parentrally. They include drugs which are given intravenously to rapidly induce anesthesia in a patient. Single or combinations of drugs usually administered intramuscularly to patients which are difficult to handle. Injectable agents generally require less equipment and are easier to administer than inhalation anesthetics, but it must be remembered that once they are given to a patient they cannot be removed.

Constant volume infusion pumps and microprocessor controlled syringe pumps are now being used to administer drug doses calculated to achieve constant serum levels over a long period of time. This, in large measure, enables one to avoid the problems of drug accumulation in the tissues which often occurs with intermittent injection techniques. However, constant infusion techniques are generally used together with oxygen administration via an endotracheal tube and also often involve IPPV (controlled ventilation). This means that a ventilator is required and thus, except for the vaporizer, very similar equipment to that required for inhalation anesthesia.

---

* Dr. Adarsh Kumar

Advantages/Disadvantages of Injectable Anesthetic Agents

Advantages

1. Simple to administered.
2. Generally have a rapid onset of action.
3. Little apparatus required.
4. No explosion or pollution hazard.
5. Non-irritant to airways.

Disadvantages

1. Possible tissue irritation.
2. Once injected, cannot be removed.
3. Drug may be cumulative.
4. During recovery excitement/ hallucinations possible.
5. Induction apnea possible.

The disadvantages no. 4 and 5 are really the result of poor anesthetic technique rather than an inherent disadvantage of the method.

Routes of Administration

If the injectable drug is to be used as an induction agent then the aim is to use routes which rapidly result in high blood and brain concentrations. It is advantageous for the patient to pass through the first two stages of anesthesia quickly, because these stages are unpleasant for the patient and the anesthetist.

1. *Intravenous* : This route provides a more immediate effect since the drug is deposited directly into the bloodstream. It is easier to titrate the final effects, because they occur almost immediately after the injection. For induction agents and for ease of titration, drugs should be selected which have an action in one 'injection site to brain' circulation time, for example thiopental has a more immediate effect than pentobarbital which requires the drug to be passed through the CNS several times for its effects. Injections which are irritant to the tissues should be administered by this route (preferably through an indwelling catheter). This route require more restraint, asepsis and experience.
2. *Intramuscular* : This is a commonly used route for administering premedication drugs, but is also useful for using anesthetic combinations in difficult patients as this route does not require as much restraint, precision and experience. It is difficult to titrate the final effect and this

can be extremely variable. Muscle has a good blood supply for absorption, but if the drug is deposited along fascial planes then the rate of absorption can be slowed.

3. *Other Routes* : Subcutaneous, oral, intraperitoneal and rectal routes are generally too slow for use in anesthesia. These routes can be used with some drugs in very small or difficult patients.

When to Use Injectable Anesthetics?

They are more commonly used for inducing anesthesia in a patient to avoid the struggling which can occur as the patient passes through the first two stages of anesthesia. Injectable agents have a faster effect when given in the correct dose. Once laryngeal reflexes are lost the patient's trachea can then be intubated and anesthesia maintained with an inhalation anesthetic agent. If necessary, short procedures can be maintained with more of the injectable agent. If this is to be done, then short-acting drugs with little accumulation in body depots should be chosen to avoid lengthy recoveries.

If the patient rapidly awakens from inhalation anesthesia because of sudden, intense surgical stimulation when in a light plane of anesthesia, small increments of an injectable anesthetic agent can be given intravenously to deepen the plane of anesthesia. Turning up the vaporizer may not deepen anesthesia rapidly enough, especially in horses. Increased analgesia can also be provided by the use of injectable analgesic agents. These are thre two examples of the role of injectable drugs as a supplementation to inhalation anesthesia.

Some of the intravenous anesthetic agents also have a medical role in the treatment of status epilepticus and poisonings because of their immediate effects of controlling convulsions.

Equipment Used for Injectable Anesthesia

Syringes : These should be of good quality, sterile and of an appropriate size. Syringes larger than 10 mL are easier to use if they have eccentrically placed nozzles so the needle can be positioned alongside the patient's body more easily. It is physically difficult to handle more than 50-60 mL of an injectable agent, so more concentrated solutions may be required. This becomes important when using thiobarbiturates for anesthetizing large horses. Otherwise the drug can be administered as an infusion. e.g. Guaifenesin in horses and cattle.

Hypodermic needles : These must be sharp and their points must have a short bevel to reduce the risk of transfixing the vein. Disposable needles are now used and good quality ones are ideal. An appropriate gauge (G) and length needle should be chosen *e.g.* 25-22 G, 2.0 cm needle is ideal for venepuncture of cats, 22-18 G, 2.0 - 2.5 cm for dogs and 18-16 G, 3.75 - 5.0 cm for larger animals.

If extra increments of the drug are required during surgery an access port to the venous system is required. Using a needle taped to the skin overlying the vein is not an ideal way of providing this port, neither it is an ideal way of providing intra-operative fluids. Movement between the skin and the vein will dislodge the needle so that injectate enters the surrounding tissues. This can result in hematoma formation, severe inflammation and skin necrosis and sloughing if the injectate is irritant.

Butterfly Needles : These are needles with plastic wings on the proximal end of the needle so they can be secured with tape to the skin overlying the vein. They also have a short length of tubing between the wings and the hub so there is flexibility in the system allowing some movement between the needle and bag of intravenous fluids or the syringe. Although they are better than using a hypodermic needle, the disadvantages are the same because of the rigid nature of the needle. They are suitable for short term use, but the patient must be supervised in case the needle becomes dislodged from the vein. The narrow diameter and the length of the tubing also confer resistance to the fluid to be injected.

Catheters : They are available in two types :

1. Through the needle
2. Over the needle

The first type is used for long term administration of fluids. They are long catheters often placed in the jugular vein through surgical cut-down. They are not commonly used in veterinary anesthesia.

The second type is almost always used. The plastic catheter is introduced into the vein while on a stylet (the needle). Once blood is seen in the viewing chamber the stylet and catheter are pushed in a fraction more so the distal end of the catheter is introduced into the vein. Once this has been done (blood should still be flowing, and it helps to still have the vein 'raised') the stylet should be kept still while the catheter is threaded into the vein. It does take practice to use these catheters, but the advantages far outweigh the disadvantages of their expense and of having to gain skill in their use. There is a lot of flexibility and the catheter rarely becomes dislodged while the patient is moving. This ensures that the injectate is being introduced into the vein and not into the tissues.

They must be placed as aseptically as possible especially if they are to remain in place for 24-48 hours. Phlebitis usually occurs after this time so, unless they are made of the less thrombogenic silastic, they should be removed after 48 hours. Do not forget to flush the catheter with heparinised saline if they are to be taped in place for use later on otherwise they will become blocked with blood clots. If this occurs, the clot should be *aspirated* out of the catheter into the syringe and *not irrigated into the circulation.*

Be very careful about replacing the stylet into the catheter if problems are experienced during placement, because the sharp end of the stylet can shear the end of the catheter and it is then lost into the circulation. Also, be careful when cutting tape which has secured the catheter in place, in case the plastic catheter or the IV tubing is cut.

Use 12-16 G, 5 1/4" catheters in large animals and 18-22 G, 1 1/2"- 2" in small animals. The longer the catheter, the more secure it is once positioned. Catheters coated with Teflon slide into place more easily.

Infusion Apparatus : This may be required when administering large volumes e.g. Guaifenesin, or drugs over a long period of time e.g. intravenous fluids.

The simplest device is an inverted bottle and flutter valve which lets air into the system. These are non-collapsible and can let air into the venous system if they are not closely monitored. Commercially prepared intravenous fluids are supplied in plastic, disposable collapsible containers.

Be aware of the pharmacokinetics behind administering boluses of an anesthetic drug compared to continuous administration (infusion techniques). Sometimes the use of injectable agents to provide anesthesia is termed 'Total Intravenous Anesthesia'. This means that all components of anesthesia are provided i.e. Analgesia; Muscle Relaxation; Narcosis. More than one drug may be employed.

Injectable Anesthetic Agents :

i. Barbiturates

ii. Dissociative Agents (Cyclohexamines)

iii. Steroid Anesthetics

iv. Imidazole Derivatives

v. Alkyl phenols

vi. Potent Synthetic Opioid Analgesics

Pharmacology and Clinical use of Injectable Agents

Factors which Affect Intravenous Anesthesia

Following the intravenous administration of a bolus of an anesthetic agent, mixing occurs in the blood with subsequent uptake in the brain and the production of the anesthetic effect.

The anesthetic effect is determined by :

1. Blood flow to the brain and other tissues.
2. Amount of non-ionized drug. (In this form the drug most readily crosses the cellular boundaries). When the pH of the blood = pKa, 50% of the drug will be in the non-ionized form.
3. Protein binding. e.g. 70-80% of thiopental is bound to plasma albumin. The amount is pH dependent.
4. Oil/water solubility. Lipid soluble drugs cross cellular membranes.
5. Distribution to, and absorption by, other body tissues.
6. Metabolism.
7. Excretion.

Dissociative Agents (Cyclohexamines)

This group of drugs produces depression, immobilization, analgesia, and dissociative anesthesia. This dissociative state is believed to be caused by the interruption of central nervous system impulses and the differential depression and activation of various areas of the brain. Impulses are not perceived in the cortical areas of the brain. Ocular, oral, laryngeal and pharyngeal reflexes remain active. Eyes remain open, salivation increases and muscle tone is pronounced. These drugs produce muscle rigidity (catatonia) rather than muscle relaxation together with an apneustic pattern of breathing, extensor rigidity, tonic spasticity and occasional convulsions. They are good somatic, but not visceral analgesics. Hallucinations and excitement commonly occur. To avoid excitement and to improve muscle relaxation they are generally used in combination with other drugs.

1. Ketamine HCl

- Ketamine molecule exists as two optical isomers.
- Ketamine is one of the most popularly used drugs in veterinary practice due to its margin of safety and compatibility with other anesthetics.
- Chloremphenicol prolongs recovery.

- It rapidly crosses the placental barrier.
- It does not produce skeletal muscle relaxation.
- Ketamine increases blood pressure and intracranial pressure so it should not be used in head injuries or intraocular surgery.
- Eyes remain open with the pupil dilated so the eye should be protected with an ophthalmic ointment to prevent exposure keratitis.
- The pharyngeal and laryngeal reflexes remain active.
- After its administration respiration becomes apneustic in nature.
- It increases heart rate (tachycardia) and blood pressure.
- It produces convulsions in dogs. For this reason it should never be used alone but always in conjunction with drugs such as diazepam, xylazine or acepromazine.
- Ketamine and its metabolites are excreted via kidney and therefore should not be used in animals with renal impairment.
- It may cause seizures when given alone.
- Physostigmine salicylate is a ketamine antidote. Mixture of 4-aminopyridine and yohimbine can be used.
- Katamine should be used in combination with or after premeditation. *Dose* : Dog and Cat : 10-12 mg/kg IM, Horse : 2.2 mg/kg IM.

2. Phencyclidine

- This was the original cyclohexamine, but became an abused drug; therefore, it has since been withdrawn.
- It was used primarily in subhuman primates.

3. Tiletamine

- This drug is marketed combined with a benzodiazepine, zolazepam, in the product *Telazol* or *Zolatil.*
- The combination is used for induction and restraint of wildlife.
- Higher doses provide anesthesia, but there is a wide dose range and the dose chosen should reflect the condition of the patient and procedure to be performed.
- Licensed in USA, and continental Europe.
- *Dose* : Dogs; 2-13 mg/kg, Cats : 2-15 mg/kg

Other combinations of ketamine used for general anesthesia : The major goals of combining drugs with ketamine are to :

1. Eliminate unwanted "side effects" (salivation, delirium, etc.)
2. Produce good skeletal muscle relaxation.
3. Improve analgesia (visceral).
4. Prolong the period of anesthesia and immobilization.
5. Decrease the amount of ketamine needed.

Drugs Commonly Used in Combination with Ketamine

1. Acepromazine
2. Diazepam
3. Guaifenesin
4. Xylazine
5. Inhalation agents

1. Xylazine-Ketamine Drug Combinations

- Xylazine-ketamine drug mixtures are among the most popular means of producing large animal anesthesia.
- Length of anesthesia depends on species, dose and route of administration.
- There is good analgesia, muscle relaxation and sedation.
- When xylazine and ketamine are given *intravenously* there are significant changes in ventilation, myocardial O_2 demand, cardiac output and cardiac contractility.
- In small animals the *intravenous a*dministration of 1 mg/kg xylazine and 10 mg/kg ketamine simultaneously causes hypoventilation (hypoxemia), tachycardia, initial hypertension, and decreases in cardiac output and cardiac contractility and increases in total systemic vascular resistance. At these doses fatal hypoxemia and cardiac depression might occur. Similar results however, have not been obtained when xylazine and ketamine are administered separately, or when reduced doses of either or both drugs are employed.
- Fatalities can occur when halothane is administered following this combination.
- Both xylazine and ketamine increase myocardial sensitization to arrythmias and this drug combination should not be used in patients with preexisting cardiac arrhythmias, or any other cardiac problems.

Clinical Applications of Xylazine / Ketamine

Cats

- Used for fractious young, healthy cats. Given IM. Induction time, depth of anesthesia and duration of action are dose and route related.
- *Doses* : 5 - 22 mg/kg ketamine and 0.3 - 1 mg/kg xylazine.
- Higher dose combinations used for surgery, but recovery can be prolonged. Cat can become hypoxemic at high doses if supplemental O_2 is not administered. Mixture is preferably not administered IV. *High dose* xylazine together with Ketamine should be avoided due to the potential for cardiac arrhythmias.
- Ketamine and its metabolites are excreted via the kidneys and therefore should *not* be used in animals with renal impairment. Ketamine should also be *avoided* in hepatic disease.

Dogs

- A major disadvantage to the use of ketamine in dogs is the production of convulsions and for that reason it is preferable *not* to use it by the intramuscular route and it should *never be used alone,* but always in conjunction with drugs such as diazepam, xylazine or acepromazine.
- Dogs can be anesthetized with xylazine/ketamine, but this method of anesthesia is not recommended by veterinary anesthesiologists. Severe cardiopulmonary depression occurs which *may not* cause death due to the body's compensatory mechanisms, but could lead to organ damage, that may not become apparent until much later. If the combination is used, O_2 and IV fluids should be provided.

Pigs

- Ketamine is *not* a good agent to use *alone* in pigs certainly not by the intramuscular route.
- Pain on injection, hypersalivation and excitement during recovery are disadvantages.
- *Dose:* 2.0-5.0 mg/kg ketamine IV following xylazine at 1-2 mg/kg (Innovar-Vet).

Goat

- Suitable for castrations, dehorning and minor orthopedic procedures.
- At higher dose rates recovery may be prolonged.
- Goats are sensitive to xylazine.
- *Dose*: 5-10 mg/kg ketamine IM together with xylazine 0.05-0.10 mg/kg IM.

Cattle

- Ketamine can be expensive to use in adult cattle, but is used IV, in calf.
- *Calves* : Xylazine 0.1-0.2 mg/kg IM and Ketamine 5.0-10.0 mg/kg Xylazine 0.1 mg/kg IV Ketamine 2.0 mg/kg.

Horses

- Ketamine is used *only* by the intravenous route in the horse, and only after the administration of sedatives usually in conjunction with xylazine.
- The addition of diazepam (0.02 mg/kg) between xylazine and ketamine gives a smoother induction.
- This combination is expensive compared to thiopental induction, but induction and recovery is smoother.
- Occasionally a horse can become excited, this is usually due to poor sedation, noisy surroundings or inadvertent intra-carotid injection (use catheters).
- *Dose* : Xylazine 1-1.25 mg/kg IV. When horse is properly sedated (2-3 minutes) *then* ketamine (2-2.25 mg/kg IV) is administered. (Diazepam at 0.02 mg/kg IV can be given 2 minutes after Xylazine).
- Onset of action is slow taking about 50-60 seconds following administration of the ketamine. The horse sits on its haunches and then rolls quietly over to one side.
- Analgesia lasts for 10 to 15 minutes and recumbency is for 15 to 20 minutes.
- The horse gives no warning of recovery but rolls quietly into sternal recumbency and remains in that position until able to rise.
- Anesthesia may be prolonged by additional doses of 1/4 to 1/2 of the original dose of ketamine, or of both ketamine and xylazine.

2. G-X-K (SuperDrip)

- This is a very useful mixture to use for maintenance for horses if inhalation anesthesia is not available e.g. for surgery on cryptorchids.
- Horses tend to maintain a "snappier" palpebral reflex during surgical planes of anesthesia compared to inhalation anesthesia.
- Mixture

  Guaifenesin (GGE) 5.0% 50 mg/mL (w 5% dextrose) (1L)

  Xylazine (Rompum) 0.05% 0.5 mg/mL (5 mL/L)

  Ketamine 0.1% 1.0 mg/mL (10 mL/L)

  Dose : 1.1 mL/kg for induction (500 mL per 450 kg).

- Much better to induce with xylazine/ketamine separately as above, then continue with SuperDrip as maintenance.
- Maintenance
  i. Continuous infusion of 2.75 mL/kg/h (1.2L per 450 kg) Minimum cardiovascular depression.
  ii. Anesthesia can be maintained for up to 2 h or longer however, oxygenation is essential if anesthesia is prolonged beyond 20 minutes
- Ketamine, 1 g in 1L 5% Guaifenesin, may also be used for maintenance.

3. Benzodiazepine/Ketamine Mixtures

Dogs

- The two drugs may be mixed in the same syringe immediately before administration.
- Gives a period of surgical anesthesia from five to ten minutes with a recovery time of 30 minutes to 1 hour.
- Diazepam/ketamine IV can be used to induce anesthesia and allow intubation.
- Anesthesia should be maintained with an inhalational technique.
- For minor procedures e.g. for radiographs, suturing wounds, biopsies, etc., anesthesia can be maintained with 'top-ups' of a third to half the induction dose.
- Relaxation and analgesia is good. Cardiovascular depression is minimal
- Ketamine/benzodiazepine combinations produce smoother induction and recovery if used after premedication with acepromazine/opioid.
- *Dose* : 0.5-1.0 mg / kg diazepam (or midazolam) + 5.0-10.0 mg ketamine IV.

Cats

- The same doses as for dogs can be used in cats IV or IM.
- There is minimal cardiopulmonary depression and the mixture is effective for chemically restraining fractious cats.
- If the IM route is to be used, it is better to use midazolam rather than diazepam.
- *Intramuscular dose* : Midazolam 0.3 mg/kg with ketamine 10 mg/kg. The combination only provides enough anesthesia/sedation for minor procedures.

- Diazepam/ketamine IV can be used to induce anesthesia and allow intubation.
- The effects do rapidly wane so anesthesia should be maintained with an inhalational technique. For minor procedures e.g. for radiographs, suturing wounds, biopsies, etc., anesthesia can be maintained with 'top-ups' of a third to half the induction dose.
- Ketamine/benzodiazepine combinations produce smoother induction and recovery if used after premedication with acepromazine/opioid.
- Also used in ferrets, birds, rabbits.

Steroid Anesthetics

Saffan or Althesin

- It is a combination of two steroids (Alphaxalone + Alphadolone acetate) in a surfactant Cremaphor EL. The vehicle may cause massive histamine release in dogs and *contraindicated* in this species.
- It is used for inducing anesthesia in cats and maintenance for short procedures e.g. castration.
- The advantages of this drug are that it provides rapid smooth induction, good analgesia; good muscle relaxation and supplementary doses do not prolong recovery very much.
- Xylazine should not be used as a premedicant since severe respiratory depression may follow.
- Transient edema of feet, ears and muzzle, occurs in dogs and cats.
- Horse develops violent paddling and galloping movements during recovery. These could be suppressed by xylazine.
- *Dose* :
  Cat : 3-9 mg/kg IV
  Pig : 6 mg/kg IV
  Reptiles : 12-18 mg/kg IM

Imidazole Derivatives

Metomidate (1% or 5% solution)

- It is a hypnotic agent with muscle relaxant properties.
- It induces sleep without analgesia
- General anesthesia can be produced by combining it with neuroleptics or analgesics.

- Metomidate can be used for caesarean section in sows.
- It is painful on injection.

Etomidate

- Used in poor risk patients because it does not depress the cardiovascular and respiratory systems or release histamine.

Alkylphenol

Propofol

- It is a substituted phenol derivative (2, 6-diisopropyl phenol) which is a relatively new short acting intravenous anesthetic agent.
- It is slightly water soluble and is marketed as an emulsion containing vehicle "Intralipid", a parentral nutritional agent which contains 100 mg of soyabean oil, 22.5 mg of glycerol, 12 mg of egg lecithin and 10 mg of propofol / ml.
- It is marketed in sterile glass vials/ampoules and contains no preservatives. Since the vehicle is capable of supporting microbial growth and endotoxin production. Any remaining content of the opened vial / ampoule must be discarded within 6-10 hours. It should not be kept overnight for use on next day.
- Propofol causes rapid loss of consciousness in 20-40 sec following intravenous administration. Rapid onset is caused by rapid CNS uptake.
- A single bolus dose of propofol provides approximately 10 minutes of anesthesia.
- Dog and cats completely recovered within 20-30 minutes.
- Its short duration of action and rapid recovery time is due to rapid redistribution from the brain to other tissues and organs as occurs with thiopental.
- Recovery is faster after propofol administration because the drug's rate of metabolism is 10 times more rapid than that of thiopental.
- It causes CNS depression by decreasing the brain's metabolic activity and by enhancing the effects of the neurotransmitter GABA.
- It produces respiratory depression and apnea as in thiopental anesthesia.
- Cardiovascular effects are very much similar to thiopental. Hypotension is primarily caused by arterial and venous vasodilatation.
- It causes significant decrease in intraocular pressure and therefore it can be used in ophthalmic procedures.

- Myoclonic twitching, muscle tremors and muscle movement have been reported during induction and maintenance of anesthesia. This muscle reaction may be due to Intralipid. Use of preanesthetic decrease the incidence of these muscle reactions.
- Heinz body formation has been reported after repeated administration of propofol over several days.
- It is suitable for patients with renal or hepatic impairment.
- It does not causes tissue damage when accidentally injected perivascularly.
- Short surgical procedures can be performed after a single bolus injection.
- Single bolus injection is also used for induction of general anesthesia to allow intubation and the use of inhalant anesthesia.
- Pain after injection is evident which can be minimized by:
  - i. Premedication with Opioid or $alfa_2$ agonists.
  - ii. Lidocaine @ 0.5 mg/kg body weight intravenously should be given with a rubber tourniquet on the limb, 30-120 seconds before the injection of propofol.
- Apnea of short duration can occur on induction with propofol which is of longer duration than with thiopental. The incidence and duration of apnea may be decreased by giving the dose of propofol over 30-90 seconds i.e. slower than thiopental.
- It can be used for maintenance of anesthesia either by intermittent bolus or continuous infusion. The rate of infusion depends on the preanesthetic drug administered and the degree of surgical stimulation.
  - i. Continuous infusion rate- 0.22-0.44 mg/kg/min.
  - ii. Intermittent bolus technique- 0.44-2.2 mg/kg. The dose is administered when needed 'to effect'. It should be given slowly over a period of 30-60 seconds to decrease the incidence of respiratory depression and apnea.
- *Dose* : Dogs and Cat :
  - i. 6-8 mg/kg without premedication.
  - ii. 2.2-4.4 mg/kg after premedication with sedatives, tranquilizers or opioid.
  - iii. The calculated dose should be given slowly till effect and approximately one third of the dose is given every 30 seconds.

- Disadvantages :
  i. It can produce hypotension.
  ii. It is a potent respiratory depressant.

Miscellaneous Agents

Chloral hydrate :

- Liebrich (1969) introduced chloral hydrate as a hypnotic.
- It may be administered orally or solution may be injected intravenously or intraperitonially.
- It irritates the gastric mucosa and may cause vomiting.
- Chloral hydrate reduced to trichlorethyl alcohol (less potent hypnotic) which converts the glucuronic acid in to urochloralic acid (no hypnotic properly)
- Chloral hydrate depresses the cerebrum with loss of reflex excitability.
- It is a good hypnotic, but poor anesthetic.
- Anesthetic doses depress vasomotor center (resulting in fall in blood pressure) and respiratory control.
- Death from chloral hydrate is caused by progressive depression of the respiratory center.
- The margin of safety is less so it is not a satisfactory surgical anesthetic.
- 7-12% w/v an aquous solution is generally used dose -22 gram/100kg b.wt., I.V. till effects.
- The chief disadvantage is that the dose required to induce general anaesthesia is such that recovery is prolonged.

Chloral Hydrate and $MgSO_4$ (Chlormag) (Ratio1 :1, 2 :1, 3 :1)

- Advantages :
  i. It results in more rapid and quicker induction.
  ii. It increases the anesthetic depth.
  iii. It reduces the toxicity of the chloral hydrate and is less irritant.

Chloral Hydrate, $MgSO_4$ and Pentobarbital sodium (Equithesin)

- Used for induction and maintenance of anesthesia in horses.
- Composition :
  i. Chloral hydrate - 28 gram
  ii. Magnesium sulfate - 14 gram
  iii. Pentobarbitone sodium - 6.5 gram
  iv. Distill water - 1000 ml

- *Dose :* In horse – 670 ml/450 kg body weight intravenously.
- Advantages :
  - i. No excitement during induction
  - ii. Complete immobility during the anesthesia.
  - iii. A wide margin of safety
  - iv. Economic
  - v. Good muscle relaxation
  - vi. No struggling during the recovery period.

Chlorobutanol (Chloretone)

- Used for anesthesia of lab animals.
- It can be administrated orally or intravenously.

Chloralose (a and b form)

- Prepared by heating and glucose and trichloroacetaldehyde on a water bath.
- α-Chloralose is the active form.
- Dose for dogs : 0.11 gram/kg I.V.

Urethane

- Prepared by heating urea with alcohol under pressure
- Used as an anesthetic in lab animals and fish
- It is mutagenic, carcinostatic and carcinogenic.

Paraldehyde

- It has wide margin of safety because it depress only the cerebrum and not the medullary center.

Magnesium Sulfate

- Dilute aqueous solutions of $MgSO_4$ can be used to produce surgical anesthesia in small animals.
- It depresses all parts of CNS and may cause fatal respiratory arrest.

Tricaine Methane Sulfonate

- Used as an anesthetic to immobilize amphibians, fish and other cold-blooded animals by complete bathing of small subjects, by gill spraying in large fish, or by injecting in larger species.
- 1 :1000 solutions can be autoclaved without loss of narcotic properties.

Electronarcosis

- Electrical stimulation of the brain can activate either opiate or nonopiate pain control pathways or both.
- Direct current (DC), pulsating direct and Alternating current (AC) have been used to produce electro narcosis.
- AC of 700 cycles, 35-50 milliamperes and 40 volts has been employed.
- Profuse salivation occurs.
- Hyperthermia is commonly seen.
- Photomotor reflex is the best mean of determining the anesthesia.

Barbiturates

This group of drugs is still a popular choice for anesthetic agents in veterinary practice. The drugs are based on the molecule of barbituric acid. The barbiturates contain a pyrimidine nucleus resulting from the condensation of malonic acid and urea.

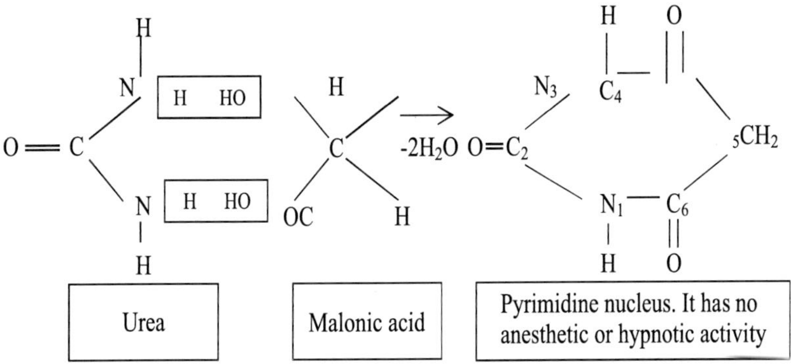

Structure activity relationship : There is relationship between the chemical structure and pharmacologic response of barbiturates. Substitutions on three key parts of the pyrimidine nucleus, four distinct subgroups of barbiturates with a wide variety of actions are formed.

1. *Oxybarbiturates* : e.g. Pentobarbital. Both hydrogen atoms at C5 must be replaced by alkyl or aryl group to form drugs with sedative and hypnotic properties. Unsaturated C-chains are more readily oxidized and hence are short acting. Short chains are more stable and hence are long acting.
2. *Methylated Oxybarbiturates* : e.g. Methohexital. Methylation of the N1 atom increases lipid solubility and shortens the duration of action. It also confers convulsive activity.

3. *Thiobarbiturates* : e.g. Thiopental and Thiamylal. Substitution of oxygen at C_2 by sulpher increases lipid solubility and shortens the duration of action.
4. *Methylated thiobarbiturates* : These are not used because of severe convulsions.

Mechanism of action : The principal effect of a barbiturate is depression of CNS by interference with passage of impulses to the cerebral cortex. Barbiturates act directly on CNS neurons in manners similar to that of the inhibitory transmitter GABA. Barbiturate anesthesia is produced by enhanced inhibition and diminished excitation.

- Over dose produces respiratory paralysis and death. Overdose is treated by ventilatory support, inotropic agents, warmth and production of diuresis with intravenous fluids to increase excretion.
- With anesthetic doses there is cardiovascular depression, both centrally and peripherally with a fall in blood pressure.
- BMR is depressed, resulting in lowered body temperature.
- Barbiturates are poor analgesics and there is no true antidote.

Classification : All anesthetic barbiturates are sodium salts. These agents can also be classified according to their length of action.

S. No.	Duration of action	Barbiturates	Action
1.	Long acting	Barbital sodium, Mephobarbital, Phenobarbital	For sedation and control convulsions
2.	Intermediate acting	Butobarbital, amobarbital	Used for clinical anesthesia
3.	Short acting	Pentobarbital, Secobarbital	
4.	Ultra short acting (Onset 20-30 second and duration of action is 10-15 min.).	Thiopental, Hexobarbital, Thiamylal	

Oxybarbiturates

Pentobarbital Sodium

- Usually available in solutions containing 50 mg/ml or 65 mg/ml. The standard solution should be diluted to half strength with sterile distilled water or physiological normal saline for administration in very small animals.

- Use is restricted to small animals and swine.
- Onset of action is slow.
- It is not irritant if injected perivascularly.
- *Dose :*

  Dogs and cats :

  - Without premedication

    20 mg/kg for light surgical anesthesia

    30 mg/kg for deep surgical anesthesia
  - With premedication, the dose is generally lowered by about ¼ to ½.

  Horses and cattle : It is not used alone in equines as recovery is slow and accompanied by excitement.

  Pigs : It may be given intravenously @ 20-30 mg/kg body weight to effect.

Thiobarbiturates

Thiopental Sodium (Pentothal)

- It is a yellow crystalline powder that is unstable in aqueous solution and when exposed to air. For this reason the powder is buffered with Na_2CO_3 and sealed.
- The powder can be dissolved in distill water or saline to make concentrations like 1.25%, 2.5, 5.0%, 10% before use. In small animals a 2.5% solution and in large animals a 5% solution of thiopental is used.
- It should be stored in a refrigerator at 5^0-6^0C to retard deterioration.
- One third of the calculated dose should be administered rapidly intravenously within 15 seconds to get over the initial excitement associated with second stage of anesthesia. Remainder is administered slowly "to effect". Surgical anesthesia is reached when the pedal reflex is abolished. Additional doses may be given to prolong anesthesia.
- Generally 4 stages are seen:

  i. Unable to raise head- Deep narcosis.

  ii. Complete relaxation of jaws and inability to move tongue, pedal reflex present - Light anesthesia.

  iii. Sluggish pedal reflex- Medium anesthesia.

  iv. Loss of pedal reflex-Deep anesthesia.

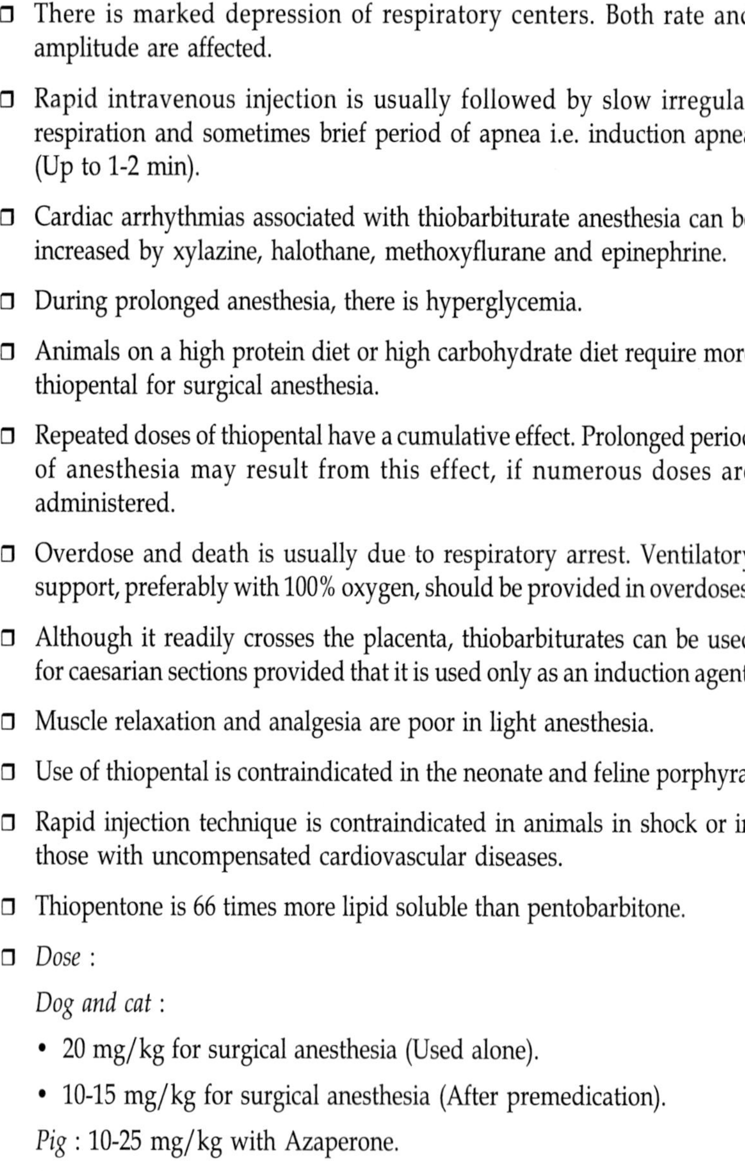

- There is marked depression of respiratory centers. Both rate and amplitude are affected.
- Rapid intravenous injection is usually followed by slow irregular respiration and sometimes brief period of apnea i.e. induction apnea (Up to 1-2 min).
- Cardiac arrhythmias associated with thiobarbiturate anesthesia can be increased by xylazine, halothane, methoxyflurane and epinephrine.
- During prolonged anesthesia, there is hyperglycemia.
- Animals on a high protein diet or high carbohydrate diet require more thiopental for surgical anesthesia.
- Repeated doses of thiopental have a cumulative effect. Prolonged period of anesthesia may result from this effect, if numerous doses are administered.
- Overdose and death is usually due to respiratory arrest. Ventilatory support, preferably with 100% oxygen, should be provided in overdoses.
- Although it readily crosses the placenta, thiobarbiturates can be used for caesarian sections provided that it is used only as an induction agent.
- Muscle relaxation and analgesia are poor in light anesthesia.
- Use of thiopental is contraindicated in the neonate and feline porphyra.
- Rapid injection technique is contraindicated in animals in shock or in those with uncompensated cardiovascular diseases.
- Thiopentone is 66 times more lipid soluble than pentobarbitone.
- *Dose* :

  Dog and cat :

  - 20 mg/kg for surgical anesthesia (Used alone).
  - 10-15 mg/kg for surgical anesthesia (After premedication).

  Pig : 10-25 mg/kg with Azaperone.

  Horse :

  - Acepromazine (0.5 mg/kg I.V.) followed by Thiopental @ 8 mg/kg I.V.
  - Xylazine (0.5 mg/kg I.V.) followed by Thiopental @ 6-7 mg/kg I.V.
  - Xylazine (1.0 mg/kg I.V.) followed by Thiopental @ 4-5 mg/kg I.V.

Thiamylal Sodium : pH 10.3 (in 2.5% Solution)

- In dogs the anesthetic potency of thiamylal is 1.5 times that of thiopental. It is less cumulative than thiopental.
- Because of its arrhythmogenic effect, thiamylal is contraindicated in any dog with impaired cardiac function.
- Because of low toxicity, it can be used in young, aged are poor risk patients.
- *Dose :*

  Dog and cat : 20-30 mg/kg for surgical anesthesia (Used alone).

  Pig : 10-18 mg/kg body weight.

Methylated Barbiturates

Methohexital

- It is not used in common practice, but good if quick recoveries are desired.
- Potency is about twice that of thiopental and duration of action is shorter than thiopental.
- More rapid recovery to full alertness even after prolonged anesthesia.
- It can be used in both large and small animals, however, the duration of effect is very short from a single induction dose.
- Use of Methohexital without premedication can have very rough recoveries with paddling, head shaking etc.
- Generally 1% solution is used in small animals. Induction is smooth followed by a period of apnea.
- Contraindicated for patients with epilepsy.
- *Dose :* Dog and cat- 5 mg/kg I.V. with premedication.

Administration of Barbiturates

- Thiopental sodium can be administered by intravenous and intraperitoneal (disadvantage of intraperitoneal route is that the dose cannot be as accurately controlled) routes.
- Under unusual circumstances animals can be anaesthetized by intramuscular, intrathoracic or subcutaneous routes. But because of high alkalinity, there is tendency for tissue necrosis.

Barbiturate Slough

- During induction of barbiturate anesthesia, some of the drug may be administered perivascularly. Because of high pH, barbiturate solution is irritant to tissue and if administered perivascularly may produce phlebitis and tissue necrosis. This should be avoided otherwise a tissue slough may develop. Slough caused by an anesthesia requires 2-4 weeks to heal.
- If it is suspected that barbiturate solution has been injected perivascularly, the area should be infiltrated with 1-2 ml of 2% procaine solution. Local anesthetics are effective for two reasons.

  i. They are vasodilators and prevent vasospasm in the area and thus aid in dilution and absorption of barbiturate.

  ii. They are broken down in alkaline medium and this reaction neutralizes the alkali (barbiturate).
- Injection of corticosteroid or $NSAID_S$ or hot pack or hydrotherapy or infiltration of the area with saline is beneficial.

Glucose Effect

- If glucose is given to animal during recovery period from thiopental anesthesia, the animal becomes reanesthetized. This effect is known as glucose effect. This effect occurs with most barbiturates and thiobarbiturates.
- The immediates of glycolysis of glucose and in the Krebs's cycle have the same effect.
- The susceptible animals are guinea pig and rabbits. Dogs are also susceptible.
- *Mechanism of action* : Glucose causes a decrease in activity of the components of the microsomal electron chain, resulting in decreased microsomal metabolism.
- Epinephrine given intravenously to dogs or mice also causes a return of sleep on awakening from hexobarbital or chloral hydrate anesthesia. This is mainly caused by increased glucose levels in the blood.

Chapter 20

INHALANT ANESTHETICS

Advantages

1. These agents are primarily exhaled through the lungs and recovery is not dependent upon redistribution within the body and detoxification mechanisms. This is helpful in poor risk patient.
2. Anesthesiologist has good control over the anesthesia.
3. Early recovery of the patient.
4. Closed system available for thoracic surgery.

Disadvantages

1. They require constant surveillance by an anesthesiologist during administration.
2. Some are explosive and inflammable
3. Some irritate body tissues.
4. Chronic exposure to operating room personnel is hazardous.

   - Cyclopropane and isoflurane are less toxic than halothane or methoxyflurane.

Methods of Administration

Inhalant anesthetics

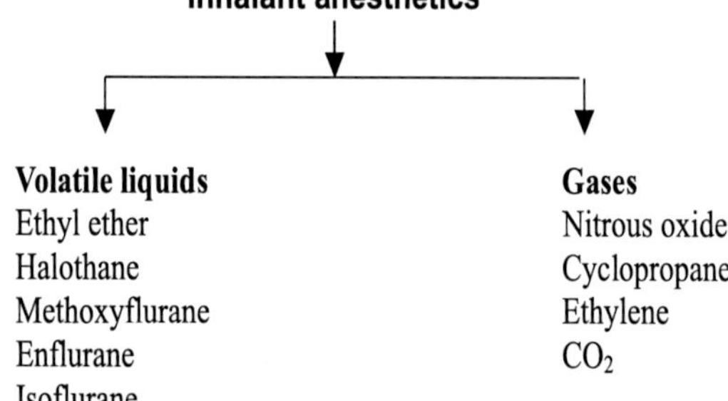

Administered by

Insufflations	Closed
Open non-rebreathing	Semi closed
Semi open	or
Semi closed	Semi open system
Closed system	

Volatile Liquid Anesthetics

Ether

- It is a colorless, highly volatile, pungent and highly inflammable agent. The vapors are 2.6 times heavier than air.
- Ether is stored in sealed metal containers coated inside with copper or another metal that combines with O_2 to prevent oxidation.
- The concentration necessary for anesthesia is 3.5–4.5% by volume in inhaled mixture. 6.7–8% causes respiratory failure.
- Ether irritates all tissues. Irritation of the airways leads to a slow induction.
- The flow of saliva and mucus increases which may interfere with respiration. Premedication with anticholinergics is desirable.
- It increases susceptibility to postoperative pneumonia.
- Ether irritates kidney tissues and reduces urine output. Albuminurea and tubular casts are common in the post anesthetic period.
- In the stage of medullary paralysis the centers are affected in the following order - respiratory, vasomotor and cardiac.
- Minimal Alveolar Concentration (MAC) -1.92%
- Extrasystoles frequently occur, particularly on induction.

- Recovery is slow because of high blood/gas (12:1) coefficient.
- Ventilation is stimulated at light level of anesthesia, but depressed at deeper levels.
- It causes hyperglycemia, vasodilatation and bronchodilatation.
- *Contra indications*
  1. Acute or chronic respiratory infections.
  2. Acidosis.
  3. Kidney or liver disease.
  4. Shock.
  5. Lack of equipment and facilities for an explosive anesthetic.
- *Advantages*
  1. Good muscle relaxation and analgesia.
  2. Wide margin of safety.
  3. It is initially a respiratory stimulant.
  4. Does not depress circulation at usual level of anesthesia.
  5. Stable, easily preserved, relatively inexpensive & can be administered with minimal equipment.
- *Disadvantages*
  1. Long induction period accompanied by excitement.
  2. Slow recovery.

Methoxyflurane

- It is a nonflammable agent with a fruity odour having high blood/gas coefficient (13).
- It has low latent heat of vaporization, but with high boiling point (104°C) the maximum available concentration from a vaporizer is 3.3%.
- Maintenance of anesthesia can be accomplished with concentration of 0.4-1.0%.
- It is highly rubber soluble. Both induction and recovery may be prolonged due to uptake and release of methoxyflurane from rubber in the anesthetic circuit.
- It reacts with metal in anesthetic circuits and is unstable in light.
- It causes a dose dependent depression of the cardiopulmonary system. The heart rate and blood pressure generally remains stable due to the release of endogenous catecholamine.

- The eye remains in a central position at surgical planes of anesthesia in cats and dogs.
- It produces good analgesia and muscle relaxation.
- It potentiates the action of curariform drugs.
- Salivation not stimulated.
- Respiratory acidosis occurs if anesthesia is maintained over long periods.
- The heart is sensitized to epinephrine (catecholamine) but to a much smaller degree than with halothane.
- It produces renally toxic fluoride ions so it should not be used with renally excreted drugs such as tetracycline and flunixin.
- *Advantages*:
    i. Non-explosive.
    ii. Good muscle relaxation.
    iii. Free from side effects and toxicity.
    iv. High margin of safety.
    v. Analgesia extending in to post-anesthetic period.
- *Disadvantages*:
    i. It crosses the placental barrier.
    ii. Slower induction recovery period.
    iii. Depression of blood pressure.
    iv. Respiratory acidosis.

Enflurane

- It is a nonflammable agent.
- Induction and recovery are rapid.
- It does not stimulate excess salivation or tracheobronchial secretion.
- Maintenance concentration should not exceed 3%.
- Muscle relaxation is generally good. But becomes poor with increasing concentrations.
- At high concentrations (> 3.5%) there is increased central stimulation and seizures like activity on the electroencephalogram. So it should be avoided in seizure prone patients.
- Enflurane slightly sensitizes the myocardium to circulating catecholamines, but does so more than isoflurane.

- The non-depolarizing relaxants are markedly potentiated.
- Enflurane is safe in pregnant animals.
- The MAC value is 2.2 in dogs.

Halothane

- It is non-explosive and non-flammable agent which is stable with soda lime.
- It decomposes in presence of light so the liquid is stabilized by addition of 0.01% (w/W) thymol and stored in amber glass bottles.
- Halothane in concentration of 2-4% produces stage III, plane 2-3 anesthesia in dogs.
- Surgical anesthesia is maintained by inhalation of 0.8-1.2% mixtures.
- Halothane is about twice as potent as chloroform and 4 times as potent as diethyl ether.
- There is dose dependent depression of the cardiopulmonary system with halothane and the blood pressure is lowered by direct myocardial depression as well as vasodilatation through depression of the vasomotor tone center of the medulla.
- It produces hypotension.
- Halothane sensitizes the myocardial conduction system to the action of epinephrine and nor-epinephrine. Arrhythmias may result.
- Halothane is safe anesthetic during severe anemia.
- Salivary, mucous and bronchial secretions are absent during halothane anesthesia.
- Concurrent use of succinylcholine is contraindicated in horses.
- MAC in dogs is 0.86%.

Isoflurane

- It is a non-flammable and non-explosive anesthetic agent.
- It is a stable compound that does not break down in contact with soda lime or in the presence of light.
- It is less potent than halothane or methoxyflurane and relatively insoluble leading to fast induction and recovery.
- The MAC for isoflurane does not change with duration of anesthesia. MAC for the dog is 1.28% and for cats is 1.63%.

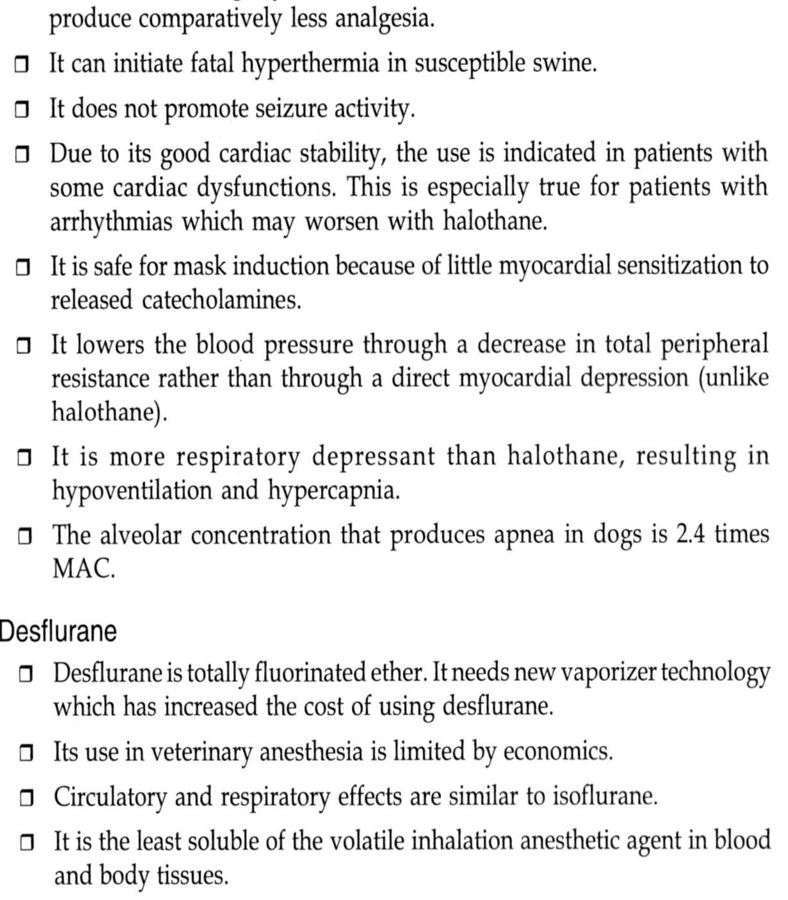

- It has fewer tendencies to sensitize the heart to catecholamine than halothane.
- It is a profound respiratory depressant in dogs and cats.
- Isoflurane has slightly better muscle relaxation than halothane and produce comparatively less analgesia.
- It can initiate fatal hyperthermia in susceptible swine.
- It does not promote seizure activity.
- Due to its good cardiac stability, the use is indicated in patients with some cardiac dysfunctions. This is especially true for patients with arrhythmias which may worsen with halothane.
- It is safe for mask induction because of little myocardial sensitization to released catecholamines.
- It lowers the blood pressure through a decrease in total peripheral resistance rather than through a direct myocardial depression (unlike halothane).
- It is more respiratory depressant than halothane, resulting in hypoventilation and hypercapnia.
- The alveolar concentration that produces apnea in dogs is 2.4 times MAC.

Desflurane

- Desflurane is totally fluorinated ether. It needs new vaporizer technology which has increased the cost of using desflurane.
- Its use in veterinary anesthesia is limited by economics.
- Circulatory and respiratory effects are similar to isoflurane.
- It is the least soluble of the volatile inhalation anesthetic agent in blood and body tissues.
- MAC in dogs is 7.2%.

Sevoflurane

- Sevoflurane is still undergoing toxicity tests regarding breakdown products produced on contact with soda lime.
- It is halogenated ether that is non flammable and non explosive at commonly used concentration.
- It should be used only in precision, agent specific, out of circuit vaporizers.

- CNS and cardiovascular effects are similar to isoflurane and desflurane.
  i. Dose dependent decrease in cardiac output and blood pressure.
  ii. It does not sensitize the myocardium to catecholamines.
  iii. Dose dependent CNS depression.
- MAC in dogs is 2.36 % and in cats is 2.58%.

Chloroform

- Because of cardiovascular, hepatic and renal toxicity, it is not longer used in clinical anesthesia.
- 1% alcohol is added to chloroform to prevent production of phosgene gas.

Trichloroethylene

- It is a sweet smelling anesthetic agent similar to chloroform.
- It is less potent and toxic than chloroform but there is still high myocardial sensitization.
- It is broken down to trichloroetanol in the body and it is this metabolic product that expresses the anesthetic effect.
- Muscle relaxation is poor but produces good analgesia.
- It is administered in concentration of 0.6%.
- It produces toxic gases with soda lime. So it should never be used with soda lime.
- Disadvantages
  i. Cardiotoxicity
  ii. Poor muscle relaxation and
  iii. Sensitization to epinephrine.

Nitrous oxide (N_2O)

- It is non-flammable, non-explosive and non-irritating inert gas. The gas is quickly absorbed and eliminated from the body.
- It is stored as a liquid under pressure at 750 Psi in blue cylinders.
- It is administered with a semi closed or closed system with O_2.
- It can not be given as the sole anesthetic agent.
- The analgesia produced is mediated through the opiate receptor system.
- It has minimal cardiopulmonary effects.

- It has no muscle relaxant property.
- The liquid continuously vaporizes to form the gas at a constant pressure.
- It is exhaled unaltered from the lungs.
- It is teratogenic in rats.
- N_2O must be given in at least 80% concentration to produce anesthesia. It has a much higher MAC in animals i. e. 188% for dogs and 255% in cats.
- Common cause of death from N_2O is failure to add sufficient O_2 to the anesthetic mixture.
- *Diffusion hypoxia / anoxia* – Diffusion hypoxia / anoxia is possible with low solubility agents which are administered in high concentration e.g. N_2O. Diffusion of nitrous oxide into the alveoli during recovery from prolonged N_2O administration may induce hypoxia by dilution of the alveolar O_2 concentration. This phenomenon is termed as diffusion anoxia. If the patient is breathing room air, hypoxia may result. To avoid this, the patient is given 100 % oxygen for a few minutes after the nitrous oxide has turned off.
- *Second gas effect* – This effect occurs when a relatively insoluble gas is present in high concentration with a gas of greater solubility e.g. N_2O and halothane in O_2. The relatively insoluble gas (because the partial pressure is greater) crosses into the blood stream quickly, thus, decreases the volume of the alveoli and therefore concentrates the remaining gases. This raises their partial pressures and therefore enhances their uptake into the blood stream. Clinically, this effect can be used to speed the induction of a patient with an inhalation agent.
- *Denitrogenization* – It is important to understand this concept particularly if nitrous oxide is to be used since N_2O is used in high concentrations. The patient's body is normally in equilibrium with the gas it is breathing. Therefore, a patient who has been just connected to a breathing circuit containing 100% O_2 will continuously release the nitrogen in its body, until the body is in a new equilibrium with 100% O_2. It is important to displace nitrogen from the lungs to obtain a sufficiently high alveolar concentration of the induction agent, and to prevent hypoxic inspired gas mixtures. Non-rebreathing anesthetic circuits already have high fresh gas flows, and there is no rebreathing of exhaled gases (and nitrogen) so denitrogenization takes place rapidly. In rebreathing systems the process can be hastened by using high fresh gas flows and opening the exhaust valve. In these circuits a hypoxic mixture is more likely if low fresh gas

flows are used initially, especially if using nitrous oxide, and N_2 is not 'flushed' from the circuit. The gas in the rebreathing bag of the anesthetic circuit can be periodically `dumped' to atmosphere and filled with fresh gas from the anesthetic machine. This increases the rate of denitrogenization. High fresh gas flows are usually run for 15 minutes in rebreathing circuits to flush N_2. Using higher fresh gas flows during the early part of anesthesia also maintains the concentration of the anesthetic agent in the circuit with an out-of-circle vaporizer and speeds induction.

Cyclopropane

- It is a potent drug since it is a relatively insoluble gives rapid induction and recovery.
- It is highly explosive and has now been withdrawn.
- Clinically there is a dose dependent ventillatory depression and capillary oozing is seen due to resulting hypercapnia. If it is used, it is advisable to ventilate the patient to prevent hypercapnia.
- Cyclopropane can cause cardiac arrhythmias especially in presence of hypercapnia.

Ethylene: Ethylene is flammable and explosive.

Carbon dioxide : CO_2 used as an anesthetic gas for laboratory animals.

Cylinder color : Cylinder color of each gas to enable quick recognition of cylinder content is recommended by Bureau of standard.

Kind of gas	Cylinder color
Oxygen	Green
CO_2	Gray
N_2O	Light blue
Cyclopropane	Orange
Helium	Brown
Ethylien	Red
CO_2 +O_2	Gray and green

Minimum Alveolar Concentration (MAC)

- The minimum concentration of the inhalation agent in the alveoli to keep 50% of a population from responding with a gross purposeful movement to a painful stimulus.

- It is a measure of anesthetic potency. Higher the MAC, the less potent is the anesthetic and vice versa.
- Anesthetic doses can be expressed in multiples of MAC.
- This value gives an indication of the concentration to set on the vaporizer. It is still essential to monitor the patient for anesthetic depth because of individual variation in response to drugs.
- Surgical anesthesia is usually obtained by delivering 1.5 to 2.0 times MAC to the patient but this can vary according to the condition of the patient and concurrent medication.
- Factors affecting MAC:
  - i. Intraspecies and interspecies variation.
  - ii. Circadian rhythms- MAC will vary in the same animal when measured at different times. MAC will increase during the period of greatest metabolic activity.
  - iii. Hypocarbia and hypercarbia- Hypocarbia after MAC vary slightly, whereas hypercarbia above 95 mm Hg is depressant and therefore will lower the MAC.
  - iv. Metabolic acidosis- Changes in arterial pH have little or no effect on MAC.
  - v. Concurrent use of opioids and other analgesics and sedatives will lower the MAC value.

MAC of various inhalation agents

S.No.	Agent	Dog	Cat	Horse
1.	Halothane	0.86	0.98	0.88
2.	Enflurane	2.2	2.37	2.12
3.	Isoflurane	1.28	1.63	1.31
4.	Methoxyflurane	0.23	0.23	NA
5.	Nitrous oxide	188.0	255.0	NA
6.	Desflurane	7.2	NA	NA

Anesthetic Index

- The alveolar concentration required to produce at least 60 seconds of apnea divided by MAC.

Chapter 21

Anesthetic Emergencies and Their Management

A sound understanding of general anesthetic emergencies and surgical techniques is vital for all practicing veterinarians. In most of the veterinary practices, after induction of anesthesia, no one is assigned the task of anesthetist to monitor anesthesia and occurrence of complications during surgery which may lead to the development of anesthetic emergencies. Onset of general anesthesia disturbs the physiological equilibrium of patient and increase the threshold of harmful events. The harmful events of anesthesia includes:

- Decrease in cardiac output and blood pressure.
- Decrease in alveolar ventilation.
- Alteration in peripheral perfusion.
- Alteration in temperature regulation mechanism.
- Increase in intracranial pressure etc.

The main anesthetic emergencies are:

- Respiratory insufficiency and arrest.
- Cardiovascular insufficiency and arrest
- Regurgitation and vomition.
- Anesthetic overdose
- Temperature regulation.

Untreated respiratory failure leads to circulatory failure. Irreversible brain damage occurs 4-6 minutes after respiratory arrest and 2-4 minutes after circulatory arrest.

The combined detrimental consequences of surgery and anesthesia leads to anesthetic emergencies and accidents. Most anesthetic emergencies and complications are related to:

Human Error

- Most of the human errors are because of not familiar with the equipment and anesthetic drug and its action.
- Miscalculation of anesthetic drug dose.
- Misidentification of drugs and accidental use of wrong medication.
- Administration of anesthetic by an incorrect route e.g. extravascular administration of barbiturates causes barbiturate slough.
- Impaction of epiglottis in larynx during intubation can cause serious obstruction.
- Faulty intubation leading in to one bronchus can also be serious consequence, since the other drug will act as arterio-venous shunt leading to cyanosis, inspite of 100% oxygen supply.

Equipment Problems

- Failure of oxygen delivery to patient due to respiratory obstruction.
- Use of defective anesthetic machine.
- Empty gas cylinders.
- Misconnected breathing system.
- Kinked or plugged endotracheal tube.
- Improper inflation of cuff of endotracheal tube.

Respiratory Insufficiency and Arrest

Causes

1. Drug Depression

- Depression of central nervous system is most serious cause of apnea due to drug overdose or deep plane of anesthesia.
- Apnea is common during induction of anesthesia with thiobarbiturates or propofol which is caused by relative overdose or a fast bolus injection.

2. *Airway Obstruction*

- Airway obstruction may be due to human error or equipment problem.
- Brachycephalic breeds are more prone to airway obstruction because of relaxing effect of sedative preanesthetics or anesthetics.
- If the obstruction of nasal passage (nasal tumor) obstruct the airway, the oral pathway must be kept open.
- Kinked or plugged endotracheal tube may cause airway obstruction.
- Forcibly intubation can lead to laryngeal edema thus further increase in chances of respiratory obstruction.

3. *Low Level of Inspired Oxygen*

- Apnea and airway obstructions leading to hypoxia commonly encountered during induction of anesthesia.

4. *Laryngeal or Bronchial Spasm*

- Laryngospasm can occur in all animals but is common in cat after administration of thiobarbiturates.
- Laryngospasm also occur in ether anesthesia due to more salivation and irritation of mucosa.
- Administration of muscle relaxants drug like suxamethonium @ 3mg/kg intravenous or 2% lidocaine should be applied to arytenoids cartilage prior to endotracheal intubation.

5. *Aspiration of Material from Stomach and Esophagus*

- Aspiration occurs if anesthesia is induced in recently fed animals leading to regurgitation and development of respiratory obstruction and bronchoalveolar pneumonia.
- During anesthesia gastric or esophageal contents are forced in to the pharynx.
- Dogs with megaesophagus are susceptible to regurgitation.
- Aspiration can be prevented by keeping the animal off fed prior to induction of anesthesia, positioning the animal with the head lower than the esophagus and protect the airway with an endotracheal tube.

6. *Faulty positioning of the animals.*
7. *Mechanical interference with the movement of thoracic wall or diaphragm.*
8. *Disease of respiratory and /or cardiovascular system.*

Recognition of Respiratory Insufficiency and Arrest

- Both tidal volume and rate of respiration decreases.
- In deep anesthesia, the intercostals muscles become paralyzed and the thoracic wall moves inward rather than outward during inspiration which is known as paradoxical respiration and a sign of anesthetic over dosage.
- Cyanosis, a sign of inadequate oxygenation is present.
- Increased heart rate, cardiac output and blood pressure due to sympathetic stimulation.

Treatment of Respiratory Insufficiency and Arrest

- Inhalant anesthetic if being given should be removed from the circuit and administer high level of O_2.
- If the respiratory depression is due to injectable anesthetics, it can be treated by specific antagonists. e.g. If partial or complete respiratory failure occurs due to narcotic agents, nalorphine or levellorphan should be given intravenously to effect.
- Controlled ventilation/ artificial respiration should be provided. Artificial respiration with compression of chest can be given in the absence of any equipment. AMBU bag (assisted manual breathing unit) can be used for this purpose.
- Airway patency and circulatory adequacy should be checked.
- If reflex respiratory failure occurs due to endotracheal intubations, the tube should be removed and larynx should be totally desensitized with topical anesthetic.
- Voluntary breath holding can occur in cases of light anesthesia. So anesthetic depth should be checked clinically by monitoring other reflexes like lateral and medial palpebral reflexes, position of the eyeball, corneal reflex, heart rate and presence or absence of pulse. If the animal is found to be in light plane of anesthesia, it should be brought in to correct plane of anesthesia
- Bronchial spasm may require treatment with aminophylline or thiophylline @ 1-2 mg /kg body weight in dogs.
- Treatment of drug over dosage is best treated by maintaining artificial ventilation. In case of volatile agents, they can be removed by ventilation.

- Analeptics increase O_2 requirements of the brain if used repeatedly may exhaust nerve cells. Over dosage may lead to convulsions and severe hypotension. It is therefore, desirable to oxygenate the animal properly prior to and following analeptic administration. e.g.

  Doxapram @ 2 mg/kg body wt, IV or IM,

  Leptazole @ 2-4 mg/kg body wt

  Nikethamide @ 0.5-2.0 mg/kg body wt
- If the cause of respiratory obstruction is not known emergency tracheostomy can be performed. A 14 Gauze needle can be put subcutaneously in to trachea in cat. 10 Gauze catheter can be used in dogs.

Cardiovascular Insufficiency and Arrest

Cardiovascular insufficiency is the failure of circulatory system to provide adequate tissue oxygenation, nutrient supply and waste removal. This may be due to reduced cardiac output. Cardiac insufficiency or arrest leads to sudden failure of O_2 supply to vital organs.

Causes

- *Over dosages of anesthetics:* Deep halothane anesthesia causes vasodilatation of vascular bed.
- *Severe hypotension:* Vascular smooth muscles are relaxed by inhalation anesthetics leading to hypotension.
- *Hemorrhage/ Hypovolaemia:* Incidence of life threatening hemorrhage during surgical procedures is low.
- *Cardiac dysrhythmias:* Cardiac dysrhythmias may occur as a result of administration of premedications, induction of anesthesia and maintenance agent and surgical stimulation.
- *Cardiac arrest:* It is really a true emergency condition, which should be treated immediately within 2-3 minutes. The brain is the most susceptible organ to hypoxia-ischemia. Severe injury develops after 4-5 minutes of cardiac arrest. The signs of cardiac arrest are:

  i. No palpable heart beat/ no auscultable heart sounds.

  ii. No palpable pulse and apnea.

  iii. Lack of surgical hemorrhage

  iv. Cyanosis of the mucous membrane.

  v. Dilated pupils.

  vi. No muscle tone and unconsciousness.

- Peripheral vasoconstriction (traumatic shock) or vasodilatation (septic shock).
- Deleterious reflex response like endotracheal intubations or mechanical manipulation of meninges, eye, diaphragm, or mesentry.
- Obstruction of venous return, intermittent positive pressure ventilation, excess intra-abdominal pressure.
- Hypoxia, hypercapnia.
- Severe electrolyte imbalance.

Recognition of Cardiac Insufficiency

- *By clinical signs* - like sudden change in respiratory pattern, cyanosis of mucous membrane or surgical site, reduced bleeding at the surgical site, increased CRT, complete loss of peripheral arterial pulse, decrease in intensity of heart sounds, progressive and persistent tachycardia or bradycardia and pulse.
- *ECG* - ventricular premature contraction, atrial flutter, atrial fibrillation, atrioventricular block and ventricular tachycardia.
- Auscultation of heart.

Treatment : When any or all of these signs are present, The traditional ABCD protocol for treatment of cardiac arrest must be started immediately

- *Airway:*
  1. Always confirm a patient airway for an animal previously intubated for general anesthesia. Endotracheal intubation is the best method of insuring a patent airway.
  2. The head must be extended.
  3. Examine for possible obstruction of the airway with food materials or kinked endotracheal tube. In emergency, tracheostomy can be done to maintain patent airway.
  4. In case of bronchospasm treat the animal with bronchodilators like aminophylline.
- *Breathing:*
  1. Supply high concentration of oxygen to the alveoli and to eliminate carbon dioxide.
  2. Artificial respiration using rebreathing bag or mechanical ventilators @ 12-20 breaths/ minutes or use AMBU type resuscitation bag or mouth to endotracheal procedures to maintain breathing. Analeptic agents like doxapram can be administered.
  3. External thoracic massage results in some alveolar gas exchange.

- *Circulation/ cardiac massage:*
  i. Cardiac massage can be done either external (thoracic) or internal.
  ii. External cardiac massage by chest compression @ 90-120/minute.
  iii. Open cardiac massage is done @ 60-100/minute.
  iv. Defibrillation is done by using external or internal paddles of cardiac defibrillators.
  v. *Treatment of cardiac arrest*
     - Cardiopulmonary resuscitation (CPR) with external cardiac massage is ineffective in protecting the brain from injury and should only be the part of the initial resuscitation. CPR performed for more than 3-4 minutes often results in significant neurologic injury.
     - At 50 mm Hg systolic blood pressure, thoracic heart beat and peripheral pulse can not be palpated. A non palpable weak heart beat along with regular electric rhythm is known as electric mechanical dissociation (EMD).
     - Cardiac massage and it should be accompanied by simultaneous artificial ventilation. Adequate cardio-pulmonary resuscitation results in constriction of pupil and detection of pulse in major artery.
  vi. Cardiac dysrhythmias can be treated by
     - Increasing the depth of anesthesia.
     - Intravenous administration of acepromazine (0.01 mg/kg) or lidocaine (0.5 mg/kg)
- *Definitive treatment*
  i. Remove the cause e.g. overdoses of inhalant anesthetics can be prevented by maintaining the vaporizer setting near the MAC of the anesthetic being used.
  ii. Epinephrine @ 0.05-0.1 mg/kg IV should be given immediately because access to the central vein may be difficult. It may be administered in to peripheral vein, Intrabronchial (0.05-0.1 mg/kg diluted in 2-3 ml volume with normal saline) or directly in to the ventricle (0.025-0.05 mg/kg).
  iii. Lidocaine should be given as a bolus injection @ 0.5 mg/kg IV.
  iv. Atropine @ 0.02-0.04 mg/kg IV will protect against bradycardia.
  v. Sodium bicarbonate should be administered as per requirement mEq of HCO_3 = 0.3 X Base deficit (mEq/L) X Body weight

vi. Calcium gluconate 10% solution @ 0.5 mg/kg IV.

vii. Doxapram @ 0.55 mg/kg IV

viii. Dobutamine @ 2.5-20 mg/kg/min in small animals. @ 1-5 mg/kg/min in large animals.

ix. Corticosteroids are indicated in shock and malignant hyperthermia.

x. Infusion of blood or plasma expander or balanced electrolyte solution low in potassium. Normally it is recommended to give crystalloid fluids 3 times the volume of blood lost. Colloids are recommended when blood loss is severe enough to produce hypovolemic shock but should be given carefully as they interfere with blood clotting.

xi. Some anesthetics sensitize the heart muscles to catecholamine release. So if anesthesia is induced in a frightened animal, it can lead to severe dysrrhythmias e.g. halothane. These dysrrhythmias can be successfully managed by epinephrine, lidocaine and dopamine respectively.

Regurgitation and Vomition

Regurgitation - it is the passive discharge of stomach contents.

Vomition – It is the active discharge of stomach contents.

Regurgitation into pharynx occurs during anesthesia due to relaxation of cardiac in dorso-ventral recumbency in small animals and due to pressure of rumen and relaxation of cardia in large animals. Following steps should be taken into consideration to minimize the hazards of regurgitation.

i. Endotracheal intubations should be done. It should be done under topical anesthesia to suppress laryngeal and tracheal reflexes. Cuff should be inflated, if laryngospasm is suspected.

ii. Sternal recumbency with head down is preferred.

iii. As soon as retching movements occur after vomiting in small animals, the operating table should be tilted so that the patient is positioned with its head down and 100% O_2 should be given.

iv. Pharynx should be cleared off from vomitus manually or through suction. O_2 administration should be continued.

v. If gastric juice goes into trachea, following drug therapy is indicated to support the patient and to prevent infection and inflammation of respiratory tract.

   a. Corticosteroids should be given intratracheally or intravenously followed by IM injection for 3 days.

b. Broad spectrum antibiotics should be administered for 5 days or more.
c. O_2 administration
d. Use of Bronchodilator
e. Use of expectorant.

Anesthetic Overdose

- Inhalation anesthetic can be removed from the body by controlled ventilation.
- Barbiturates over dosages cause respiratory depression and respiratory acidosis. Following measures should be taken to manage patients with barbiturates over dosage.
  i. Hyperventilation to reduce CO_2 tension.
  ii. $NaHCO_3$ is given IV to increase pH and for ionization of barbiturates (α-adrenergic blockade).
  iii. Phenothiazine tranquilizers are given to maintain tissue perfusion and prevent anaerobic metabolism with lactic acid formation.
  iv. Normal saline with diuretics should be given intravenously.
  v. Hypostatic congestion of lungs is prevented by frequent turning of animal.
  vi. Peritoneal dialysis may be done to remove barbiturate form the system.

Temperature Regulation

- Intraoperative hypothermia is common after general anesthesia. Regulation of body temperature abolished during anesthesia. Hypothermia results if heat production is less than heat loss. Heat loss occurs generally through convection and radiation from the skin and surgical incision.
- Operation theatre temperature should be at least 100^0F and animal should be kept warm during anesthesia by lamps, warming pads etc.
- Intravenous fluid being administered should be warmed to body temperature.
- Because dogs and cats use panting as a method of reducing body temperature. The use of a circle anesthesia system, which traps expirated heat, can contribute to *hyperthermia*. Removal of carbon dioxide by soda lime produces heat as a byproduct in circle system of anesthesia. This hyperthermia is temporary and subsided after recovery from anesthesia.

- *Malignant hyperthermia:* It is a syndrome which includes muscle rigidity, tachycardia and fever. It is common in pigs but may affect other animals like dog, cat and horses. Susceptible patients should be anesthetized with nitrous oxide, barbiturates, opiates, tranquilizers and non depolarizing muscle relaxants. The potent inhalation anesthetics and the depolarizing muscle relaxants should be avoided.

Injuries During Anesthesia

1. For surgery, the animal is restrained in supine position with the leg tied to the surgery table. If the ties are too tight enough to inhibit venous drainage of distal legs, the feet become edematous.
2. *Corneal dehydration* : Most anesthetics reduce tear formation and eliminate the palpebral and corneal reflexes. Making artificial tears is an important component of anesthesia protocol.
3. *Careless endotracheal intubation* : The tube should be chosen by comparing the length of the tube with the distance from the muzzle to the thoracic inlet when the head and neck are in the natural position (*Not overextended or flexed*).
4. *Inflation of the endotracheal tube cuff* : Overinflation of the cuff causes injury to the tracheal epithelium.
5. *Anesthetic machine* : High atmospheric pressure induces injury or volotrauma, is always a possibility when semiclosed or high oxygen flow anesthesia system is used. When the oxygen flow rate is greater than 4-6 ml/kg, the pop off valve must always be open unless assisted or controlled ventilation is applied.

Chapter 22

Endotracheal Intubation*

- Endotracheal intubation is the placement of a tube in the trachea to provide a patent airway.
- It is a valuable technique that enables to attach an animal to a breathing circuit or, just as importantly, to secure an airway during an emergency such as respiratory or cardiac arrest.
- It is important that time be taken to learn the anatomy of the laryngeal area and the skill of intubation so that intubation may be performed quickly and with little chance of misplacement.

Indications and Advantages

- Maintenance of a patent airway - preventing obstruction, aspiration, and laryngospasm.
- Prevents aspiration pneumonia if an inflated cuff is used.
- Allows controlled ventilation (minimizing atelectasis, permitting intra-thoracic surgery).
- Correct size tube minimizes dead space.
- Economy of gases with inhalation anesthesia.

* Dr. Adarsh Kumar

Possible Unfavourable Complications

- Laryngitis, tracheitis (trauma).
- Laryngeal edema (trauma).
- Increased resistance to ventilation (too narrow a tube).
- Obstruction of tube (bending of tube, occlusion by biting).
- Intubation of esophagus.
- Bronchial intubation.
- Dislodgment of tube (improperly fastened).
- Laryngospasm, particularly likely to occur in lightly anesthetized cat-remove tube while anesthesia still moderately deep. Other species remove tube after swallowing reflex returns.
- Over-inflation of cuff leading to damage to the tracheal mucosa.
- Lack of sterility.
- Contamination with disinfectants leading to a chemical tracheitis.

Endotracheal Tubes

There are many endotracheal tube types, and they basically consist of a tube, generally curved except for large animal tubes, with a beveled end and an adapter for attachment to the anesthetic circuit (given below).

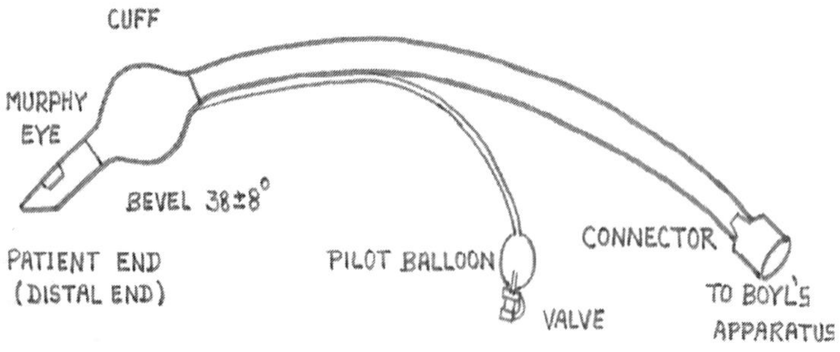

Endotreched tube

1. Diameter

- Tube diameter is used to indicate size.
- The modern standard diameter gives the internal diameter (ID) in millimeters.

- Other methods include a French unit (external diameter in millimeters multiplied by 3) which approximates the external tube circumference.
- The ID method does not give any indication of external diameter which varies with the tube type.
- The larger the internal diameter the lower the resistance to breathing.
- This is critical in very small sizes used in cats, puppies and rodents.
- One should use the largest tube that can be placed through the larynx without force.

2. Length

- Avoid the use of excessively long tubes, especially in very small animals, as they will increase resistance and may increase apparatus dead space if the tube is allowed to protrude out of the mouth.
- Tubes for human use have external length markings to assist placement.
- A tube which is too long may accidentally enter one bronchus, allowing ventilation of only one lung.

3. Curvature

- Based on use in man, the tubes have 14 cm radius of curvature for oral insertion with a 20 cm curvature in nasal tubes.
- Some larger small animal tubes (size 11 or greater) or large animal tubes made for veterinary use have no curve.

4. Bevel Angle

- Most tubes are beveled to facilitate slipping the tube between the vocal folds.
- Some armoured tubes do not have any bevel.

5. Murphy Eye

- A hole through the tube wall near the bevel end on the opposite side to the bevel.
- The purpose of the eye is to allow passage of gas if the bevel is tight against the tracheal wall or otherwise occluded.

6. Construction Material

- This covers a wide gamut from metal, synthetic and natural rubber, polyethylene, polyvinyl chloride, silicone, and the other plastics.

- The material is tested for inertness and safety – indicated by markings on tube wall "IT" (implant tested) or "Z-79" (Committee Z-79 of the USA Standards Institute).

7. Wall Reinforcement

- Some tubes have their walls reinforced with coiled wire or heavy nylon thread to prevent collapse or kinking.
- These often have no bevel and may be quite flexible, mandating the use of a stylet for placement.

8. Cuff

- Tubes may be cuffed or uncuffed.
- The cuff is inflated with air to create a seal against the underlying tracheal mucosa. This seal facilitates positive pressure ventilation and prevents pulmonary aspiration.
- Cuffs are classified as high pressure, low residual volume or low pressure, high residual volume.
- Low volume cuffs must be inflated to high intraluminal cuff pressures (180-250 mm Hg) before they expand enough to create a seal. This high cuff pressure is partially transmitted to the underlying tracheal mucosa. Ischemia may occur wherever the pressure on the tracheal mucosa exceeds capillary arteriolar pressure (about 32 mm Hg).
- High volume, low pressure cuffs inflate symmetrically adapting to the contour of the tracheal wall with low intraluminal cuff pressure (15-30 mm Hg). These cuffs decrease but do not prevent tracheal injury at the cuff site.

9. Adapters

- Connect the tube (patient) to the breathing circuit. 15 mm outer diameter at the machine end.
- These should be tightly attached to the endotracheal tube, and secured to the jaw by a length of gauze bandage.

10. Special Designs

- There are many of these but some that veterinarians are more likely to encounter are:

a. *Cole Tubes* : These tubes are uncuffed and the distal end is tapered. The smaller portion is inserted into the trachea and the larger portion wedged against the arytenoid cartilages to form a seal.

b. *Endobronchial Tubes* : Designed to allow differential ventilation of the lungs by intubating each bronchus.

Care of Tubes

- Mechanical cleaning both internally and externally to remove mucus and saliva.
- Sterilization (autoclave, chemical, or ethylene oxide).
- Storage (packaged, labeled, and dust-free).
- Sterilization and storage are not commonly carried out in veterinary practices. Beware of chemical contamination of rubber tubes.

Laryngoscopes

- The laryngoscope is useful in providing a direct light source to visualize the laryngeal structures.
- Many veterinarians do not use laryngoscopes, but those that do are able to intubate animals with fewer traumas, greater ease, and more assurance of correct placement.
- The laryngoscope consists of a battery powered handle and a blade or spatula with a light source attached.
- There is a wide variety of blade types, usually designed for use with human patients. There are two principle designs:
  1. Curved blade (Macintosh): It is used to exert pressure on the base of the tongue in front of the larynx. It does not touch the epiglottis, but if used correctly will displace the epiglottis ventrally to allow visualization of the arytenoid cartilages, vocal folds, and rima glottides.
  2. Straight blade (Miller): Most blades have a side flange on the back part of the blade that serves as a tongue deflector for use in the human patient in dorsal recumbency. Since dogs and cats are commonly intubated in sternal recumbency, the flanges tend to be in the way and some people will purchase blades (such as a Michael's blade) which have no flange.
- Care of laryngoscopes consists of cleaning the blades, keeping charged batteries and having a spare light bulb available.

- Special flexible guides are available to increase endotracheal rigidity to facilitate intubation. When used they introduce an additional risk of trauma and may be difficult to withdraw. They should not protrude beyond the patient end of the endotracheal tube.

Anatomy

- Knowledge of the anatomy of the structures surrounding the laryngeal opening will make intubation much easier. The following structures should be visualized.
  1. Soft Palate
  2. Epiglottis
  3. Glottis
  4. Vocals folds
  5. Rima glottides
  6. Lateral ventricles
  7. Cuneiform and corniculate processes of the arytenoid cartilages
- Note the position of the larynx and cranial trachea in relation to the esophagus. The larynx is ventral to the esophagus, thus extending the head and neck will facilitate intubation.
- The cuneiform and corniculate processes project out cranially on both sides of the laryngeal opening and the endotracheal tube will often "hang up" on these structures.
- Note the position of the soft palate in relation to the epiglottis in the resting animal. The most caudal end of the soft palate usually lies ventral to the tip of the epiglottis and must be displace dorsally during intubation.
- The vocal folds are pulled laterally during inspiration, making intubation easier at this time, particularly in cats and horses. Horses which are "roarers" may be more difficult to intubate and require a smaller size tube than would normally be required.

Preoperative Evaluation : Prior to anesthetizing an animal, the preoperative exam should include an assessment of the animal's mouth and airway.

- Can the mouth be opened wide enough to allow intubation? Certain conditions such as tumours or diseases of the temporomandibular joint or myositis may prevent the animal or you from opening its mouth. These conditions may be so severe that even under anesthesia the mouth cannot be opened wide enough to permit intubation, and an alternative must be found (e.g. nasotracheal intubation or a tracheotomy).

- Are there any fractures of the head or neck region of which you need to be careful during intubation?
- Is the animal's airway normal e.g. hypoplastic trachea, elongated soft palate, roarers, oral or laryngeal tumours, etc.?
- Is the animal likely to vomit or regurgitate during intubation? Animals with a megaesophagus should have the esophagus suctioned out prior to intubation.

Method of Intubation

1. Patient

- State of mouth and ability to open.
- Patent nares.
- Palpate trachea.

2. Select Tube

- Size.
- Type.
- Test cuff.
- Measure length against outside of patient.

3. Other Equipment Ready

- Laryngoscope
- Lubricant (sterile).
- Mouth gag. The necessity of a mouth gag and the style of gag will depend on the species and the individual animal.
- Gauze bandage to tie in the endotracheal tube.
- Air syringe to inflate the cuff.
- Emergency equipment (suction, relaxant).
- Stylet

4. Prepare Patient

- Wash mouth in horses.
- Preoxygenate if necessary.

5. Intubate

- Inflate cuff.
- Secure tube.
- Observe reservoir bag and or check lung sounds.
- Do not use external thoracic compression as a routine check for tube placement.

6. Maintenance

- Check position and patency.
- Check cuff "pressure" periodically.

7. Extubation

- Suction pharynx if necessary.
- Cuff deflated - only partially if foreign material in pharynx.
- Remove tube.
- KY Jelly or lidocaine ointment is used to lubricate the tube but it should not be allowed to dry out on the tube.
- Secure the tube so it does not move during anesthesia as this increases trauma. Usually the tube is secured to the maxilla in dogs and the mandible in horses. In cats, the gauze is tied around the head behind the ears.
- Be careful to avoid contaminating the endotracheal tube (e.g. don't put it on the table beside the animal).
- Inflate the cuff after closing the pop-off valve and while squeezing the reservoir bag. Fill the cuff just to the point that air ceases to escape as evidenced by cessation of sound at the mouth. Do not forget to reopen the pop-off. The cuff volume/pressure will increase as the gases warm up and nitrous oxide diffuses into the air filled cuff. Readjust cuff inflation after 15-30 minutes. Pilot balloon inflation may be a guide when over inflation occurs.

Causes for Failure at Intubation Include

- Insufficient depth of anesthesia
- Inexperience
- Trauma, neoplasia, or inflammation of the laryngopharyngeal region
- Inability to open the mouth or extend the head.

- Inappropriate choice of tube size. It is essential that, in the face of failure, one neither forces the tube nor traumatizes the oral cavity. Instead, consider nasotracheal intubation, tracheostomy or wake up the patient or choose a method for the conduct of anesthesia.

Intubation for Individual Species

Canine

Dogs are the easiest species to intubate. After induction of anesthesia, the patient is positioned in either sternal or lateral recumbency. The head is extended and the mouth opened and the tongue brought forward. The laryngoscope is used to obtain a good view of the vocal folds and the laryngeal opening. The laryngoscope or the tip of the endotracheal tube can be used to dislodge the epiglottis from the soft palate. The bevel of the E/T tube is then gently slipped between the vocal folds. Occasionally the tube will "catch" on the processes of the arytenoid cartilage on a vocal fold. Do not force the tube to advance. Retract the tube slightly and rotate the position of the tube so the beveled end slips between the folds easily.

It is wise to learn to intubate without putting your fingers into the dog's mouth. This avoids the risk of injury. One-person intubation is possible in a deeply anesthetized dog; preferably using a mouth gag then passing the tube.

Feline

Cats are difficult to intubate because of the deep position of the larynx in the neck and the propensity of cats to have laryngospasms. The use of local anesthetic sprays help by decreasing the tactile perception to start spasm.

Intubation is easiest with the cat in sternal recumbency and with the assistant holding the head and neck up by grasping the cat's zygomatic arches Then open the mouth and pull the tongue forward. Use a small laryngoscope blade to visualize the larynx and slowly and gently pass a tube between the arytenoids when they are open. The tube must not be forced through nor allowed to touch the larynx prior to intubation.

Inhalation anesthesia makes intubation easier compared to light thiobarbiturate anesthesia which seems to increase spasm. Ketamine, either as a premedication or induction agent, makes intubation easier despite the fact that laryngeal reflexes are supposed to remain intact. Laryngeal spasm does not occur during deep general anesthesia. However, very deep anesthesia is not recommended as a routine procedure for intubation. Should several attempts at intubation fail, the anesthetized cat may be paralyzed by the administration of a relaxant drug such as succinylcholine after it has inhaled 100% oxygen for 1 to 2 min. to prevent hypoxia during the subsequent intubation. The cat must be ventilated until spontaneous respiration returns.

Equine

The primary problems are an inability to visualize the larynx and the high seating of the epiglottis. Oral (or nasal) intubation is done blindly with repeated but gentle passes at the larynx. Position the horse in lateral recumbency with the head extended. The mouth is opened and a gag or block inserted. The tongue is held down and to the side to allow tube to pass over the dorsum of the tongue and engage the larynx. If the tube has much of a curve, another technique is to turn the concave side towards the hard palate until the tip pushes up the soft palate & is over the epiglottis. Then by rotating the tube 180 degrees pass it into the larynx. When the tube passes into the trachea it should meet no resistance. If it does it is either in the esophagus or "caught" on the arytenoids or vocal folds. The tube is withdrawn 2-6 cm, rotated slightly and passed forward again. Nasal intubation is fairly easy in horses but requires a tube one to two sizes smaller than for oral intubation.

Bovine

Except for small cows or calves, laryngeal visualization is not possible. Intubation is carried out blindly or by manual guidance. The technique of blind intubation is not easy and has the animal at increased risk of aspiration. The more common method is to put in a strong and secure mouth gag (Hauptner or Bayer's) and use one arm to enter the pharynx and identify the laryngeal glottis. The tube is passes up beside or under the arm and guided into the trachea. It is a tight fit for both arm and the tube and it is important to avoid tearing the cuff on the teeth. A variation of the manual method is to place a 3-5 mm polypropylene or nylon guide into the trachea and then to pass the tube over the guide. The guide must be at least three times longer than the endotracheal tube or it will be lost inside the tube.

If regurgitation occurs during intubation, an endotracheal tube should be put quickly into the esophagus, inflating the cuff, and guiding ruminal contents out of the mouth via the tube.

Ovine and Caprine

In sheep and goats (and calves) endotracheal intubation is best performed by blind intubation which is simpler with these animals than with adult cattle. Sometimes the tube needs to be stiffened with a stylet and given a good curve to get over the back of the tongue. Intubation is also possible under direct vision with the aid of a laryngoscope.

Porcine

Pigs are probably the hardest domestic species to intubate. The rima glottis is small and the larynx is set at an the angle to the trachea, making it difficult to pass a the tube beyond the cricoid ring. A curved tube tends to get lodged into the ventral diverticulum of the larynx. Intubation is made easier with a small diameter long tube that has been straightened with a stylet. Use a laryngoscope if possible and rotate the tube 180 degrees as it passes through the larynx.

Avian

Intubation is very easy in birds with the larynx visible in the base of the tongue when the mouth opens. The main danger is over inflation of the cuff and tracheal damage. The trachea of birds is not flexible due to complete tracheal rings in most species.

Lagomorphs and Rodents

These are difficult species in which to visualize the very small larynx. Intubate rabbits blindly. Once anesthetized, position the animal in sternal recumbency and extend the head in a vertical position as much as possible and pass the tube down to the larynx. (Do not pull the tongue out). Listen for respiratory sounds through the tube and gently rotate until the tube passes into the trachea. Guinea pigs and hamsters are even more difficult with the additional problem of food pouches. Use an otoscope or small laryngoscope blade to try and visualize the larynx.

Llamas

Llamas have a very deep-seated larynx and a very narrow jaw (somewhat similar to rabbits). They are extremely difficult to intubate. A further complication is their tendency to regurgitate if the larynx is stimulated under light anesthesia. Make sure that anesthesia is adequate and *keep the llama in sternal recumbency* until an endotracheal tube has been correctly placed and the cuff inflated. The head should be extended vertically on the neck. Blind intubation may be accomplished (similar to the rabbit) or a long-bladed laryngoscope may be used to visualize the larynx. Direct intubation may be possible or a long stylet passed into the trachea and the endotracheal tube passed over it.

Complications of Endotracheal Intubation

Laryngoscopy and Intubation

- Trauma.
- Hypertension and tachycardia.
- Dysrhythmias.
- Aspiration.
- Trauma to handlers.
- Aggravation of spinal injuries.

Tube in Place

- Misplacement (endobronchial or esophageal).
- Obstruction (foreign body, kink, cuff, bevel).
- Accidental extubation.
- Aspiration.
- Bronchospasm.
- Tracheal epithelial ischemia.
- Aspiration of tube.

Immediate and Delayed Complications following Extubation

- Laryngospasm.
- Aspiration.
- Laryngeal edema or ulceration.
- Tracheitis.
- Introduction or bacteria or foreign matter into lung.
- Vocal cord damage.
- Webs or stenosis secondary to tracheitis.

Manufacturers and Suppliers

Tubes

- Bivona Surgical Inc., Gary, IN.
- National Catheter Co., Argyle, NY.
- Portex, Wilmington, MA.
- Snyder Laboratory, New Philadelphia, OH.

Laryngoscopes

- North American Drager, Telford, Penn.
- Foregger Co. Inc., Roslyn Heights, NY.
- Ohio Medical Products, Madison, Wisconsin.
- Rusch Inc., New York, NY.
- Suggested Tube Sizes.

Canine

2-4 kg	4-5 mm
7 kg	6.0 mm
9 kg	7.0 mm
12-14 kg	9-10 mm
16-18 kg	11-12 mm
20-25 kg	12-14 mm

Feline		
Kittens	2-3 mm	Cole or uncuffed
Adults	3 - 4.5 mm	Cuffed
Equine		
Foals	9 - 14 mm	
Small Ponies	14 - 16 mm	
Thoroughbreds	26 - 30 mm	
Draft Horses	30 - 36 mm	
Bovine		
Calves 3 months	9 - 12 mm	
Calves 6 months	14 - 18 mm	
Yearling cows	22 mm	
Mature cows	26 mm	
Large Bulls	30 mm	
Caprine and Ovine		
Adults	7 - 9 mm	
Porcine		
25 kg	6 mm	
50 kg	9 mm	
Large sows and boars	10 - 14 mm	
Rodents and Lagomorphs		
Rabbits	2 - 4 mm	
Guinea Pigs	2 - 3 mm	

Chapter 23

Muscle Relaxants

Historical Aspect

- Curare was the first known muscle relaxant which was used by South American Indians to immobilize wild animals. Hence the term curariform has been applied to the action of this group of drugs.
- In year 1958, a plant alkaloid alcuronium was introduced but there were difficulties in reversing the action of this drug.
- Succinylcholine was first used in 1906. However, its paralyzing property was discovered in year 1949.
- Pancuronium was introduced in 1964.

Muscle Relaxation can be Effected in Three Ways

1. Administration of drugs acting centrally, such as intravenous or Inhalant anesthetics. These drugs depress the CNS.
2. Local anesthetics produce muscle relaxation if injected directly into a muscle or around the nerve that supplies it.
3. A third means of producing muscle relaxations with drugs known as muscle relaxants. All muscle relaxants produce their effect on neuromuscular junction, except mephenesin and guaifenesin, which act upon synapses in the spinal cord.

Indications

- To provide the muscle relaxant component of the anesthesia without having to give higher doses of more CNS depressant drugs in a very sick or geriatric patient.
- To facilitate endotracheal intubation of those species which are prone to laryngospasm.
- To paralyze respiratory muscle so that artificial respiration can easily be controlled. Surgeries requiring mechanical ventilation include thoracotomies, repair of ruptured diaphragm, surgery for severe trauma to thoracic wall; animals with pneumothorax, hydrothorax and hemothorax may require positive pressure ventilation.
- To ensure immobility of the patient during delicate surgery and stabilize a central eye position for ophthalmic surgery. Non depolarizing muscle relaxants maintain the eye in central position without raising intraocular pressure.
- To help removal of foreign bodies from the proximal portion of the esophagus which is composed of striated muscles.
- To facilitate surgical access to difficult anatomic regions.
- To facilitate fracture reduction and aid in relocating the luxated joints. This is more useful if the luxation is less than 48 hours old.
- As a part of balanced anesthesia procedures to produce the amount of general anesthetic required.

Rules for Using Neuromuscular Blockade

- There must be facilities to ventilate the patient. The respiratory muscles will be paralyzed and so the patient will not be able to breathe. An anesthetic machine can be used for ventilation.
- If you have any doubts about your ability to monitor the patient and are not very confident of the techniques; do not use.
- Do not use these drugs as a substitute for sedation or analgesia for they do not provide either component. It is inhumane for the patient to remain awake and feeling pain and yet be incapable of moving.
- The patient must be anesthetized before their use.

Classification of Muscle Relaxants

1. Depolarizing Agents

a. Decamethonium
b. Suxamethonium (succinylcholine)

2. Non-depolarizing Agents

a. Tubocurarine chloride
b. Metocurine iodide
c. Gallamine
d. Benzoquinonium
e. Hexafluorenium
f. Pancuronium
g. Rapacuronium
h. Vecuronium
i. Alcuronium
j. Atracurium
k. Pipercuronium
l. Doxacurium
m. Mivacurium and
n. Rocuronium

3. Miscellaneous

a. Mephenesin
b. Guaifenesin
c. Baclofen
d. Dantrolene

Mechanism of action : Transmission of nerve impulse may be interfered if -

1. Anything that interferes with release of acetylcholine (Ach) interferes with transmission of the nerve impulse. Procaine, Mg^{++} or deficiency of calcium ions will slow or stop production of Ach at the nerve terminal.
2. Delay in breakdown of Ach at the end plate region causes persistent depolarization of the membrane and transmission of subsequent impulse is impossible. Delay of breakdown can be caused by anticholinesterase drugs such as neostigmine and edrophonium.

Classification of the neuromuscular blocking drugs according to their duration of action:

S.No.	Duration	Drug	Dose (mg/kg)	Onset (min)	Duration of effect (min)	Recovery index (min)	Cardio-vascular effects
1.	Ultrashort	Succinylcholine	1.0	1-1.5	7-12	3-4	++
2.	Short	i. Rapacuronium	2.0	1-1.5	15-25	5-7	++
		ii. Mivacurium	0.2	3-5	15-25	6-8	++
3.	Intermediate	i. Atracurium	0.5	3-4	35-45	10-15	++
		ii. Cisatracurium	0.1	4-6	40-50	10-15	-
		iii. Rocuronium	0.6	1.5-3	30-40	10-15	+
		iv. Vecuronium	0.1	3-4	35-45	10-15	-
4.	Long	i. Doxacurium	0.05	5-7	90-120	30-45	-
		ii. Pancuronium	0.15	3-5	90-120	30-45	+++
		iii. Pipercuroneum	0.10	3-5	90-120	30-45	-

3. Agents that produce depolarization and continue to persist at the end plate will stop transmission of impulses at the neuromuscular junction e.g. decamethonium and succinylcholine.
4. The drugs of this group (tubocurarine, gallamine etc) compete with Ach for the cholinergic receptors. This block is referred to as competitive inhibition since these drugs compete with Ach for the end plate receptor sites. The term non-depolarizaiton block is used to describe the action of these agents. The result is a flaccid paralysis.

a. In all species of animals, relaxant drugs produce approximately the same sequence of muscle relaxation. The recovery pattern is in reverse order.

b. When diaphragm is paralyzed artificial respiration should be given.
   - O_2 should always be available when these drugs are used.
   - With the exception of Guaifenesin none of the muscle relaxants produce analgesia. For this reason, analgesics or anesthetics should be administered concurrently.
   - Tubocurarine, gallamine and succinylcholine are transmitted across the placenta whereas decamethonium is not.

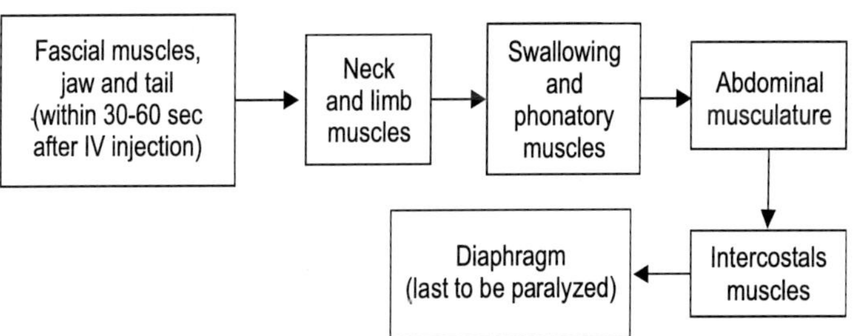

Doxapram test : This test is performed for differential diagnosis of apnea following the use of general anesthesia (due to central depression) or muscle relaxants (due to peripheral neuromuscular blockade).

In apnetic patients, injection of 2 mg/kg of doxapram evokes marked respiratory response if the cause of apnea is central depression. If there is no response, the cause is persistent neuromuscular blockade.

Side Effects of Muscle Relexants

- Among all side effects, cardiovascular effects are of great importance.
- At present Doxacurium, Cisatracurium, Vecuronium and Rocuronium are devoid of cardiovascular side effects in normal clinical doses.

- Rapacuronium produces bronchospasm or increased airway pressure after tracheal intubation.
- Succinylcholine has a long list of side effects like profound cardiovascular effects, increase in intraocular, intragastric and intracranial pressure, hyperkalemia, myoglobinemia and malignant hyperthermia.
- Gallamine have the greatest vagotonic action (tachycardia). Other blockers with this potential in decreasing order are:

  d-Tubocurarine> Pancuronium> Alcuronium> Metocurine> Atracurium > Vecuronium

  d-Tubocurarine is the most potent liberator of histamine. Other agents with this potential in decreasing order are:

  d-ubocurarine> Atracurium> Alcuronium> Succinylcholine> Vecuronium > Pancuronium.
- Neuromuscular blocking drugs cross the placenta from the maternal to fetal circulation very slowly. These agents can be used safely in cesarean section without any side effects.
  - d-Tubocurarine produces marked hypotension in dogs and cats.

Precautions

- These agents block neuromuscular function to skeletal muscles, preventing the animal from breathing. So some method of artificial ventilation must be available.
- These agents have no central depressant or analgesic effects. So the patient should receive appropriate analgesia for the surgical procedure intended.

Factors Affecting Neuromuscular Block

The duration and intensity of neuromuscular blocks are influenced by a number of factors:

1. Hepatic Diseases

- Impaired liver function (liver cirrhosis, obstructive liver disease) may prolong relaxant metabolism (because plasma cholinesterase is synthesized by the liver).
- Atracurium is the agent of choice in liver diseases because it metabolizes through other routes.

2. Renal Diseases

- The agents rely predominately on urinary elimination should not be given in patients having renal disease e.g. Gallamine, Pancuronium and Pipercuronium.
- Atracurium is the drug of choice in these patients.

3. Anesthetic Drugs

- Volatile inhalant anesthetics cause a dose related potentiation of the duration and intensity of muscle relaxants.
- Enflurane and isoflurane have a greater effect than halothane on reducing the dose of d-Tubocurarine, Vecuronium and Pancuronium for producing muscle relaxation.
- Injectable anesthetics have very little or no effect on the relaxation properties of muscle relaxants.

4. Acid base Disturbances

- Respiratory acidosis potentiate the action of d-Tubocurarine, Vecuronium and Pancuronium.
- Respiratory alkalosis antagonizes the action of above drugs.

5. Electrolyte Disturbances

- Changes in serum concentration of K, Mg and Ca influences the duration of action of muscle relaxants.
- Hypokalemia prolong the duration of action of non depolarizing muscle relaxants.
- Hypercalcemia antagonizes the action of muscle relaxants.
- Increased Mg concentration potentiates the neuromuscular block by non depolarizing muscle relaxants by inhibiting the presynaptic release of the transmitter.

6. Hypothermia

The effect of hypothermia on muscle relaxant is variable.

- It prolongs the d-tubocurarine and pancuronium neuromuscular block.

7. Age

Age influences the dose requirement of the muscle relaxant.

- Neonates are slightly more sensitive to atracurium and pancuronium.
- The duration of action of non depolarizing muscle relaxants is prolonged in older patients.

8. Interaction with Drugs

- Antibiotics
  - i. Administration of "mycin" drugs (Aminoglycoside antibiotics) e.g. Neomycin, Geantamicin, Streptomycin, Kanamycin drugs will potentiate the effects of neuromuscular blocking agents by the following mechanisms:
    - Decreases the availability of Ca++ at the axonal terminals and thus interferes with the excitation - secretion-coupling process.
    - Reduces its sensitivity to Ach by competitively blocking the nicotinic cholinergic receptor.
  - ii. Polymixins have both pre and post junctional actions including depression of muscle action potential. This effect is unresponsive to calcium and neostigmine.
  - iii. Tetracyclines, lincomycin and clindamycin have a pre junctional action and may directly depress muscle contractility. This effect is responsive to calcium and neostigmine.
- Other drugs- reduction in presynaptic release of acetylcholine by certain drugs potentiate the action of neuromuscular blocking agents. These drugs are- Local anesthetics, propranolol, barbiturates etc.

Depolarizing Muscle Relaxants

Succinylcholine chloride

- Chloride salt is 1 ½ times as potent as the iodide salt.
- Succinylcholine is sometimes referred to as diaectylcholine (because two acetyl choline molecules are joined back to back).
- The chief disadvantage is that the effective dose and duration of effect are inconsistent between individuals.
- Succinylcholine is hydrolyzed by plasma cholinesterase or pseudo cholinesterase.
- Acetyl cholinesterase, true cholinesterase of erythrocyte, can't hydrolyze succinylcholine.
- In liver diseases, administration of succinylcholine may produce prolonged apnea (because plasma cholinesterase is synthesized by liver).
- Succinylcholine is contraindicated in digitalized patients (both produce cardiac arrhythmia).

- Use of this drug is also contraindicated if any of the following have been administrated or applied within 30 days.
  - i. Any organic phosphate anthelmentic.
  - ii. Amino glycoside antibiotics ('Mycin' drugs).
  - iii. Any organic phosphate insecticide.
  - iv. Any other cholinesterase inhibitors.
  - v. Procaine.
  - vi. Patient suffering from respiratory or liver disease.
  - vii. In glaucoma (increase in intraocular pressure due to contracture of extraocular muscles).
- *Doses:*

  Horse: 0.12-0.15 mg/kg, IV.

  Dog: 0.3 mg/kg, IV.

  Cat: 1.0 mg/kg, IV.

  Cattle and sheep: 0.02 mg/kg, IV.

Non Depolarizing Muscle Relaxants

1. Tubocurarine Chloride

- Obtained from plant *Chondodendron tomentosum*
- Aquous solutions can be stored for long periods or even autoclaved without serious decomposition.
- In cats, antagonism of tubocurarine and pancuronium induced blockade is opposed by respiratory acidosis and metabolic alkalosis.
- Both amide and ester type of local anesthetics enhance the effect of tubocurarine.
- Drugs which increases the duration and intensity of blockade are :
  - i. Lidocaine
  - ii. Propranolol
  - iii. Quinidine
  - iv. Ketamine
  - v. Furosemide
- It causes release of histamine.
- *Antagonist:* Neostigmine methylsulfate (1:2000)

- *Doses:*
  Dog: 0.4 mg/kg body wt, IV.
  Horse: 0.2 mg/kg body wt, IV.
  Ruminants: 0.05 mg/kg body wt, IV.

2. Metocurine Iodide

- It is the iodide of dimethyl tubocurarine.
- More potent than tubocurarine (2-3 times) but duration is slightly shorter.

3. Gallamine Triethiodide

- 7 mg ≈ 1 mg of tubocurarine in action.
- It does not produce histamine release in dog. In addition it also produces some vegal block.
- Contraindicated in animals suffering from renal failure, but may be used in animals with compensated chronic nephritis.
- Prior administration of gallamine prevents the rise in intraocular pressure, following succinylcholine injection.
- Gallamine extensively used for immobilizing wild animals.
- *Antidote*: Neostigmine.

4. Pancuronium Bromide

It is an aminosteroid which is free from hormonal action.

- Pancuronium is metabolized in to 3-hydroxypancuronium, 17- hydroxy pancuronium and 2, 17 hydroxy pancuronium.
- It is longer acting than gallamine and has no histaminic effect.
- *Antidote*: Neostigmine or pyridostigmine and atropine.
- *Dose* : Dog, Cat, Swine and Goats 0.01-0.05 mg/lb body wt.

5. Alcuronium

It is a long acting semi synthetic muscle relaxant.

6. Atracurium

- It is a synthetic bisquaternary isoquinoline compound metabolized by esterases and Hofmann elimination.

$$\text{Atracurium} \xrightarrow[\text{elimination}]{\text{Hofmann}} \text{Laudanosine (In higher doses it causes seizure activity in dogs)}$$

7. Vecuronium

Vecuronium was developed to avoid the undesirable actions of pancuronium namely ganglionic blocking and the indirect sympathomimetic effects.

8. Pipercuronium

It has higher potency than pancuronium.

9. Doxacurium

It is slightly more potent than pipercuronium and much more potent than pancuronium.

10. Mivacurium

Its potency is about one third to one half that of atracurium.

11. Rocuronium

It is a derivative of vecuronium and is less potent (1/8 to 1/10).

12. Cisatracurium

It is 4 times more potent than atracurium.

13. Rapacuronium

- It is a new muscle relaxant having rapid onset of action.
- It is metabolized to its 3 hydroxy metabolites (org 9488) which is 2.5 times more potent than the parent compound and is cleared slowly by the kidney. Hence, there is risk of more prolonged block.
- It has $1/20^{th}$ the potency of vecuronium.

Miscellaneous Muscle Relaxants

Guaifenesin (Antitussive)

- It is extensively used in horses.
- Its unique advantage is that it produces muscle relaxation with little effect on respiration.

Anticurariform Agents

- Edrophonium- 0.5-1.0 mg/kg body wt, IV.
- Neostigmine- 0.03-1 mg/kg body wt, IV.
- Pyridostigmine- 0.2 mg/kg body wt, IV.

All are anticholinesterases.

- Action of these drugs is due to their inhibitory effect on Ach hydrolysis, thus intensifying Ach effects.
- Salivation, bronchial secretion, intestinal hypermotility, bradycardia.
- Atropine should be given concurrently to prevent side effects.

Chapter 24

LOCAL ANESTHETICS

These are the drugs that reversibly block the propagation of action potentials along nerve axons. General anesthesia may be advantageous where complete immobilization and relaxation of the patients required. However, local anesthetic techniques are advantageous for providing surgical anesthesia in animals that are considered at risk for inhalant or intravenous anesthesia. These drugs are injected directly at the target site.

History

- Cocaine was the first local anesthetic to be discovered. It is an alkaloid present in the leaves of *Erythroxylon coca.*

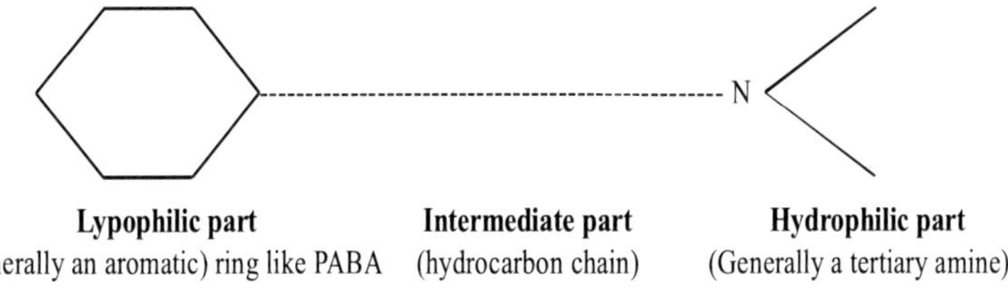

Basic Molecular Structure of Local Anesthetics

- A basic local anesthetics molecule has three parts.
  - i. A hydrophilic end.
  - ii. A lipophilic end.
  - iii An intermediate hydrocarbon chain connecting the both ends.
- Most of the local anesthetic are weakly basic tertiary amines (Nitrogen atom attached with 3 organic groups).
- Hexylcaine and prilocaine - secondary amines.
- Benzocaine lacks the hydrophilic tail and is nearly insoluble in water, thus used for topical application.
- Addition of butyl group to the lipophilic end of procaine yields tetracaine. It is more lipids soluble and intrinsically more potent than procaine.

General Properties

- Local anesthetic techniques are simple, safe, economical and do not require sophisticated equipments.
- Poor surgical risk patient can withstand local anesthetic without major complications.
- Many surgical procedures can be carried out satisfactorily under local anesthesia *e.g.* caesarian section.
- In adult bovines, many operations can be performed on standing animals to eliminate the danger of forcible casting and restraint and prolonged recumbency.
- Local anesthetics in effective concentration abolish both sensory and motor sensation without any apparent damage to the nervous tissue.
- Time of effect, potency and duration of action of local anesthetics depends upon the physicochemical properties of their molecular structure. Lipid solubility is a major determinant of intrinsic local anesthetic potency because axonal membranes are highly lipid in composition, local anesthetics act strongly on these structures.
- Slower onset and poor quality local anesthesia is produced when local anesthesia is injected in to an acidic infected area (pus).
- Protein binding is the primary determinant of local anesthetic duration.
- Amides are mainly metabolized by the liver. Patients with severe hepatic disease may be more susceptible to adverse reactions from amide local anesthetics.

Classification of Local Anesthetics

- Local anesthetics are typically classified to ester linked or amide linked, depending on the structure of the molecule's intermediate chain and on the basis of duration of action.
- *Amides drugs have 'i' in generic prefix before 'caine', Exception is piperacaine, an ester drug.*

	Potency and duration	Name of Agent	Duration of action (min)	Ester /Amide
1.	Low potency, short duration	i. Procaine (least potent L.A.) ii. Chlorprocaine	60-90 30-60	Ester (derived form Benzoic acid and Biotransforms by hydrolysis)
2.	Intermediate potency and duration	i. Mepivacaine ii. Prilocaine iii. Lidocaine	120-240 120-240 90-200	Amide (derived from aniline and biotransforms by liver microsomal enzymes)
3.	High potency, long duration	i. Tetracaine (ester) ii. Bupivacaine iii. Etidocaine	180-600 180-600 180-600	Amide (derived from aniline and biotransforms by liver microsomal enzymes)

Mechanism of Action

- Local anesthetics prevent the rapid influx of sodium into nerve axons that produces the action potential. So, it prevents the generation of propagated action potential.
- A number of theories about the mechanism of action have been given. One of the most consistent ones is that local anesthetics, in positively charged form, enter the sodium channel from inside the axon and plug the channel.
- Molecular mechanism of local anesthetic action suggests that local anesthetics act by binding to receptors located on sodium channels. Local anesthetics may differ in their ability to bind to sodium channels depending on channel status.
- Sensory nerve fibers are more readily blocked by local anesthetics than the large motor fibers.

- Thin nerve fibers are more easily blocked than thick ones.
- Myelinated fibers are more readily blocked than unmyelinated ones because of the need to produce blockade only at the node of Ranvier.
- Preganglionic sympathetic nerve fibers (β fibers) are more sensitive to local anesthetics than small sensory nerve fibers (A-δ) which are more sensitive than large motor fibers (A-α)
- β fibers > A-δ > A-α
- Local anesthetics solution does not diffuse through fascial sheets.

Pharmacokinetics of Local Anesthetics

Absorption

- Local anesthetics are not injected intravascularly to induce anesthesia except intravenous regional anesthesia (IVRA) which is used to anesthetize an anterior or posterior extremity.
- Rate of absorption is directly proportional to vascularity at the injection site. The faster the absorption rate, the shorter the duration of action of the local anesthetic and the greater the risk of systemic toxicity.
- A vasoconstrictor (epinephrine) is added to local anesthetic solution to reduce absorption rate (30%), thereby prolonging duration of action (50%) and reducing the probability of systemic toxicity. Maximum recommended dose of local anesthetic can be increased if a vasoconstrictor is added. Usual concentration of epinephrine is 1 :200,000 (5 mg /ml) or 1 :400,000 (2.5 mg/ml).
- Local anesthetics are generally ineffective when applied to unbroken skin but they are effective at broken skin, cornea or mucous membrane.
- Mixture of prilocaine and lidocaine is effective on intact skin.

Distribution

Local

- Distribution of local anesthetic at the site of injection depends upon the volume of local anesthetic solution injected and how resistant the tissue is to the spread of the local anesthetic.
- Hyaluronidase enhances the spread of local anesthetic solution at the site.
- When a local anesthetic is injected in to the subarachnoid space, the specific gravity of the solution relative to the specific gravity of the CSF influences distribution.
- Patient positioning is used to direct local anesthetic to specific sites.

Systemic

- The liver and lungs are major sites for plasma clearance of local anesthetic.
- Procaine metabolism produces p-amino benzoic acid which is excreted unchanged or as a conjugated product of urine.
- Amide linked local anesthetics are cleaved by plasma cholinesterase.

  Elimination : Local anesthetics are excreted from the body via the urine or bile.

Local Anesthetic Toxicity

- Accidental intravenous injections of local anesthetic are the most common cause of adverse reaction associated with local anesthetic administration.
- Toxic reactions to local anesthetics are not fatal if recognized early and appropriately treated.
- The most frequent reactions observed clinically are acute reactions involving the direct effects of local anesthetics on the cardiovascular system and central nervous system.
- Acute toxicity is usually associated with accidental intravascular injection of local anesthetic.
- Premeditation with diazepam increases the local anesthetic seizure threshold.
- Propofol is also effective for the treatment of seizures caused by local anesthetic toxicity.
- The toxic dose of lidocaine is about 8 mg/kg and 4 mg/kg of bupivacaine.
- General signs of overdose are initial sedation, twitching, convulsions, coma and death.

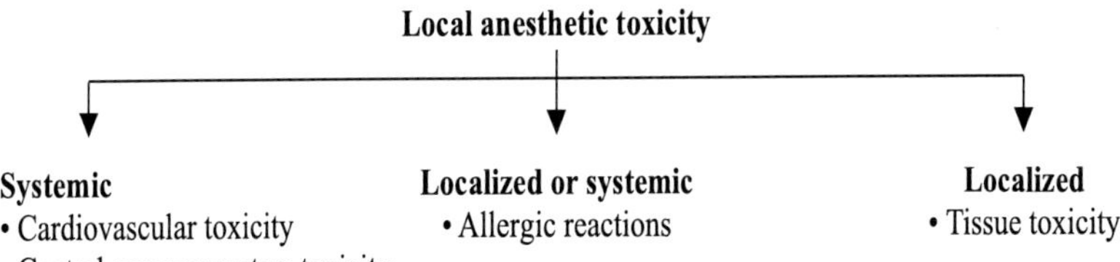

Systemic Toxicity

Central Nervous System Toxicity

- Central nervous system toxicity occurs before cardiovascular changes.

- It includes drowsiness progressing to numbness of lips, diplopia, fine tremors and seizures. Local anesthetic induced seizures originate in the limbic brain.
- Large doses produce generalized CNS depression.

Cardiovascular Toxicity

- By direct cardiac and peripheral vascular action.
- Indirectly by conduction blockade of autonomic fibers.
- Primary site of action is the myocardium. There is decrease in electric excitability, conduction rate and force of contraction. On ECG, increased PR interval and widened QRS complex is noted.
- High concentration of local anesthetics dilates blood vessels, but low concentrations my cause vasoconstriction.
- K^+ channel block may also contribute to the cardiotoxicity of local anesthetics.
- Bupivacaine is more cardiotoxic than lidocaine.

Methemoglobinemia

- Prilocaine, benzocaine, lidocaine and procaine produce methemoglobinemia. Methemoglobin is formed when ferrous ion (Fe^{++}) in hemoglobin is oxidized to the ferric ion (Fe^{+++}) form.

Localized or Systemic Allergic Reactions

- Ester linked local anesthetics causes more allergic reactions in comparison to amide linked ones. (Metabolites from ester local anesthetics, the PABA is believed to be an antigen responsible for allergic reactions).
- Methylparben, a preservative, may cause allergic reaction.
- Cutaneous and respiratory reactions are the most common indicators of anaphylaxis.

Localized Tissue Toxicity

- The potent long lasting local anesthetic with high lipid solubility appears to be more likely to cause tissue damage than other local anesthetics.
- High concentration of local anesthetic is also cytotoxic.

Tissue toxicity Includes irritation and lysis of cells. Muscles and nerves are primarily affected. Skeletal muscles are more sensitive. Local anesthetic affects the perineurium, Schwann cells and axons.

Always draw back on syringe to check not in vein before injecting local anesthetics

Local Anesthetic Agents

Procaine HCl

- It is an ester of p-amino benzoic acid.
- It is generally used in 2% concentration.
- A yellow or dark solution indicates deteriorated potency.
- Aqueous solution is heat resistant and thus can be repeatedly sterilized by boiling.
- It is lethal to parakeet.

Lidocaine HCl

- This is the most widely used local anesthetic in veterinary practice.
- It is an amide derivative of diethylamino acetic acid.
- It is available in the market with or without epinephrine, and in the form of solutions, creams, jellies, spray etc.
- Lidocaine is available with or without epinephrine (1 : 50,000 to 1 : 200,000).
- Lidocaine is also used for infiltration anesthesia (0.5-1%) and nerve block (1-2%).
- A 2-5% solution of lidocaine is used as topical anesthesia on mucous membrane. The effect produced within 5 minutes and lasts for 30 minutes.
- It is more potent than procaine.
- The solution remained stable even if boiled with acid and alkalies.
- The onset is shorter, power of penetration is more and duration of action is longer (1 h without epinephrine and 2 h with epinephrine) as compared to procaine.
- It may cause some local irritation and swelling, which is particularly a problem in the horse.

Proparacaine

- It is an excellent topical anesthetic for examination of painful eye, removal of foreign bodies and sutures, obtaining conjunctival scrapings and subconjunctival injections.
- It is used to anesthetize the cornea of the eye. It has rapid onset of action (within 1 minute) and lasts for about 15-30 minutes.
- It does not affect the size of the pupil.

Tetracaine HCl

- It is more potent than procaine.
- It should not be autoclaved.
- It is 13 times more highly bound to proteins and its anesthetic duration is 3-7 times longer than that of procaine.
- Systemic toxicity is 12-20 times and potency 10 times more than cocaine.
- Mostly used for topical anesthesia (0.2%).

Mepivacaine HCl

- Most widely used drug *in equine practice* as it causes very little swelling and edema in the area of injection, possibly due to lack of vasodilator action.
- It is 2 times more potent and 1-1.5 times more toxic than procaine.
- Its toxicity is less than lignocaine and lidocane.
- Duration of action is 2-3 times longer than procaine.
- Concentration (1-2%) for infiltration anesthesia and nerve blocks.

Bupivacaine HCl

- Bupivacaine is 15 times more lipid soluble and 4 times more potent than mepivacaine.
- It is a longer acting anesthetic agent (4-6 h) and up to 8 hours when combined with epinephrine. It is used wherever long action is required.
- 2-4 times more potent than lignocaine and mepivacaine.
- It is 15 times more lipid soluble than mepivacaine.
- 0.25% solution is used for infiltration anesthesia.
- 0.50% solution is used for nerve blocks.

Hexylcaine

- It is an ester and 4-8 times more active than cocaine.

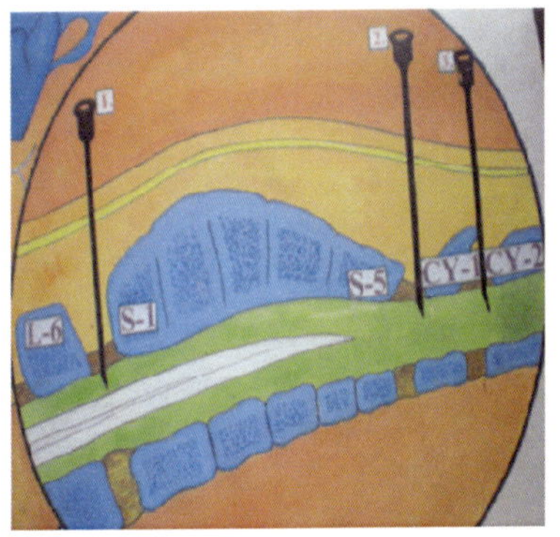

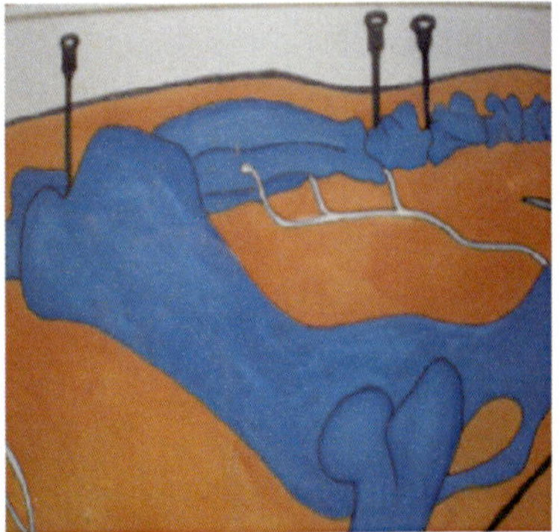

1. Epidural anesthesia in cattle

2. Epidural anesthesia in cattle

(1. Lumbosecrel, 2. Sacrococcygeal, 3. Intercoccygeal)

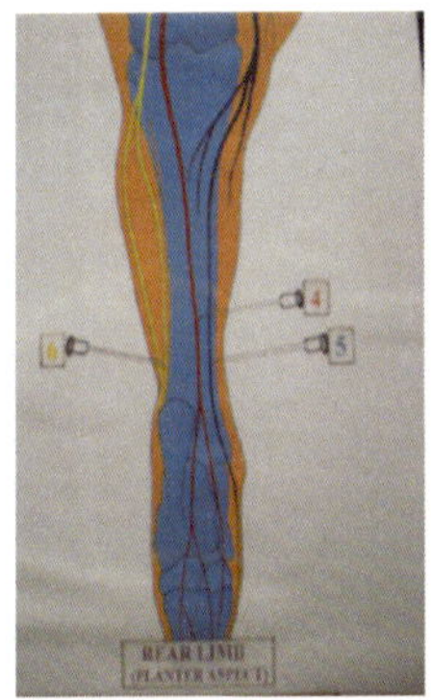

3. Needle placement for nerve block fo limbs in horse. 4. Saphenous nerve 5. Peroneal nerve, 6. Tubiel nerve

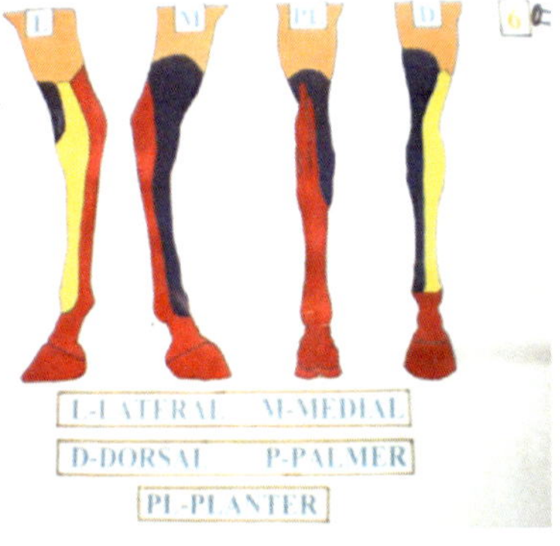

4. Desesitized area after blocking saphenous, peroneal and tebial nerve.

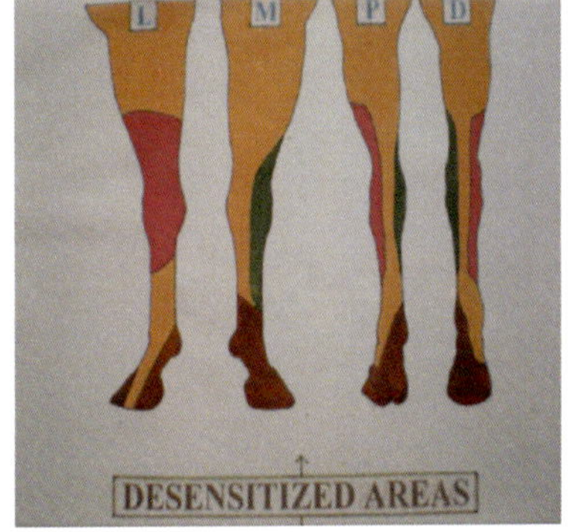

5. Desesitized area after blocking medial, under and musculocutaneous nerve.

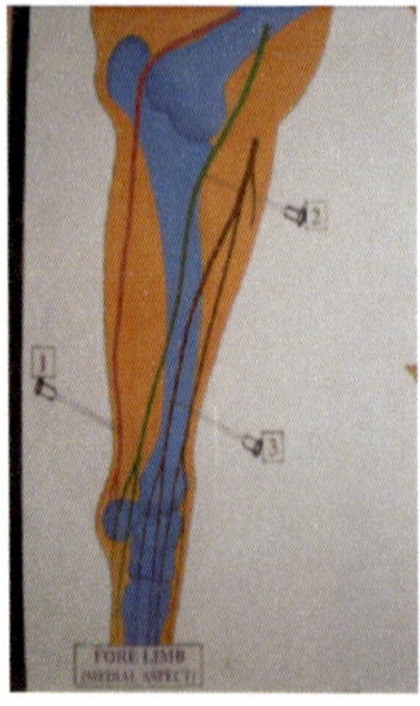

6. Needle placement for desensitilization of 1. Medien, 3. Ulnar and 3. Musculocutoneous nerve.

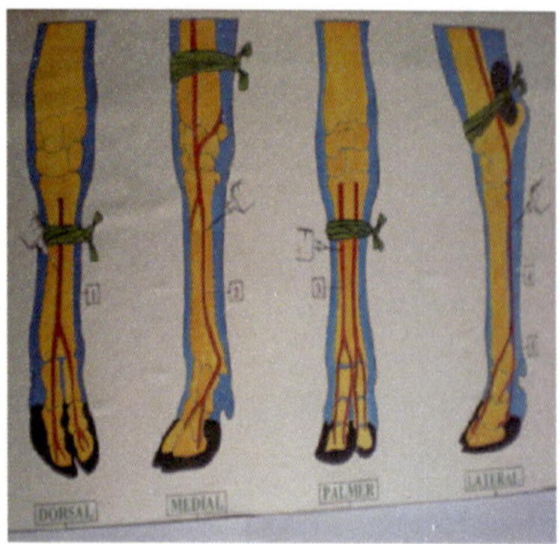

7. Torniquet and needle placement for intravenous regional anaesthia in bovines.

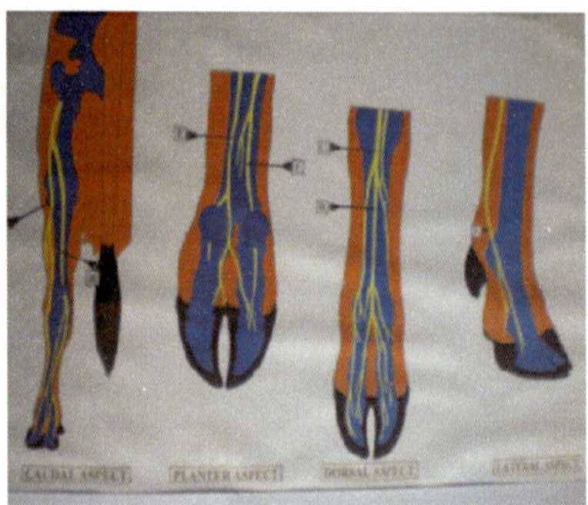

8. Needle placement for desensitilization of nerves of hind limb in cattle

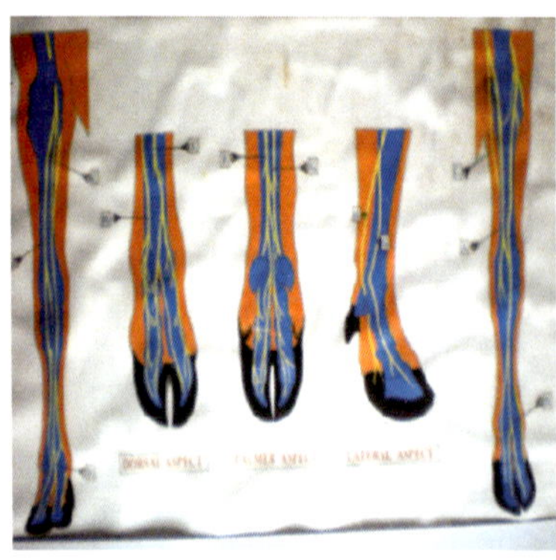

9. Needle placement for desensitilization of nerves of fore limb in cettle.

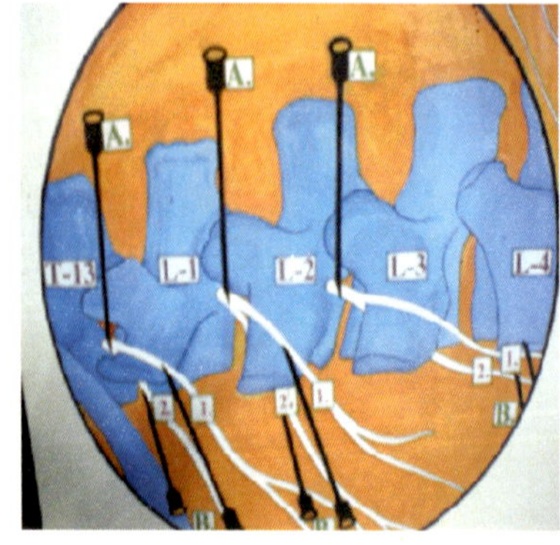

10. Needle placement for para vertebral anaesthesia in cattle.

Amethocaine

- It is well absorbed by the surface and is used on mucous membrane.

Prilocaine

- It has slower onset of action and spreads less as compared to lidocaine.
- It causes dose dependent methemoglobinaemia which limits its usefullness.

Butacaine

- It is 9 times more toxic than cocaine.

Cocaine

- It is the only local anesthetic agent which causes vasoconstriction. Other causes vasodilatation.

Ropivacaine and Lovobupivacaine

- Newer long acting local anesthetics with less cardiotoxicity.

Clinical Uses

1. *For injection* : Lidocaine, Bupivacaine, Ropivacaine, Procaine, Chlorprocaine, Mepivacaine and Tetracaine.
2. *For ophthalmology* : Benoxinate and Proparacaine.
3. *For mucous membrane and skin* : Dibucaine, Cyclonine, Paramoxine, Eutectic mixture of prilocaine and lidocaine.
4. *For sustain anesthesia* : Local anesthetics of low solubility are used for this purpose e.g. on wounds and ulcerated surface.

> *Local anesthetic containing epinephrine should not be injected in to tissues supplied by end arteries (e.g. ears, tail, and teat) because of risk of severe vasoconstriction, local ischemia and necrosis.*

Methods of Producing Local Anesthesia

1. Surface/topical anesthesia
2. Infiltration anesthesia
3. Spinal/epidural anesthesia
4. Peripheral/regional anesthesia
5. Intrasynovial anesthesia
6. Intravenous local anesthesia (IVRA)

All the local anesthetic techniques should be performed in a sterile manner. The animal should be clipped and the site surgically prepared. Sterile needles, syringes, and anesthetic solution should be used.

1. Topical Anesthesia

- The local anesthetics which are effective when placed topically on mucous membrane are known as topical anesthetics.. These agents may be used in the mouth, tracheobroncheal tree, esophagus and urogenital tract.
  - i. Lidocaine (2-5%)
  - ii. Proparacaine (0.5%)
  - iii. Tetracaine (0.5-2%)
  - iv. Butacaine (2%)
  - v. Cocaine (4-10%)
  - vi. Piperocaine (2%)
  - vii. Oxybuprocaine (0.4%)
- Used to desensitize the mucous membrane of teats, genital system, oral cavity, nasal cavity and for surface anesthesia of eye.
- Local anesthetic sprays (10% lidocaine, 14-20% benzocaine) produce anesthesia of the mucosa up to a depth of 2 mm within 1-2 minutes after application. Anesthesia lasts for about 15-20 minutes.
- Ethylene chloride can be used as topical anesthesia to freeze a small local area of skin for punctures, skin biopsy or incision of small abscesses. Surface anesthesia results from cooling (< 4^0C), which occurs during the evaporation process. Topical anesthesia of large skin areas is contraindicated because of potential for frost bite.

2. Intrasynovial Anesthesia

- Local anesthetic solution is injected in joints, bursa and tendon sheath.
- Intrasynovial anesthesia is indicated for diagnosis of lameness and for pain relief.

3. Infiltration

- Local anesthetic agents are injected extravascularly to desensitize the nerve endings.
- This method is more reliable and safest of all the local anesthetic techniques.

- It can be performed either in the form of linear (at the line of incision) or in the form of inverted 'L' or 'T' form (for desensitization of paralumbar fossa in cattle).
- Line block : Simple infiltration of the incision line (line block) by local anesthesia. Successive injections of local anesthesia are made slowly and continuously as the needle is inserted at the edge of desensitized skin for the skin and subcutaneous line block. This is followed by infiltration of muscles.
- Inverted 7 or L block : 100 ml of a 2% lidocaine HCl in adult cattle is injected into the tissue bordering the dorsocaudal aspect of last rib and ventrolateral aspect of the lumbar transverse process.
- The amount of local anesthetic used for infiltration anesthesia depends upon the size of the area to be desensitized. Approximately 2-5 mg/kg of lidocaine or mepivacaine and 4-6 mg/kg procaine may be used for infiltration. The total dose should be reduced by 30-40% in old, sick or cachetic animals or animal in poor condition.

4. Peripheral/ Regional Anaesthesia

- Injection of local anesthetic solution in to the connective tissue surrounding a nerve produces loss of sensation (sensory nerve block) and/or paralysis (motor nerve block) in the region supplied by the nerve.
- In such type of anesthesia either minor (e.g. radial) or major (e.g. brachial plexus) nerves are blocked.
- Regional anesthesia is brought about by blocking conduction in the sensory nerve or nerve innervating the region where the operation is to be performed.
- The operations field it self is not touched while its sensitivity is being abolished by depositing the local anesthetic around the nerve supplying to the operative site.
- Its major advantage over field block is that much smaller amount of agent is required to produce nerve block compared to field block, therefore reducing the dangers of toxicity.
- Disadvantage is to approximate the exact course of nerve.

5. Epidural and Spinal Anesthesia

(The detail is given in Chapter 25)

6. Field Block

- Used for producing anesthesia in a longer area than local infiltration.
- It is accomplished by making fanwise injection in certain planes of the body so as to block all the nerves which cross these planes on their way to the operation field.

7. Intravenous Regional Anesthesia (IVRA) or Bier's Block

- IVRA is an alternative method of producing analgesia of the digit.
- In cattle, a catheter is inserted in to a vein and the limb is exsanguinated by esmarchs bandage.
- A tourniquet is applied above the elbow or hock joint (for occluding the arterial blood supply of limb by applying pressure,>150 mm Hg, adequate to prevent arterial circulation).
- Local anesthesia solution (preferably without epinephrine) is injected in to the vein. Analgesia of the limb upto the lower limit of tourniquet comes on rapidly and once tourniquet is released the effect is abolished with almost equal rapidity.
- It is an ideal method for digital surgery. The amount of bleeding at the surgical site is considerably reduced.
- In adult cattle, 30 ml of a 2% lignocaine hydrochloride solution in injected as rapidly as possible. In small ruminants 3-10 ml of lidocaine is sufficient for producing anesthesia.
- Anesthesia of the limb distal to the tourniquet develops after 5 minutes, is optimal in 10 minutes.
- Complications like ischemic necrosis, severe lameness and edema are not occurred, if the tourniquet is applied for less than 2 hours.
- Chance of cardiovascular and CNS toxicity are very rare.
- The veins that can be chosen for injection site are :
    - *In thoracic limb (fore limb) :*

      i. Planter metacarpal vein

      ii. Common dorsal metacarpal vein

      iii. Radial vein
    - *In pelvic limb (hind limb) :*

      i. Cranial branch of lateral saphenous vein

      ii. Lateral planter digital vein

Chapter 25

LOCAL ANESTHETIC TECHNIQUES

Local Anesthetic Techniques of Head Region

The following nerves can be blocked in the head region for performing surgery.

1. Cornual nerve block
2. Peterson's orbital nerve block
3. Auriculopalpebral nerve block
4. Supra orbital nerve block
5. Infra orbital nerve block
6. Retro bulbar nerve block
7. Mental nerve block
8. Maxillary nerve block
9. Mandibulo alveolar nerve block

1. Cornual Nerve Block

Cornual nerve block is performed to desensitize the horn in cattle, buffalo and goats.

Indications

- Cosmetic dehorning/ disbudding in young ones.
- For treatment of horn injuries and horn cancer.

Technique

Cattle

- The Cornual nerve is a branch of the Lacrymal nerve which is a portion of Ophthalmic division of Trigeminal nerve (CLOT).
- Analgesia of the horn and base of the horn in cattle is achieved by desensitizing the cornual nerve.
- The cornual nerve passes through periorbital tissue dorsally and then runs ventral to lateral border of the frontal crest to the base of the horn.
- The needle is inserted immediately ventral to the frontal crest at a point midway between the base of the horn and the lateral canthus of the eye.
- The site is located by palpating the frontal crest where the cornual nerve passes just below the crest.
- 10 ml of 2% procaine HCl or any other local anesthetic solution is deposited subcutaneously around the nerve.
- Adult cattle and bulls with well-developed horns require extensive subcutaneous infiltration at the caudal aspect of the horn base in order to desensitize the cutaneous branches of the second cervical nerve.

Goat

- The horns and bases of the horns in goats are supplied by the cornual branches of the lacrimal and infratrochliar nerves.
- The cornual nerve is desensitized by inserting a 2.5 cm 22 gauze needle halfway between the lateral canthus of the eye and lateral base of the horn.
- 2-3 ml of a 2% lignocaine HCl solution is injected in the adult goat.
- A second injection is made midway between the medial canthus of the eye and medial base of the horn to desensitize the infratrochlear nerve.

Buffalo

- In case of buffalo the cornual nerve lies about 4 cm deep into the temporal fossa.

- To block the cornual nerve the needle is inserted midway between the lateral canthus of the eye and the base of the horn in a medio-ventral direction just below the frontal crest about 4 cm deep into temporal fossa.
- Desensitization of the area is achieved by depositing 10-15 ml of local anesthetic in a fan shape manner.

2. Peterson's Nerve Block

Eye enucleation is a fairly common procedure in cattle, and this technique will provide analgesia of the eye and orbit and immobilization of the globe.

Indications : Surgical management of conditions of eyeball, eye lid and horns.

Following nerves except for the optic nerve, pass through the orbital foramen and can be blocked by this technique..

- Auriculopalpebral branch (motor) of the facial nerve (VII).
- Oculomotor (III), trochlear (IV), and abducens (VI) nerves - motor innervation to the ocular muscles.
- Maxillary branch of the trigeminal nerve (V).– sensory, innervates lower eyelid, soft and hard palate, the nasal cavity, maxilla and adjoining bones, the maxillary sinus, and the region supplied by the infraorbital nerve.
- Ophthalmic branch of the trigeminal nerve – sensory, innervates the horn, upper eyelid, third eyelid, medial canthus, caudal part of nasal septum, cornea sclera, and frontal sinus.
- Optic nerve (II).

Technique

- Anesthetic is deposited anterior to orbital foramen.
- Locate the notch formed by the supraorbital process, the zygomatic arch, and the coronoid process of the mandible.
- Insert a 12-15 cm 18 gauge needle at this notch and direct it horizontally for 7-11 cm until it strikes the pterygopalatine fossa (make sure the needle is kept horizontal and that it is directed perpendicular to a sagittal plane through the head.) Withdraw the needle slightly and deposit 15 mL of 2% lidocaine. An additional 15 ml of lidocaine should be deposited slightly caudodorsally.

- This does not block the *auriculopalpebral nerve* so to keep the animal from blinking this nerve should be anesthetized separately.
- The animal will be blind in the blocked eye and will not blink. The upper eyelid will droop and the globe will protrude.
- If the eye is not being removed, an ophthalmic ointment should be applied to the eye.

3. Auriculopalpebral Nerve Block

The nerve is blocked to cause motor paralysis of the eyelids (orbicularis oculi muscles). Blocking this nerve will prevent blinking, but does not desensitize the eyelids.

Indications

- Since the animal is unable to close the eye following this block, the procedure facilitates examination of the eye or removal of foreign bodies.
- This block does not cause analgesia of the eyeball or the eyelids; topical anesthetics should be used for minor procedures like removal of foreign bodies or for subconjunctival injections.

Technique

- The needle is inserted in front of the base of the ear at the end of zygomatic arch and is introduced until its point lies at the dorsal border of the arch.
- 5-10 ml of local anesthetic solution is deposited medial to the process.

4. Mental Nerve Block

This technique used to anaesthetize the dental nerves of lower jaw at the mental foramen.

Indications

- For surgery of lower lip and lower jaw.

Technique

- The mental foramina is situated on the lateral aspect of the ramus in the middle of the interdental space in horse, or just behind the 4th incisor in the cow and buffalo or below the 1st molar in dog.

- The mental foramen is palpated by holding the lower jaw just below the angle of lip where the formina is felt as a shallow depression in the bone.
- The mental nerve is blocked by injecting local anesthetic solution into the canal (10-15 ml in horse and cattle and 1-2 ml in dog and cat).

5. Infraorbital Nerve Block

This technique is used to anesthetize the whole anterior half of the face (upper lip nostril, incisors and gums) including the cheek teeth as far as the second molar.

Indications

- Surgical management of condition of upper lip and nostrils e.g. removal of polyp, trephing the facial sinuses and extraction of canine or incisor tooth.

Technique

- Infra orbital nerve emerges from the infra orbital foramina and is located rostral to the facial tuberosity, dorsal to 1st molar tooth.
- A 4 cm long 20 gauze needle is inserted about 2.5 cm deep into the canal and 5-10 ml of 2% lignocaine is injected to block the nerve.

6. Supraorbital Nerve Block

Supraorbital nerve is a branch of the ophthalmic nerve and emerges through the supra orbital foramen and supplies sensory fibers to the upper eyelid and part of the skin of forehead.

Indications

- Operations above the upper eyelids.
- Suturing of the wounds in forehead region and
- Trephing of fontal sinus.

Technique

- The foramen is felt as a small depression midway across the supra orbital process on a vertical line running upwards from the medial angel of the eye.

- A 20 gauze, 2-3 cm long needle is used to deposit 5 ml of anesthetic solution at the site.
- In bovine, the frontal nerve does not emerges from the supraorbital foramina but sends several fibers along the supraorbital process.
- To block the nerve deposit the local anesthetic solution above the medial canthus and spread it laterally along the supra orbital process.

7. Mandibulo-alveolar Nerve Block

To desensitize the lower jaw along with its teeth and the lower lip.

Indications

- Surgical conditions of molar and incisors teeth, body of the mandible in the lower jaw, and lower lip.

Technique

Facial Approach

- The manidibular alveolar nerve is blocked at the mandibular foramen. In bovines, needle is inserted from the angle of the jaw along the medial surface of the ramus of mandible, at a point where an imaginary line along the masticatory surface of the lower molar teeth is crossed by another imaginary vertical line from the lateral cantus of the eye.
- About 20 ml of 2% lignocaine is injected at the site.

Through Mental Foramina

- A 7.5 cm, 20 gauge spinal needle is inserted through the mental foramina in to the mandibular canal as far as possible in a ventromedial direction.
- 10 ml of local anesthetic is deposited at the site to desensitize the nerve.

8. Retrobulbar Nerve Block

Indications

- Surgical management of conditions of eye ball (enucleation) and membrane nictitans.

Technique

- In medial canthus approach the needle is inserted in the fornix of the conjunctiva cranial to the nictitans dorso-medial to the operator's finger until the orbital apex is encountered.

- Approximately 15 ml of 2% xylocaine HCl is injected at the site.
- Structure desensitized includes:
  - i. Optic nerve
  - ii. Elevator palpebral muscle medial, ventral, dorsal rectus and inferior oblique (innervated by occulomotor nerve).
  - iii. Superior oblique muscle (by IV cranial nerve).
  - iv. Sensory part of eye and adenexa (V cranial nerve).
  - v. Retractor oculi muscle and lateral rectus muscle (VI cranial nerve).
  - vi. Orbicularis oculi muscle (VII cranial nerve).

Adverse Effects

- Orbital hemorrhage, direct pressure on globe, penetration of globe, damage to the optic nerve and globe.
- If the optic foramina is penetrated and local anesthetic is injected beneath the meningeal covering, epidural or subarachnoid anesthesia of brain may result which can be fatal. Risk of subarachnoid injection is minimized by aspiration check.

Anaesthesia for Laparotomy

Certain local anesthetic techniques are used for inducing anesthesia of the paralumbar fossa and abdominal wall in standing ruminant :

1. Paravertebral anesthesia (proximal or distal).
2. Epidural anesthesia.
3. Infiltration line block or inverted "L" block.
4. Subarachnoid anesthesia.

Indications

1. Rumenotomy
2. Cecotomy
3. Correction of gastrointestinal displacement, intestinal obstruction and volvulus.
4. Cesarean section
5. Ovariectomy
6. Liver or kidney biopsy
7. Diaphragmatic hernia

1. Paravertebral Anesthesia

It refers to the deposition of local anesthesia near the spinal nerves as they emerge from the vertebral canal through the intervertebral foramina.

Indications

- For surgical operations at the lumbar and paralumbar regions.
- Standing laparotomy surgery e.g. Caesarean section, rumenotomy, cecotomy, correction of gastrointestinal displacement, intestinal obstruction and volvulus.

Technique

Proximal Paravertebral block (Farquharson, Hall or Cambridge technique):

- The dorsal aspect of the transverse processes of the last thoracic (T-13) and first and second lumbar (L-1 and L-2) vertebrae is the site for needle placement.
- The dorsal and ventral nerves roots of the last thoracic (T-13) and first and second lumbar (L-1 and L-2) spinal nerves emerge from the intervertebral foramina are desensitized.
- 10-20 ml of 2% lidocaine is injected to each site.
- Onset occurs usually within 10 minutes of injection.
- Scoliosis towards the desensitized site indicates effective block

Dorsal and ventral branch of nerve are desensitized	Site
T-13	Front of transverse process of L-1
L-1	Front of transverse process of L-2
L-2	Front of transverse process of L-3

Distal Paravertebral Block (Magda, Cakala or Cornell Technique)

- The dorsal and ventral branches of the last thoracic (T-13) and first and second lumbar (L-1 and L-2) spinal nerves are desensitized at the distal ends of L-1, L-2 and L-4.
- A 7.5 cm, 18 gauze needle is inserted ventral to the tips of the respective transverse process where approximately 10-20 ml of a 2 % lidocaine solution is injected in fan shaped infiltration pattern.

- The needle is withdrawn and reinserted dorsal to the transverse process and local anesthetic is deposited as above.
- The procedure is repeated for the second and forth lumbar transverse processes.

Paravertebral block	Advantages	Disadvantages
1. Proximal	1. Small quantity of local anesthetic is needed so chances of local anesthetic toxicity are less. 2. Increased intestinal tone and motility.	1. Arching of the spine due to paralysis of the back muscles. 2. Risk of penetrating the aorta and thoracic longitudinal vein on the left side and the caudal vena cava on the right side.
2. Distal	1. Very less chance of penetrating major blood vessels. 2. Lack of scoliosis. 3. Minimal weakness in the hind limb and ataxia.	1. Larger doses of local anesthetics are needed.

2. Epidural Anesthesia or Spinal Anesthesia

Anesthesia caused by injection of local anesthetic out side the duramater is called epidural anesthesia. Injection into the CSF is termed as subarachnoid (subdural) or intrathecal anesthesia. The local anesthesia first desensitizes the sensory nerves followed by sacral, parasympathetic, sympathetic and motor nerves.

Anatomical Consideration

- The epidural space is the compartment between the duramater and the bony and ligamentous walls of the spinal canal.
- The spinal nerves, as they leave the duramater, cross this epidural space before exiting from the spinal canal through the intervertebral foramina.
- Injection of local anesthetic in to this space will desensitize the spinal nerves.

Indications

- Prevention of straining, reduction of prolapsed vagina, uterus and rectum.

- Treatment of parturient injuries.
- Amputation of tail.
- Urethrotomy
- Correction of atresia ani or atresia ani et recti, amputation of rectum, anal tumor surgery, anal sac extirpation.
- Repair of perineal fistula.
- Caslick's operation, laceration of vulva and vagina, recto-vaginal fistula and episiotomy etc.

Techniques

A. Hanging Drop Technique

- This technique involves filling of the hub of the needle with saline or anesthetic solution and allowing one drop to hang from the hub.
- As the needle penetrates the ligamentum flavum, the negative pressure in the epidural space will draw the drop of the anesthetic in to the needle, indicating proper placement in the epidural space.
- A popping sound is felt when the needle passed through the ligamentum flavum.

B. Lack of Resistance Technique

- Prevention of straining, reduction of prolapsed vagina, uterus and rectum. If the needle is properly placed in the epidural space, there is least resistance to the injection of local anesthetic/air.

> *After placing the needle in the epidural space, it is important to aspirate to rule out the possibility of administering drug in to the venous sinus (presence of blood) or subarachnoid space (presence of CSF)*

Site of Injection in Different Domestic Animals

- The area blocked by epidural anesthesia depends on site of injection.
- Common sites used in veterinary practice are the lumbo-sacral space, sacrococcygeal or intercoccygeal space. Segmental block by using other points can be done.
- High/anterior epidural block: If the block extends to the segment from which the sciatic nerves arises, the second sacral, and to more cranial segments.

- Low/caudal epidural block: If this segment is not reached. The extent to which the analgesia extends will depend on the amount of local anesthetic solution given. If the dose is increased, it is known as high caudal epidural block.
- The anatomical terms caudal, lumbo-sacral and thoracic epidural refers to the site of injection of the local anesthetic in to the epidural space.
  1. Cattle and buffalo - Sacro-coccygeal or 1st intercoccygial space.
  2. Sheep and goat - Sacro-coccygeal space
  3. Dog and Cat - Sacro-coccygial or 1st intercoccygeal space.
  4. Horse - 1st intercoccygeal space (because last sacral vertebrae is fused with 1st coccygeal vertebrae).

Bovine

- In bovines spinal cord ends in the region of the last lumbar vertebra, but the meningeal sac goes to the 3rd/ 4th sacral segments.
- For caudal epidural anesthesia, the injection site used is either sacro-coccygeal space or 1st intercoccygeal space.
- The site is located by raising tail in "pump handle" fashion and palpating the depression and movement between the respective vertebrae.
- In older bovines, the S_5 - Co_1 space has ossified, thus Co_1 - Co_2 is the site used for anesthesia.
- The skin over the site is prepared aseptically and desensitized with 2-3 ml of local anesthetic.
- A 5 cm long, 18 gauze needle is inserted in the center of the space either at right angle to the general contour of the croup or ventro-cranially at an angle of approximately 10^0 to vertical.
- A maximum dose of 1.0 ml/ kg body weight will give analgesia to the middle of the sacrum, over the perineum and the inner aspect of the thigh.
- Onset of paralysis of tail should occur in 1-2 minutes. The block lasts for 1-2 hours.
- Larger doses will produce increasingly anterior effects like posterior ataxia.
- A high caudal epidural using 10 ml/ 100 kg (2% lidocaine) with maximum dose of 120 ml is sufficient for surgery of hind limbs, mammary tissue, flanks and abdominal wall.

- Epidural xylazine alone may be suitable for analgesia for laparotomies in cows. The dose used is 0.07 mg/kg diluted to a volume of 7 ml with normal saline.
- Injection of local anesthetic can be carried out at the lumbo-sacral junction in order to produce an anterior block with less anesthetic.

Equine

- The site for injection is the first coccygeal interspace (Co_1 - Co_2). It is the first movable joint caudal to the sacrum.
- The site is located by raising tail in "pump handle" fashion and palpating the depression.
- A 7.5 cm, 18 gauge spinal needle is inserted in the center of the intercoccygeal space at an angle of about 30^0 to the horizontal until it strikes the floor of the vertebral canal.
- The needle is then withdrawn slightly and injection is made.
- A 500 kg horse will require 5-7 ml of 2% lidocaine with epinephrine to desensitize the rectum, vagina, bladder and urethra.
- If more than 10 ml is given it may block motor supply to the hind limbs and the horse will go down.
- The time of onset is 10-30 minutes (longer than bovines because of more amount of epidural fat).
- High epidural is not used in the horse because of the danger of the horse becoming excited when it losses motor control of the hind limbs.

Dogs and Cats

- Epidurals in dogs and cats are also performed at the lumbosacral space.
- Place the animal on its sternum with the hind legs tucked underneath or in lateral recumbency with the legs extended and pulled forward to open up the space.
- The site for needle placement is on the midline, just caudal to a transverse line between the cranial prominences of the wing of the ileum on either side.
- Make sure to aspirate before injecting. Strict asepsis is essential.
- A 24 to 20 ga, 3.75 to 5 cm needle is used. The needle can be felt to penetrate the interarcuate ligament and there is lack of resistance to injection. Sometimes a small quantity of air is injected first to ensure that the needle is in the correct position.

- A dose of 1 mL of lidocaine or 0.5% bupivacaine for 5 kg body weight will give analgesia up to about T_{11} or T_{12}. This is adequate for operations on the limbs or for a laparotomy.
- The epidural route is now being used for the administration of opioids for post-operative analgesia. This route has many advantages over intravenous or intramuscular administration.

Complications

- Infection- all the procedure should be done aseptically.
- Some times subarachnoid injection causes irritation which may lead to spinal damage.
- In large animals motor paralysis of the hind limbs may occur.
- Injections should be made slowly in epidural anesthesia. Sometimes severe hypotension may occur specially in ruminants when sympathetic vasoconstrictor fibers to the abdominal viscera are blocked.
- Severe respiratory depression with hypotension may occur if local anesthesia is deposited into subarachroid cavity accidentally. Controlled or assisted ventilation together with intravenous injection of vasopressor drugs is essential if convulsions occur, intravenous injection of thiobarbiturates is indicated.

Advantages

- It is safe in pregnant animals or there is no effect of anesthetic on the fetus.
- No respiratory assistance is required.
- Single injection provides excellent analgesia, muscular relaxation and reduced bleeding during operation in lumbo-sacral analgesia.
- Meningitis and other neurological sequlae are less common as compared to subarachnoid injections.

Segmental Dorsolumbar Epidural Anesthesia or Arthur Block

Indications

- Induction of anesthesia and relaxation of the abdominal wall and flank for operations such as rumenotomy, cesarean section with the animal maintaining in standing position.
- Laparotomy, nephrectomy, abdominal or ventral hernia and spleenectomy etc.

Technique

- The anesthetic agent is injected in the epidural space either between the first and second lumbar (L_1 and L_2) vertebra or less commonly between the T_{13} and L_1 in cattle to desensitize the right and left flank without causing the hind limb paralysis.
- The first lumbar (L_1 - L_2) intervertebral space in cattle is located 1.5-2.0 cm caudal to an imaginary line drawn across the back from the cranial edge of the transverse process of the L_2.
- The needle is advanced through the interossious canal until an abrupt reduction in needle passage is noted. At this point the needle has reached the epidural space.
- Approximately 8 ml of 2% Lignocaine HCl in an average 500 kg cow are injected. Analgesia develops within 7-20 minutes and persists for 45 to 120 minutes.
- The epidural intervertebral space at T_{13} – L_1 or L_1 – L_2 in cattle can not be reached by the spinal needle if the interarcuate ligament is ossified due to old age (> 8 years).
- Rapid onset and duration of anesthesia can be increased by increasing concentration of the anesthetic.

3 a. Infiltration Line Block

- In any species analgesia can be provided by infiltration of the surgical site with local anesthetic.
- The volume used will depend on the size of the animal and the area to be blocked.
- The advantages of this technique are that it requires no great skill or knowledge of anatomy.
- It does have disadvantages which include having large volumes of anesthetic in the tissues to be incised and sutured.
- Epinephrine in the anesthetic solution may also interfere with the blood supply and retard healing.
- If a flank laparotomy is being done local anesthetic must not only be infiltrated subcutaneously but into the muscles and fascia as well.

b. Inverted 'L' Block

- This technique (done for flank laparotomies) is a nonspecific regional analgesic technique in which all the nerves entering the surgical field are desensitized.

- Lidocaine is injected into the tissues bordering the dorsocaudal aspect of the last rib and ventrolateral aspect of the lumbar transverse processes.
- Advantages include deposition of the anesthetic away from the surgical site thus decreasing edema and hematoma formation from the block.
- Disadvantages include incomplete analgesia and muscle relaxation of the deeper layers of the abdominal wall.

Local Anaesthesia of Limbs

1. Brachial Plexus Block

Nerves arise from the plexus are :

- Suprascapular nerve.
- Subscapular nerve.
- Anterior thoracic nerve.
- Posterior thoracic nerve.
- Long thoracic nerve.
- Thoracodorsal nerve.
- Axillary nerve.
- Musculocutaneous nerve.
- Median nerve.
- Ulnar nerve.
- Radial nerve.

Indications

Surgical conditions at or below the elbow joint.

Technique

- It can be blocked in standing position or in lateral recumbency keeping the side to be anaesthetized upper most.
- Long needles are required.
- The position of the shoulder joint and the costo-chondral junction of the first rib are located. The forelimb may be drawn backward during this process. The needle is inserted in the triangular depression bounded by supraspinatous muscle to the level of spine of scapula and local anesthetic is injected at this site.
- Dose - 3-5 ml of 2% procaine in dog and 20-30 ml in cattle.

- Before injecting the local anaesthetic agent the syringe should be aspirated to make sure that no blood vessel is punctured.
- The characteristics posture adopted by the animal after successful block of brachial plexus is of radial paralysis.

2. Radial Nerve Block

Indications : Surgical condition below the elbow joint.

Technique

- The nerve is blocked as it spirals around the humerus from medial to lateral surface at a point midway between the olecranon and the acromian process.
- The needle is penetrated in the depression felt between the long and lateral heads of the triceps brachii muscle which is located on the posterior aspect of upper 3rd of humerus.
- 2-4 ml of 2% lignocaine is injected at the site.

3. Median Nerve Block

- Median nerve is sensory nerve to the medial and dorsal surfaces of the digit except for a narrow band on the lateral aspect which is supplied by ulnar nerve.
- It innervates to :
  - i. Flexor carpi radialis.
  - ii. Superficial and deep digital flexors.
  - iii. Pronator teres.
  - iv. Pronator quadratus.
- The nerve lies 1-2 cm deep between the flexor carpi radialis muscle and the radius bone below the insertion of the anterior superficial pectoral muscle.

  Indication : Median neurectomy.

Technique

- In cattle, the median nerve is located on the medial aspect of the elbow joint covered only by the skin and fascia, a little cranial to the medial epicondyle of the humorous.
- About 10-20 ml of 2% lignocaine solution is injected at the site.

4. Ulnar Nerve Block

- Ulnar nerve is the sensory nerve to the caudomedial and caudolateal parts of the forearm and the lactarl aspect of digits.
- It supplies innervations to the flexor carpi ulnaris, superficial and deep flexors and intrinsic muscles of digits.

  Indications : Tenotomy.

Technique

- This nerve is located behind the medial epicondyle of the humerus.
- It is blocked about 7-8 cm above the accessory carpal bone in the depression between the muscle ulnaris lateralis and flexor carpi ulnaris.
- About 10 ml of 2% lignocaine is deposited at the site.

5. Musculocutaneous Nerve Block

- It is a sensory nerve to the major part of the medial side of forearm (some part of upper fore arm is also supplied by axillary nerve) and partly to the medial aspect of fetlock along with the median nerve.

  Indications : Operations on medial and dorso anterior aspect of the carpus.

Technique

- In cattle, the needle is inserted about 6-8 cm above the proximal end of the carpus on the dorsal surface of forearm, medial to the tendon sheath of extensor carpi radialis up to the depth of radius bone and then the needle is directed medially over the bone.
- 10-15 ml of 2% lignocaine is deposited at the site.

6. Peroneal Nerve Block

- The peroneal nerve innervates tiblia, long medial and lateral digital extensors and peroneus longus muscle.
- This block desensitizes the antero-lateral part of leg and antero-medial part of fetlock joint.

  Indications : Diagnosis of lameness.

Technique

- This nerve is blocked immediately behind the posterior edge of the lateral condyle of tibia.
- 20 ml 2% lignocaine is deposited at the site.

7. Tibial Nerve Block

- The tibial nerve supplies the innervations to the muscle gastronemius, superficial and deep digital flexors, popliteus and tibialis posterior muscles.
- The tibial nerve block will desensitize the posteromedial and posterolateral aspect little above the hock.

  Indications : Diagnosis of lameness and tibial neurectomy.

Technique

- The nerve is blocked by inserting the needle about 10 cm above the hock between the tendo achilles and digital extensor on the medial aspect of the limb.
- 15-20 ml of 2% lignocaine is deposited under the fascia.

Miscellaneous Local Anesthetic Techniques

Analgesia of the Interdigital Space

- The procedure is similar for both fore and hind limbs.
- The axial digital nerves on the dorsal aspect of the limb are blocked immediately below the level of the fetlock.
- A 2.5 cm 21g-auge needle is inserted subcutaneously and 5 ml of a 2% solution of lidocaine with epinephrine injected.
- Following this injection a 10 cm 18 or 16 gauge needle is inserted perpendicularly through the skin immediately above the interdigital cleft and pushed through until the point of the needle can be felt behind the foot, again immediately above the interdigital space 10 to 15 mL of a 2% solution of lidocaine with epinephrine is injected as the needle is withdrawn.
- The interdigital space is desensitized, allowing for surgery for such operations as removal of corns.

Analgesia for Castration

- Analgesia can be provided by injecting local anesthetic solution either into the spermatic cord or directly into the testicle.
- With either technique, the incision site should be infiltrated subcutaneously with local anesthetic.
- To inject the spermatic cords, gently pull down on the scrotum to tense the cords then inject 5 mL of lidocaine with epinephrine into each cord.

- Be sure the needle is in the cord and not just subcutaneous.
- To inject into the testicle, insert a 7 cm needle midway along the posterior border of the testicle and perpendicular to the testicle.
- Insert the needle deep to the center of the testicle and inject 10-15 mL of 2% lidocaine with epinephrine.

Internal Pudendal Nerve Block in Cattle

- This technique is used most commonly for penile relaxation and analgesia.
- The lesser sciatic foramen is located by rectal palpation as a soft circumscribed depression in the sacrosciatic ligament.
- The internal pudendal nerve is found a finger's width dorsal to the pulsating pudendal artery present in the fossa.
- The skin over the ischiorectal fossa on both sides is disinfected and is then desensitized with 2-3 mL of lidocaine.
- A 8-10 cm long 8 gauge needle is inserted and directed toward the nerve. One hand is left in the rectum to palpate for the placement of the needle.
- Twenty to 25 ml of 2% lidocaine with epinephrine is injected around the nerve.
- The procedure is repeated to the opposite side.
- Penile relaxation and cutaneous analgesia over the anus, perineum, posteriomedial thigh, and urethral opening can be expected.

Teat and Udder Analgesia

- The udder is supplied primarily from nerve fibers originating from the third and fourth lumbar spinal cord segments, which form the genitofemoral nerve.
- Caudally the udder is supplied by the mammary branch of the pudendal nerve and distal cutaneous branch of the perineal nerve, which have their origin from the second, third, and fourth sacral spinal cord segments.
- The skin and some glandular tissue of the forequarters are supplied by the L1 and L2.
- Paravertebral analgesia of L1, 2, and 3 will result in analgesia to the fore udder and fore teats.

- Surgical procedures of the teat alone are generally performed with a ring block at the base of the teat.
- There is potential for the use of xylazine epidurals alone or preferably with local anesthesia supplementation for standing surgery on the teats and udder.
- General anesthesia or a high caudal epidural with local anesthetic may be necessary for major surgery on the udder.

Chapter 26

ACUPUNCTURE

Acus means needle. It is an ancient Chinese system of therapy utilizing long fine needles at specific points and their stimulation by various means to induce analgesia and to cure certain diseases. The specific points are known as acupuncture points or acupoints.

The procedure is safe. There are no post anaesthetic complications and can be used in poor surgical risk patients. The major disadvantage is poor muscle relaxation. Acupuncture has been used to produce local anaesthesia.

Acupoints : Alphanumeric code system is used to recognize the acupoints universally e.g. BL, LI, SP, GB etc means meridians of the urinary bladder, large intestine, spleen, gall bladder etc. respectively.

Various acupuncture points differ in their physiological behaviour, electrical response and therapeutic role. The acupuncture are located on the imaginary horizontal lines known as meridians which have internal connections with the organs from which the meridian or channel gets the name. More than 360 points exist in the body. The Chinese believe that the vital energy 'chi' flows through these pathways.

There are 12 organs meridians :

	Symbol	Organ	Points
1.	LU	Lung	11
2.	LI	Large intestine	20
3.	ST	Stomach	45
4.	SP	Spleen	25
5.	H	Heart	9
6.	SI	Small intestine	19
7.	BL/UB	Urinary bladder	67
8.	K	Kidney	27
9.	P	Pericardium	9
10.	TH/TW	Triheater/ Triwarmer	23
11.	GB	Gall bladder	44
12.	LIV	Liver	14

There are 2 non-organ meridians :

i. GOV (Governor vessel, 28 points)

ii. COV (Conception vessel 24 points).

- Acupuncture technique can be used to produce anaesthesia of the abdominal wall.

Acupoints

No. 1 TW-8 (Sanyangluo) : This point is located on the lateral aspect of the forelimb about 10 cm below in the lateral groove e.g. 2.5-5 cm distal to the lateral ligament of the radius. The needle at this point is inserted at an angle of 20^0 along the caudal border of the radius and passed caudomedially to a depth of 6-10 cm.

No. 2 LU-1 (Chcngfu) : This point is located at the second intercostal space just caudal to the shoulder joint.

No. 3 Tongquiao (Tongoiao) : This point is located on the dorsolateral aspect of the most proximal part of the 7th intercostal space and below the caudal angel of scapula. The needle is passed cranioventrally to a depth of 3-4 cm.

No. 4 SANTAI : This point is located on the dorsomediamline at the center of the depression between the spines of 4th and 5th thoracic vertebrae. The needle is inserted vertically to a depth of 6-8 cm.

No. 5 Tianping : This point is located on the dorsomedian line between the neural spines of the 13th thoracic and 1st lumbar vertebrae. The needle is passed vertically to a depth of 2.5-4 cm. The same point was named as T4 celestial peace (Tienping) by Klide and Kung.

No. 6 Yaopang : This is located on the dorsolateral aspect at the tip of the 1st lumbar transverse process. The needle should pass cranioventrally to a depth of 5-6 cm and allowed to slide under the wing of transverse process pointing at the body of last thoracic vertebra.

No. 7 : GOV 4 (MINGMEN) : It is located on the dorsomedian line at the center of the depression between the second and 3rd lumbar spines. The needle is inserted vertically to a depth of 3.5 –4.0 cm.

No. 8. YAOPANG-II : This point is located on the dorso lateal aspect at the tip of the second lumbar transverse process. The needle is passed cranioventrally to a depth of 5.5-6.0 cm and allowed to slide under the transverse process. The tip of the needle is pointed at the body of the 1st lumbar vertebra.

No. 9. YAOPANG-III : The point is located on the dorsolateral aspect at the tip of the 3rd lumbar transverse process. The needle at this point is passed cranioventrally to a depth of 5.5-6.0 cm and allowed to slide under the transverse process. The tip of the needle is pointed at the body of the 2nd lumbar verteibra.

No. 10. GOV-20 (BAIHUI) : This point is located on the dorsomedian line in the center of the depression between the supraspinous process of the last lumbar and 1st sacral vertebrae. Depth and direction of the needle is 3-5 cm perpendicularly penetrating the fascia, supraspinous ligament and extending up to the diameter. This point was named as No. 68 by Westermayer.

No. 11. BL-30 (BAIHUANSHU) : This point is located at the caudal part of the lateral sacral crest and about 10 cm from the mid dorsal line. Depth and direction of the needle is 1.0-1.5 cm, passed subcutaneous in a cranioventral direction.

No. 12. WEIGAN : This is a governor vessel. Meridian point located on the mid dorsal line of the tail at the center of the depression between the 2nd and 3rd coccygeal vertebrae. Depth and direction of the needle is 1-1.5 cm vertically.

No. 13. DAZHUAN : This point is located on the lateral aspect of the gluteal region, immediately above the acetabular brim. Direction and depth of the needle is 3-4 cm crani ventrally.

No. 14. LIV I4 (CHIMEM) : This point is located on the lateral aspect of the thorax at the 8th intercostal space and in level with the shoulder joint. The needle is inserted subcutaneously in a cranio-ventral direction to a depth of 3-6 cm.

NO. 15. ST 36 (TSU-SAN-LI) : This point is located at the dorsolateral aspect of the hind limb, about 5 cm distal to the head of the fibula, near the base of the tibial crest. The needle is inserted obliquely and distally through the subcutaneous tissue to a distance of 3-4 cm.

No. 16. SP-6 (SAN-YIN-JIAO) : This point is located on the medial surface of the hind limb caudal to the tibia and approximately 3.0 cm proximal to the medial malleolus. The needle is inserted subcutaneously in the proximal direction for 3-4 cm.

Acupoint	Corresponds to
No. 1 : TW-8 (SANYANGLUO)	P 4-5 (YAN YAN LO-YIE YIN) and FL-23 described by Klide and Kung.
NO. 3 : Tongquiao	Point described by Sun and colleagues for white cattle
No. 4 : Santai	Point No. 80 of Westermayer and T_2 (Three platforms santai) of Klide and Kung.
No. 5 : Tianping	Point No. 64 described by Westermayer for cattle
No. 6 : Yaopang I	Oint No. 80 of Westermayer for cattle
No. 10	Point No. 68 of Westermayer
No. 12	Identical point described by Sun in cattle and point No. 71 of Westermayer.
No. 15	Point No. 132 of Westermeyer.

Various acupoints are located with the help of a acupuncture search probe designed on the principles of low skin electrical resistance or impidance. The probe provides an audiovisual signal whenever it touches the point of least electrical impedance. A distinct sound of audio-indicator and maximum brightness of visual indicator occur when the search probe comes into contact with a acupoint.

Acupoints exhibit electric impedance

- In goats – 200 kilo ohms
- In buffalo calves – 100-200 kilo ohms.
- Non acupoint shows – one megaohms.
- If moisture content on skin is not uniform, many false point can be found.

Annexure-1

S. No.	Anesthetic agent	Canine (Dog)	Feline (Cat)	Ovine (sheep)	Caprine (Goat)	Bovine (Cattle and Buffalo)	Equine (Horse)	Swine (Pig)
1.	Atropine sulphate	0.02-0.04 S.C./I.M	0.02-0.04 S.C./I.M	0.7	0.7	0.04-0.06	-	0.06-0.08
2.	Chlorpromazine	1.0 I.V. 2.0 I.M	1.0 I.M	1.0 IV	1.0 IV	0.3 IM	-	0.2-0.3 IM/IV max dose 100 mg
3.	Triflu promazine	1-2 IV, 2-4 IM	4 I.M	1.0 IV	0.2-0.3 IM	0.1 IV max 40 mg	-	-
4.	Aupromazine maliate	0.03-0.1 Max 3 mg IV, IM or SC	0.03-0.1	-	0.5-1.0 IM	0.5-1.0 IM	0.02-0.05 IV, IM, SC	0.5-1.0 IM
5.	Diazepam	0.5-1.01 IV, 1.0-2.0 IM	0.5-1.0 I.M	0.5-1.0 IM	0.1-0.3 IM	0.1-0.03 IM	0.05-0.2 IV	2-4 IM, 1.0-2.0 IV
6.	Xylazine	1-2 IM	1-2 I.M	1-2 IM	-	10-40	1.0-2.1 IM, 0.4-1.1 IV	-
7.	Detomidine	5 20	-	-	-	-	10-40	-
8.	Thiopental Sodium	20 mg/kg IV, 15 mg/kg IV with Premedication	-	-	-	2 mg/kg IV	-	-
9.	Ketamine	2.5 mg/kg IV	-	-	-		2.2 mg/kg, IV	-

Technique

Stainless steel solid, filiform, shafted needles with silver or silver plated spirally wound handle are used. The diameter of needles ranges from 26-34 G and the length ranges from 1.5-14 cm.

Moxibustion : It is a form of point cautery, and has also been used restricted to treat chronic conditions.

- Methods used to provide stimulus for acupuncture : Mechanical, thermal, chemical, electronic and light stimulation.
- Mechanical needling and electronic stimulation are commonly used to produce anaesthesia.
- For electronic stimulation, a electro puncture unit capable of delivering biphasic square, biphasic spike and dense disperse wave forms of pulses (produce least discomfort to animal) with a frequency range of 0-323 Hz along with a pulse width of 2.2 mm is used.
- Generally a current of 35-100 mA and a frequency of 120-200 Hz is sufficient for stimulation of acupoints. The current is reduced to the level of tolerance when animal shows symptoms of uneasiness by bellowing and rapid respirations. Perfect local anaesthesia develops in 20-30 minutes.
- The exact location of acupoints is absolutely essential for successful acupuncture anaesthesia.
- Moderate muscle relaxation along with analgesia develops in 20-30 minutes after onset of stimulation.

Section-II
EXERCISES

Exercise 1

Objective :
General Consideration for Set up of an Operation Theatre

Operation theatre (OT) is a place where surgical operations are performed under the principle of aseptic surgery. An ideal operation theatre :

- Should be located near the work and intensive care areas of the hospital.
- Should be independent of general traffic. One way traffic flow is maintained to ensure sterility.
- If possible, air within the OT should be under mild positive pressure so that when the surgery room opened, air flows out of rather than into the room.
- Floors, walls and ceilings should be constructed of impervious material that can easily be cleaned and disinfected.
- The lighting of the OT should entirely be dependent on artificial light.
- Room temperature should be about 70^0F with a relative humidity of about 50% provides a better environment for the surgeon and patient.

The various components of the OT are :

1. Patient's preparation room
2. Surgeon's preparation room
3. Sterile operation room

4. Intensive care and recovery room
5. Visitors gallery

1. Patient's Preparation Room

Preparation of patient must be completed in a separate room. It should be well lighted with facilities of clipping, washing, stainless steel sink with hot and cold water supplies. For large animal surgery, an open space with facility of Trevis and restraining of animals like horse stock and cattle chute can be used. The preparation room should have space for preanaesthetics, syringes, needles, intravenous catheters, laryngoscope, endotracheal tubes and oxygen cylinder. Clippers fitted with blade should be located on the wall immediately adjacent to table. A refrigerator, a dressing bin and a suction apparatus should also be kept inside preparation room.

2. Surgeon's Preparation Room

This room should be directly connected to the operation room. It should be equipped with stainless steel washbasin with both hot and cold water supply fitted with elbow or knee operated tap. It should have the following facilities :

- Surgical scrub and brush for scrubbing hands and nails of surgical team.
- Stainless steel sink with soap dispenser.
- Hangers for hanging unsterilized clothing of surgical team.

3. Sterile Operation Room

Surgical interventions are carried out in this room. All individuals in this room should worn sterile cloths. Anyone approaching the surgical field must wear sterile cap, face mask, shoe covers, gown and gloves. This room should have the following facilities :

- Operation table
- Anaesthetic apparatus
- Shadow less lamp
- Instrument trolley
- Equipments for resuscitation
- Pulse oxymeter
- ECG machine
- X-ray viewer
- Soiled dressing bin

x. Cattle chute/stock/trevis for large animal surgery
xi. Close circuit camera assembly
xii. Equipments as per requirement.

i. *Operation table* : It should be constructed of stainless steel with hydraulic raise-lower, tilt and V-trough facilities as per requirement of surgeon and comfort to the animal. For large animal surgery, it should be padded and should have headrests.

ii. *Shadow less lamp* : It is used for proper illumination at the operation site. It originates light from different angles and converge at the site of operation without causing shadow of surgeon's head or instruments. It may be ceiling mounted or stand mounted. The light emitted should produce a maximum of 25-microwatt/cm^2 heat to minimize drying of operating site and comfort to surgeons. It should be placed one meter away from the surgical field.

iii. *Anaesthetic apparatus/ Boyl's apparatus* : It is used for maintaining inhalation anaesthesia and can be used for resuscitation or for positive pressure ventilation.

iv. *Instrument trolley* : It should be placed near the operation table for keeping surgical instruments during operation.

v. *Resuscitation apparatus* :

   i. *Ventilator* : It is used for giving artificial respiration. Bird mark 2 and 7 are mostly used for small and large animal surgery respectively.

   ii. *Cardiac defibrillator* : It is used to stimulate heartbeat at the time of cardiac failure.

   iii. *Oxygen cylinder* : It is used for giving extra oxygen during respiratory failure.

   iv. *Emergency drugs* : Anaesthetic antagonists, cardiac and respiratory stimulants.

vi. *Soiled dressing bin/kick bucket* : This is used to store waste material during operation to minimize contamination of surgical area.

vii. *X-ray viewer* : It is used to visualize radiographs of various body parts/ organs of surgical interest and should be placed at one corner of operation theatre.

viii. *Pulse oxymeter* : It is used to visualize the percent oxygen saturation of hemoglobin. It gives additional strength to the anaesthetist.

ix. *Instruments as per requirement* : For specialized surgery -
- ❒ Suction pump
- ❒ ECG machine
- ❒ Instruments for laparoscopic surgery
- ❒ Thermocautry/electroautry
- ❒ Operating microscope

4. Intensive Care and Recovery Room

This room should be directly connected to main operating room. After operation, the animal is transferred to this room and kept up to complete recovery. After starting of swallowing reflex the endotracheal tube should be removed.

For large animal, it should have well-padded floor and walls. There should be animal transportation trolley. This room should have all monitoring instruments with emergency facilities like :

a. Positive pressure ventilation
b. Fluid therapy
c. ECG equipment
d. Oscilloscope for monitoring heart rate, respiration rate and rectal temperature.
e. Emergency drugs
f. Room temperature controlling device.

5. Visitors' Gallery

This gallery is separated from the OT by a glass wall so the visitor can see the surgical procedure. Now a day, this can be done by CCTV.

Note

i. There should be a surgery room outside the OT for operating contaminated cases like pyothorax, draining of sinus tract and perianal fistula etc.
ii. The operation theatre should be cleaned daily and disinfected at least once weekly.
iii. Sterilized swabs for culture should be taken time to time from OT.

Question

1. Sketch a flow diagram of OT.

Exercise 2

Objective : Preparation of General Surgical Pack

Surgical pack : It is sterilized bundle containing the conventional surgical instruments and drapes etc. required for routine surgical operation.

Common surgical instruments: These instruments are used in routine general surgery and made up of stainless steel. Stainless steel not only has excellent strength but also resistant to corrosion. The general instruments are:

1. *Towel clamp* : It is used to hold the drape in position. It has pointed ends so that drape does not slipped away from the area of operation. Small amount of skin is grasped to secure the drape. It is of two types :

a. Backhause towel clamp

b. Cross action towel clamp

2. *Bard Parker knife / scalpel (B.P. handle with blade)* : Bard Parker knife is available as disposable knife. BP handle is available with changeable blades.

B.P. handle No.	Holds surgical blade No.
3	9,10,11,12,14,15,16,17,18
4	20, 21, 22, 23, 24

The scalpel or knife is the primary cutting instrument of the surgeon. It is used for the sharp division of the tissue to cause minimal trauma to the tissues. A single stroke is more efficient and less traumatic and more likely to produce a smooth edge than multiple small cuts. The scalpel can be used for incising, puncturing or for debridement of tissue. The longest possible blade surface should be in contact with the skin rather than the shortest. For this the angel between the tissue surface and blade should be 30-40°C. The thumb, middle of ring fingers are used to grip the handle which rests in the palm of the hand. The index finger is placed on the upper edge of the cutting blade for stability. It should neither touch the skin nor obstruct the surgeon's view of the incision line.

3. *Tissue forceps* : They are used to grasp tissue. These forceps are of following types :
   - *Allis tissue forceps* : Consist of two blades and the grasping surface or tips. Tip have teeth, which are arranged in odd manner i.e. 3/4 or 4/5 etc. It is used in pair for holding and retracting the wound edges to facilitate deeper exposure during operation.
   - *Rat tooth forceps* : Consist of two blades with jaw having rat tooth like structure. It is used on the skin and other hard tissues.
   - *Thumb forceps* : Consist of two blades with jaw having transverse serrations at their ends. It is used for holding soft tissues and viscera.
4. *Mayo's scissors* : They can be classified on the basis of shape of blades e.g. straight or curved or on the basis of blade points like blunt-blunt, sharp-sharp, sharp-blunt. Scissors are used for dissection through the subcutaneous tissue after the use of B.P. knife. Straight scissors are used close to the surface of body, whereas curved scissors are used for deep structures. Scissors are also used for blunt separation of tissue by inserting the points and opening the handle. The surgeon must hold the scissors with the ring finger and thumb inserted in the ring of the scissors with the index finger guiding the scissors by its placement over the box joint.
5. *Haemostats* : are used to clamp and hold the cut ends of blood vessels to achieve haemostasis. They vary in size, shape of jaw and in the direction of serration present on inside surface of tip.
   a. *Small haemostats* – Mosquito haemostats (i) Straight (ii) Curved
   b. *Large haemostats* – (i) Oschner's haemostate – curved with rat tooth at the tip. (ii) Coker's haemostat – straight with rat tooth at the tip.

Guideline for the use of haemostats :

a. Use the smallest haemostat as far as possible.

b. Bleeder should be grasped by the tip of instrument and grasp only as much tissue as necessary.

c. When using curved haemostat, the curved portion of the haemostat should come down to hold bleeder.

d. Apply haemostats perpendicular to the tissue.

6. *Needle holder* : It is used to hold suturing needle for suturing. It has a long shank with a locking device and short stout jaws. The jaws have transverse serration and a deep longitudinal groove in the middle of both jaws. During suturing the needle holder and suture materials are held with the shank in the plam of the hand and the index finger on the box joint. Suture needle is grasped by the middle of the needle holder jaws, about one third the distance from the eye of suturing needle. Needle holders are of three types :

   a. Mayo's hegar needle holder.

   b. Mcphail's needle holder.

   c. Gillis's needle holder cum scissors.

7. *Groove director* : It has a groove in its blades portion which facilitates incising of tissues without damaging underlying structures.

8. *Suturing needles* : Can be classified on the basis of size, shape and curvature of suturing needle.

   a. Size - 1 to 18 No.

   b. Shape - (i) Circular (non-cutting or atraumatic) (ii) Triangular (cutting or traumatic)

   c. Curvature - (i) Staight (ii) Curved - full circle, half circle, one forth, two third circle.

      - Atraumatic needles are used for suturing hypervascularized tissues e.g. visceral organs, muscular tissues etc.

      - Traumatic needles are used for suturing skin, ligaments, tendons and other hard tissues.

      - Swaged on needle (Eyeless needles) - made for single use. Suturing needle and thread size is equal.

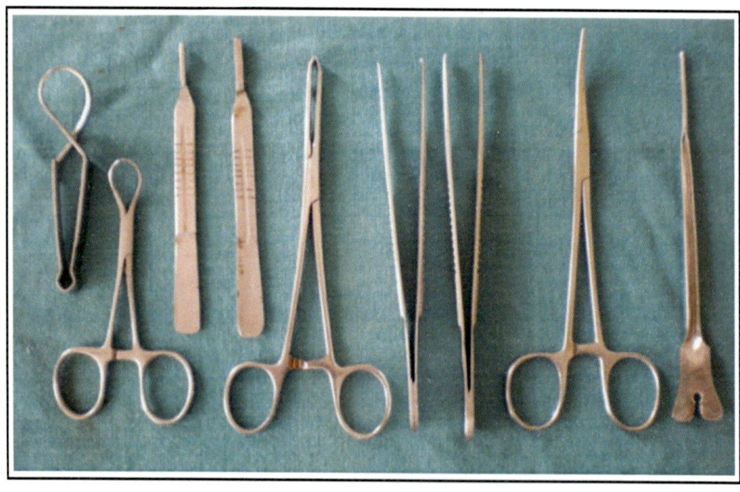

General surgical instruments

1. Cross action towel clamp
2. Backhaus towel clamp
3. Bard parker handle (B.P. handle) No. 3
4. Bard parker handle (B.P. handle) No 4
5. Alis tissue forceps
6. Rat tooth forceps
7. Thumb forceps
8. Artery forceps curved
9. Groove director

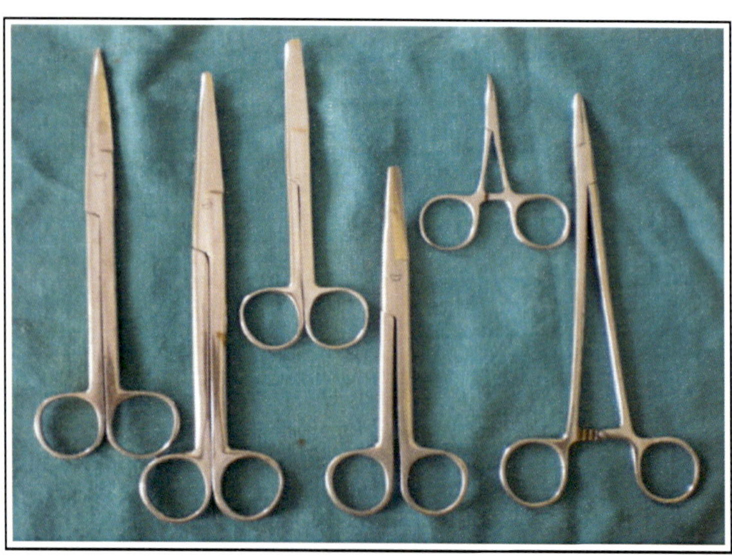

General surgical instruments

Mayo's scissors

1. Pointed-pointed
2. Blunt-blunt (8″)
3. Blunt-pointed
4. Blunt-blunt (6″)
5. Mosquito hemostat
6. Needle holder

List of instruments of a general surgical pack

S. No.	Name of instrument	Numbers required
1.	B.P. handle No. 3 and 4	One each
2.	Mayo's scissors (straight)	One
3.	Mayo's scissors (curved)	One
4.	Rat tooth forceps	One
5.	Allis tissue forceps	Two
6.	Towel clamps	Four
7.	Mosquito haemostats	Four
8.	Artery forceps (curved)	Two
9.	Artery forceps (straight)	Two
10.	Needle holder	One
11.	Groove director	One
12.	Suturing needle (traumatic and atraumatic, straight and curved of different sizes)	Two each
13.	Surgical gloves	Two pair
14.	Surgical gown	Two
16.	Slit shroud (slit in the center as per requirement)	One
17.	Shroud without slit	One
18.	Gauze sponges	Ten
19.	Surgical pack wrapper	One

Points should be Noted During Preparation of Surgical Pack

1. Arrange all the items in such a way that the article may be removed in the order in which they are used.
2. Unlock all the instruments having locking facility.
3. Surgical shrouds and other clothing should be folded in accordion fashion at 10 cm intervals.
4. Fold the surgical gown by folding it inside out with the sleeves back to back and then place the gown on the table and straightened out all the folds. Roll it up in accordion fashion.
5. Prepare gauze sponges from a single layer of cotton gauze. Loose ends of gauze should not be present.

6. Surgical gloves should be dusted with talcum powder form inside and outside. Turn the cuff of each globe back at least 5-6 cm. Keep a packet of about 2 gram of telcum powder in each pair of gloves and put these gloves in the gloves case.
7. First of all place the instruments and gauze sponges on the wrapper. Over these keep surgical shrouds with and without slit, gloves, surgical gowns and towels serially and then close the wrapper.
8. Wrap facemasks and caps and sterilize separately.

Question

1. Write down the difference between needle holder and artery forceps.

Exercise 3

Objective : Familiarization with Udder and Teat Instruments

1. *Milking tube* : It is used for milking the animal after udder or teat surgery. It can also be used for infusing intramammary medication through teat canal.
2. *Teat plug* : It is used to plug the teat in cases of leaky teats or trodden teats or following operation at teat sphincter. It can also be used for retaining medication in the teat canal.
3. *Udder infusion tube* : It is used for infusion of medication in the udder/ teat.
4. *Teat slitter with concealed blade* : For cutting any growth inside the teat canal without injury to the teat.
5. *Teat tumor extractor* : It is used for removal of teat tumour or polyps from the teat canal.
6. *Teat bistoury* : It is used for enlargement of teat canal and for removal of growth in teat canal.
7. *Litchy teat knife with sharp point* : It is used for cutting any growth inside the teat canal.
8. *Teat scissors* : it is used for closed teat surgery. This instrument can be easily inserted into the teat canal to trim the extra growth.

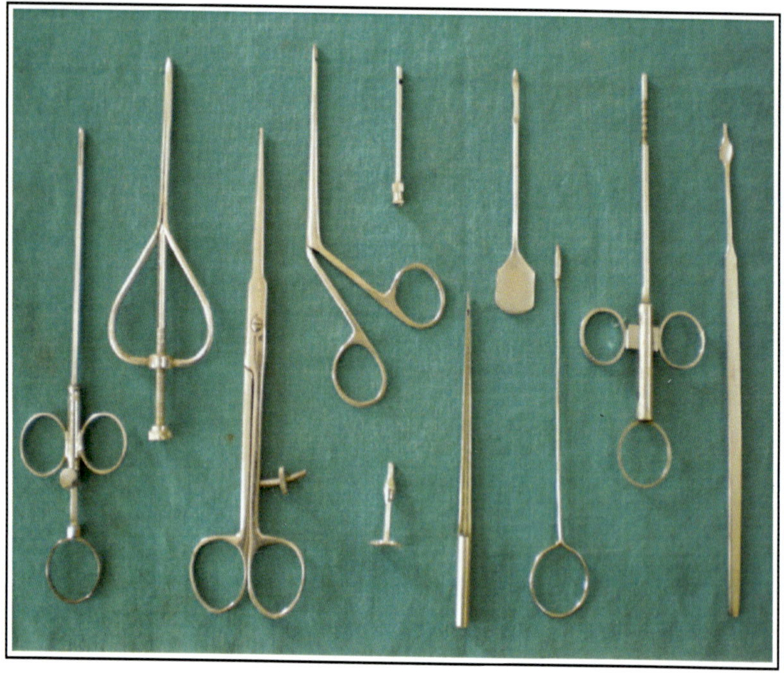

Teat Instruments

1. Teat slitter with concealed blade.
2. Teat dilator
3. Teat scissors
4. Teat plug
5. Milk tube
6. Teat scoup
7. Teat lancet
8. Teat tumor extractor
9. Teat tumor extractor
10. Teat bistoury

Exercise 4

Objective : Familiarization with Orthopedic Instruments

These specialized instruments are used for operation of skeletal system. Common instruments are as follows :

1. *Loman bone holding clamp* : It is used for holding fractured bony ends with bone plates.
2. *Bone plates* : are used for rigid immobilization of fractured fragments. Bone plates are of difference shapes, sizes and with varying number of holes. These are of following types :
    a. Dynamic compression plate.
    b. Neutralization plate.
    c. Shcrnab plate etc.
3. *Bone screws* : are either used to immobilize fractured fragments or to fix bone plates. They are of different sizes and classified in to cancellous and cortical types.
4. *Hexagonal bone screw driver* : It is used for tightening of bone screw.
5. *Kern self-retaining bone holding forceps* : It is used to hold fractured fragment and bone plate.

6. *Listen bone cutting forceps* : It is used to cut the bone ends and may be straight or curved.
7. *Still lure double action rounger* : Used to cut the bone and requires less force.
8. *Chiesel and osteotome* : They are of different sizes and used alone or with hammer to cut or shape the bone.
9. *Bone curetter* : It is used to remove necrotic bone.
10. *Gigli wire* : It is used to cut the bone.
11. *Gigli wire handle* : T handle or ball handle.
12. *Bone rasp* : It is used to rasp the sharp pointed fractured ends.
13. *Wrenches* : it is used for tightening of all nuts and bolts during application of external fixater.
14. *Bone plate bender* : It is used to shape the bone plate according to the shape of bone.
15. *Bone drill* : It is used to make hole in the bone for setting bone screw or bone pin. It may be either hand driven or power driven.
16. *Orthopaedic hammer/ mallet* : This is used to hammer bone chesel, osteotome or nail.
17. *Periosteal elevator* : It is used for raising periosteum from the shaft of bone. It is available in different sizes and shape.
18. *Orthopaedic scale* : It is used for measuring the diameter of drill bit for a particular screw.
19. *Depth gauze* : It is used for measuring the length of screw to be used.
20. *Trephine* : It is used to make a relatively large hole on the bone e.g. trephining of sinus. They have a T-shaped handle and cylindrical serrated cutting blade to cut the bone.
21. *Orthopaedic saw* : It is used for cutting the bone.
22. *Reamer* : It is used for making a hole in the bone e.g. during fixation of K-nail.
23. *Guide wire* : It is used to guide the K-nail.
24. *Intra medullary pins* : They are used for internal fixation of fractured long bone. They are of following types :

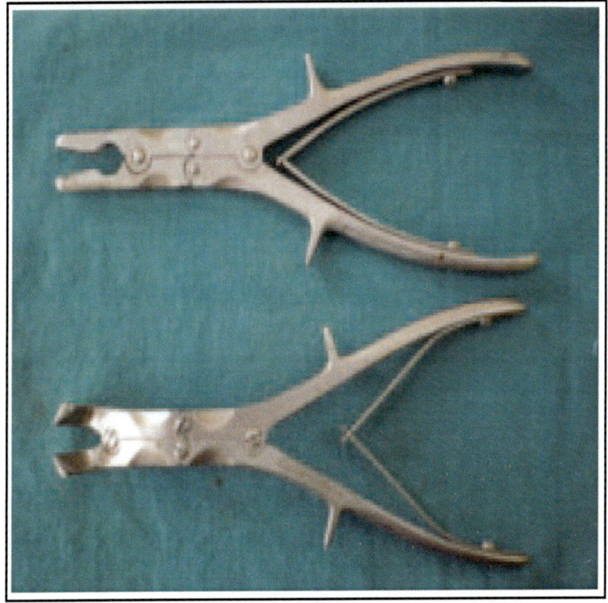

1. Still-luer double action rongeurs 2. Bone cutting forceps (curved)

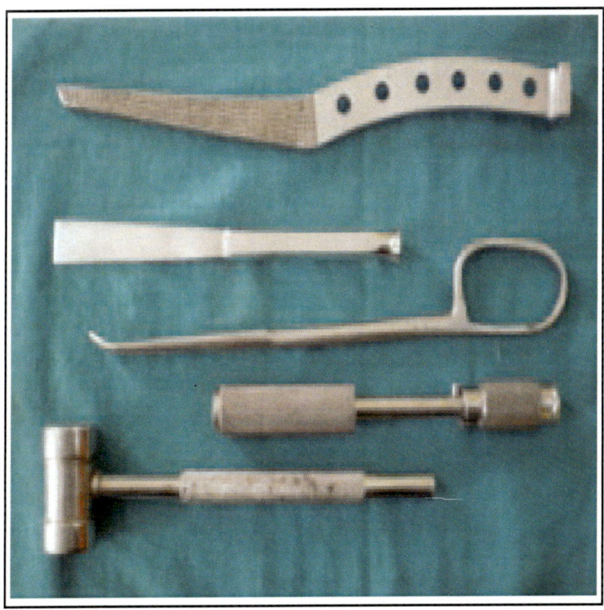

3. Bone rasp 4. Chiesel or osteotome 5. Bone elevator
6. Orthopaedic wire twister 7. Orthopaedic hammer

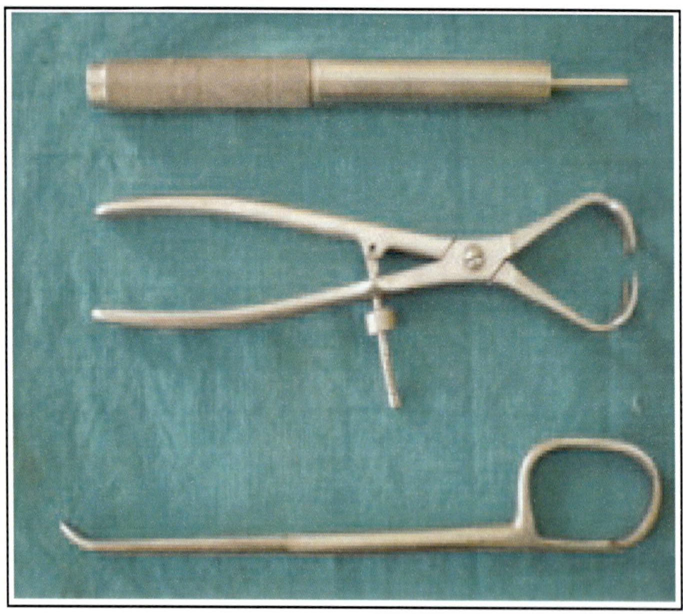

8. K nail setter 9. Bone holding forceps

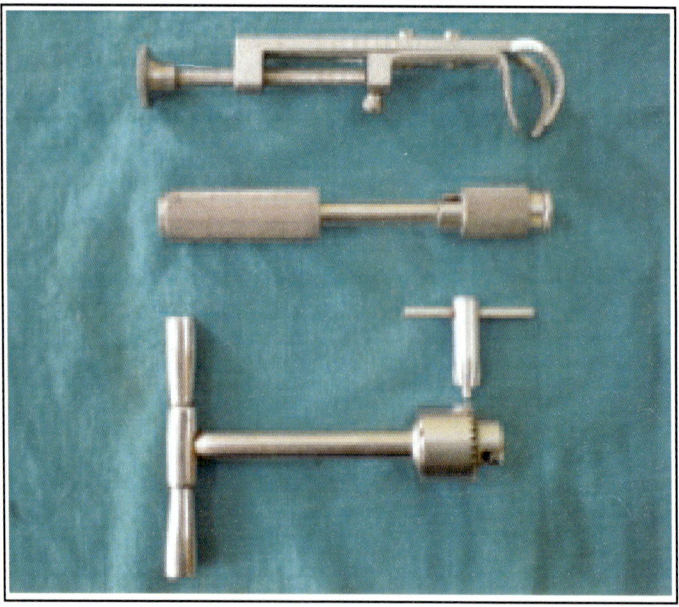

10. Loman bone holding clamp 11. Jacob's chuck with key 12. Triphine

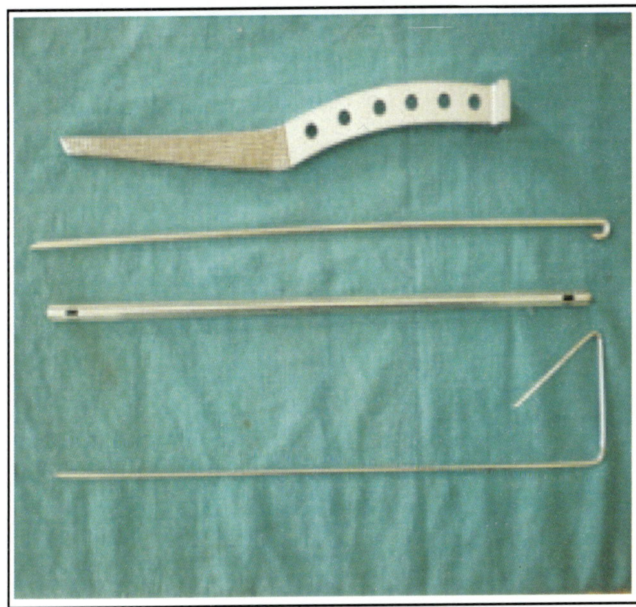

Bone rasp 13. Rush nail 14. K-Nail 15. Guide wire

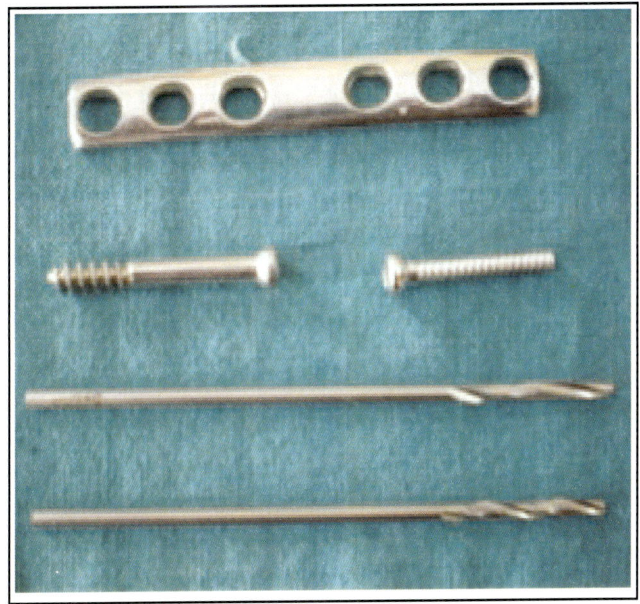

16 Bone plate 17. Cancellous screw 18. Cortical screw. 19. Drill bits.

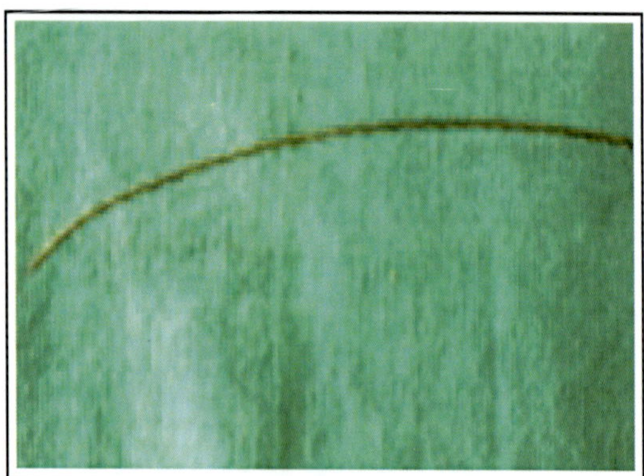

20. Gigli wire saw

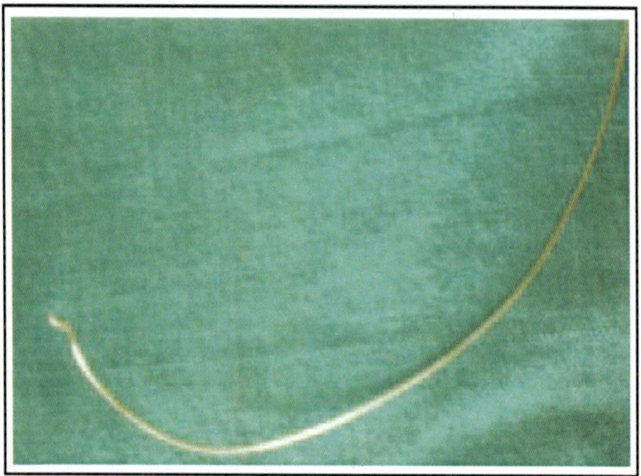

21. Orthopaedic wire

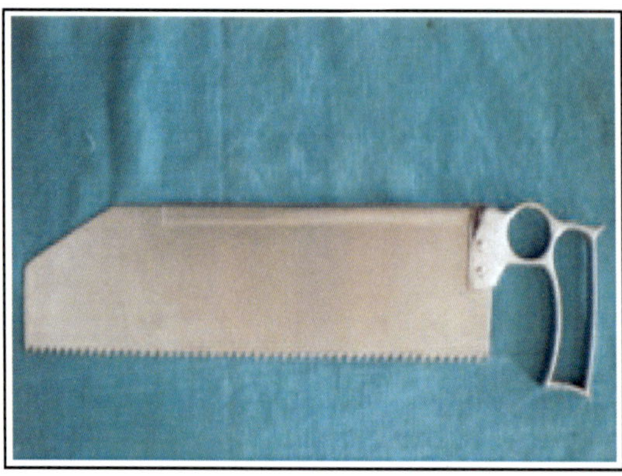

22. Orthopaedic saw

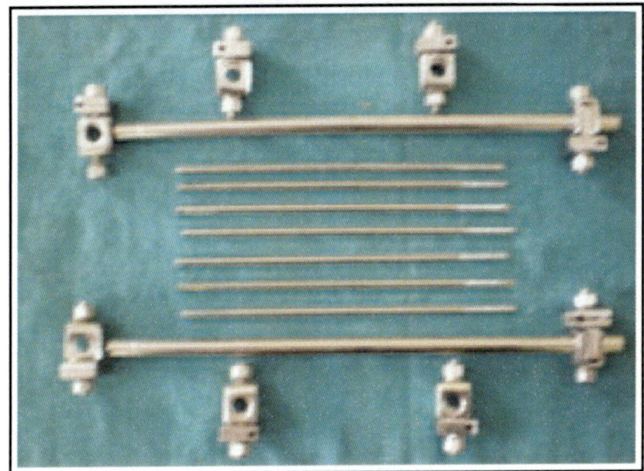

23. External fixator assembly

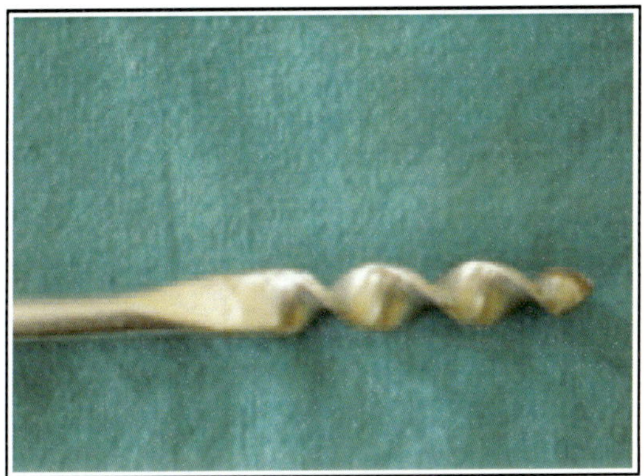

24. Bone reamer.

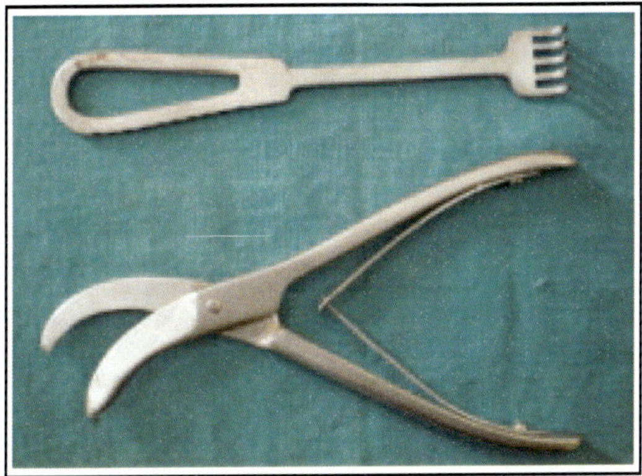

25. Volkman wound retractor 26. Plaster shear

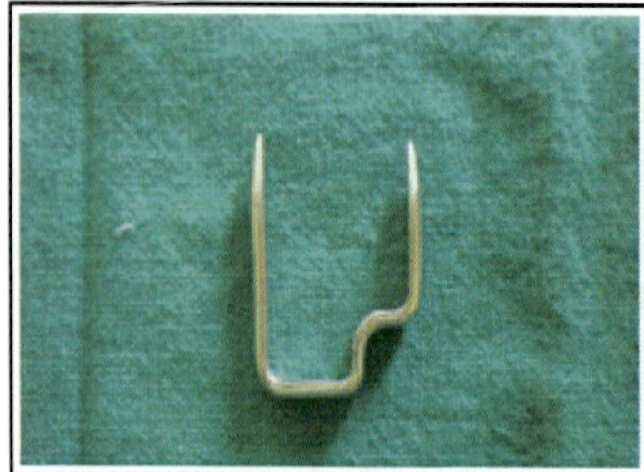

27. Bone staple

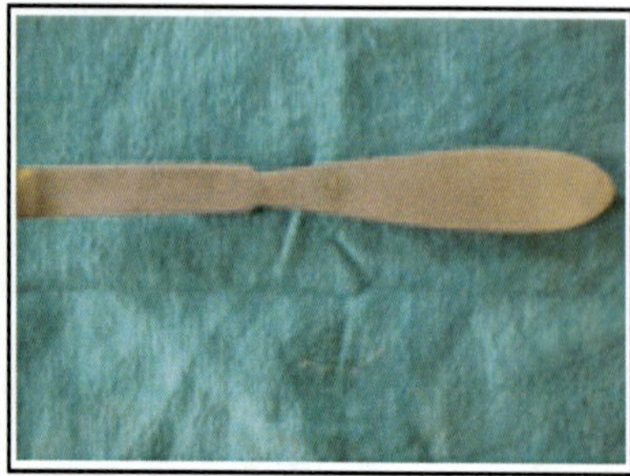

28. Periosteal elevator

a. Steinmann intramedullary pin
b. Kirschner wire, (K-wire).
c. Rush pin- having hooked end and always used in pair. The end of steinman intramedullary pin may be trocar, crow or threaded. Threaded intramedullary pin is also known as schan screw.

25. *Intramedullary pin cutter* : It is used to cut the extra length of steinmann intramedullary pin.

26. *Drill bits* : These are of different sizes and are used for drilling holes in the bone for passage of wire, screws or pins.

27. *Drill sleeves* : To check the injury to the surrounding tissue during drilling.

28. Tap : To make threads in hole for a particular size of screw.

Question

Write the name of instruments used for :

i. Plating
ii. Instramedldllay pinning
iii. K-nailing
iv. Wiring

Exercise 5

OBJECTIVE : FAMILIARIZATION WITH OPTHALMIC INSTRUMENTS

These instruments are used for surgery and need special care and attention for sterilization and storage.

1. *Strabismus scissors* : It is used for treating strabismus i.e. sectioning of affected muscle.
2. *Me Guire corneal scissors* : It is used for incising cornea
3. *Graefe's eye speculum* : It is used for retraction of eyelids for examination of eye or for ophthalmic surgery.
4. *Ziegler knife needle* : It is used for separation of ocular tissues during ophthalmic surgery.
5. *Iris hook* : It is used for handling of Iris drug ophthalmic surgery.
6. *Tenotomy scissors* : It is used either for cutting the ocular ligament of eye or for removal of ocular sutures.
7. *Dressing forceps* : It is used for manipulation of eyelids, 3rd eye lid and other tissues of the eye.
8. *Von Grafe fixation forceps* : It is used for holding ocular tissues during ophthalmic surgery.
9. *Air injection cannula* : It is used for injection of air to facilitate ophthalmic surgery.

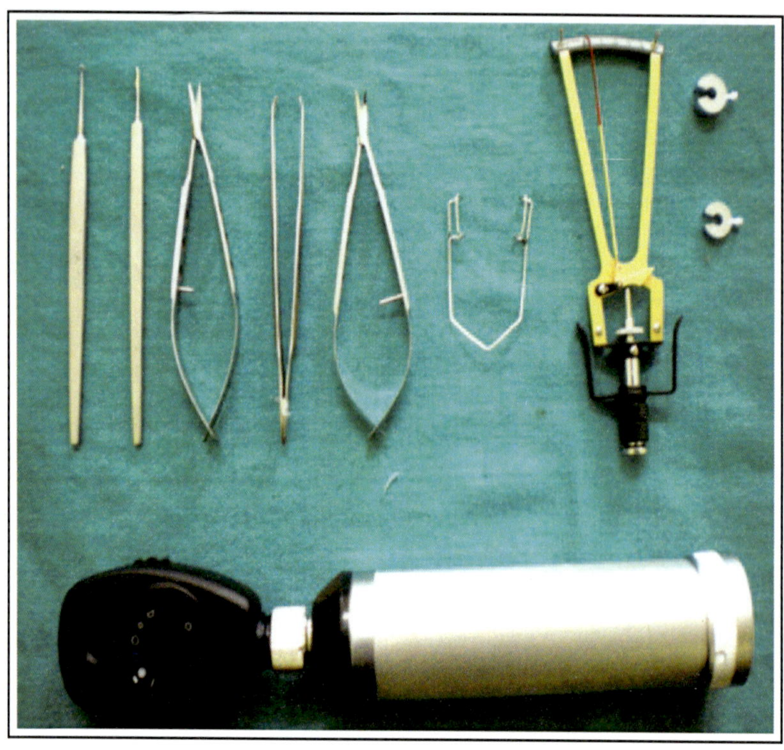

Opthalmic instruments

1. Blunt iris hook 2. Zieglar knife 3. Strabismus scissors 4. Von grafe fixation forceps 5. Mc Guire corneal scissors 6. Graef's eye speculum 7. Schioetz tonometer 8. Opthalmoscope

Exercise 6

Objective : Familiarization with Hoof Instruments

These instruments are used for different surgical conditions of hoof.

1. Drawing knife: It is used to remove excess sole and trimming of horny tissue (Fig. 6.1).
2. Hoof plane: it is used to plane the surface of the hoof.

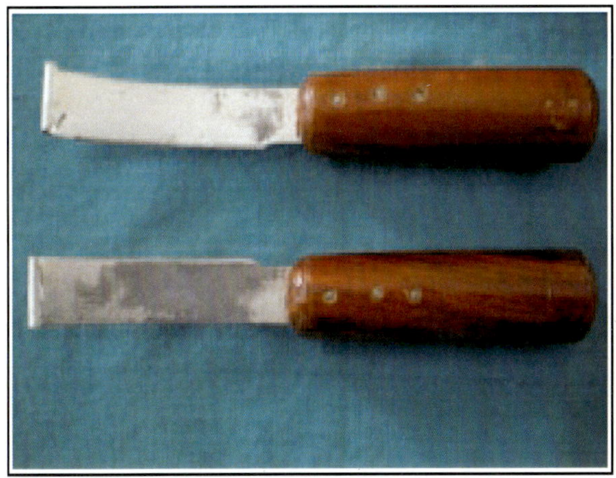

Fig. 6.1: Drawing knife

3. Hoof cutter: It is used for trimming of extra growth of hoof. (Fig. 6.2).

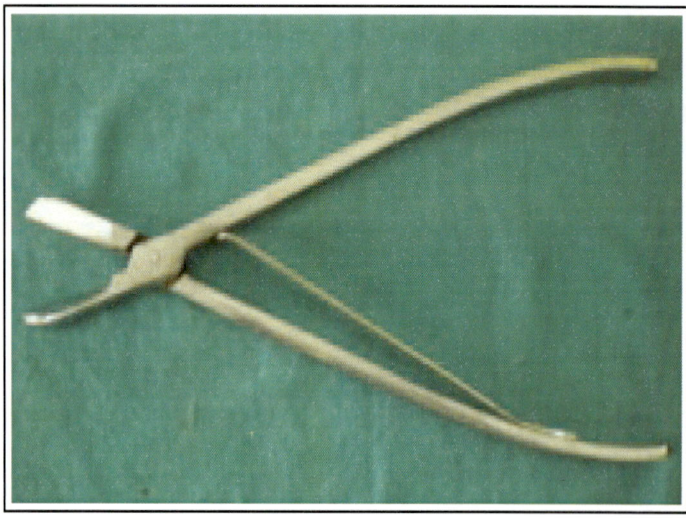

Fig. 6.2: Hoof cutter

4. *Hoof pick* : It is used to check the ground surface of the foot for any injury or any foreign particle around the frog and bars of hoof.
5. *Hoof nipper* : it is used to trim the excess of hoof wall (Fig. 6.3).

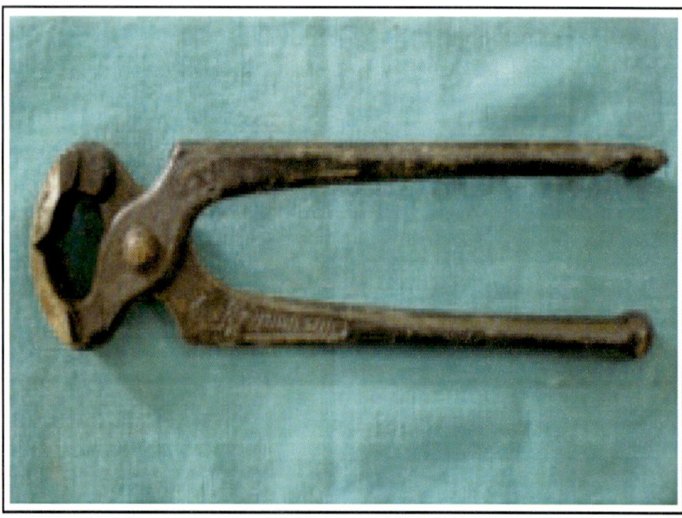

Fig. 6.3: Hoof nipper

6. *Hoof section saw* : It is used to cut the excess dead tissue (Fig. 6.4).

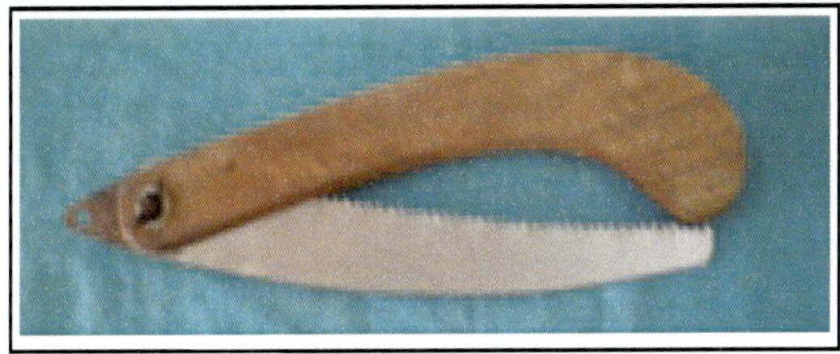

Fig. 6.4: Hoof section saw

7. *Hoof sage knife* : It is used to trim the soft flaky part of the sole.
8. *Hoof tester* : It is used to test the clinical abnormalities in the hoof and its various structures to locate the lesion (Fig. 6.5).

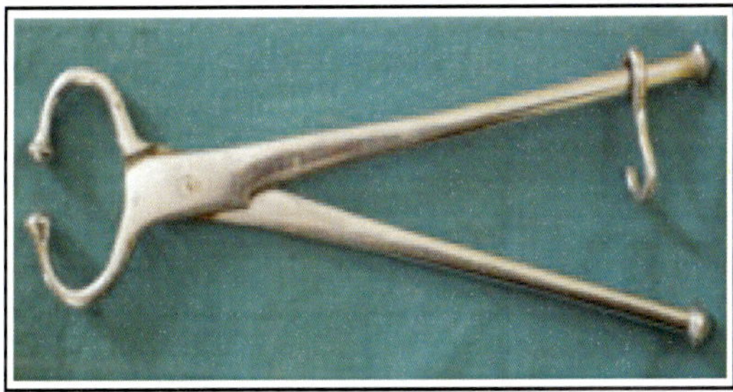

Hoof tester

9. *Hoof rasp* : It is used to rasp the hoof (Fig. 6.6).

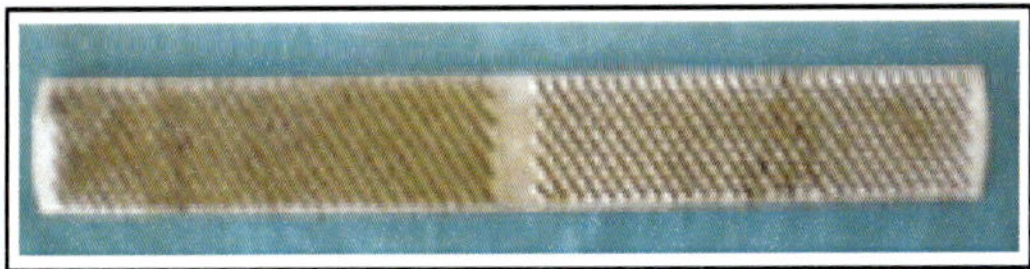

Fig. 6.6: Hoof rasp

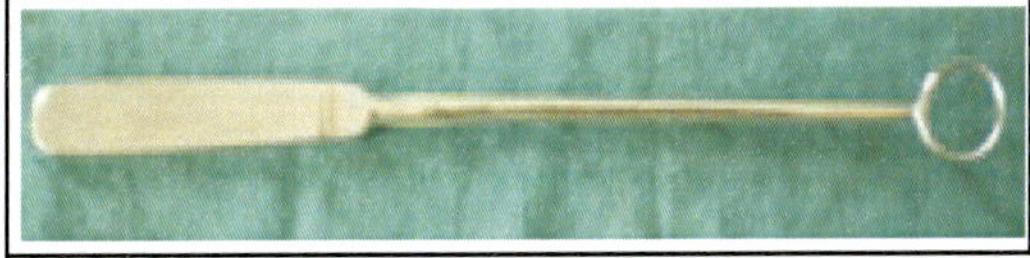

Quitter knife

Exercise 7

Objective : Familiarization with Dental Instruments

1. *Molar tooth cutter* : It is used to cut the extra sharp molar tooth in large animals (Fig. 7.1).

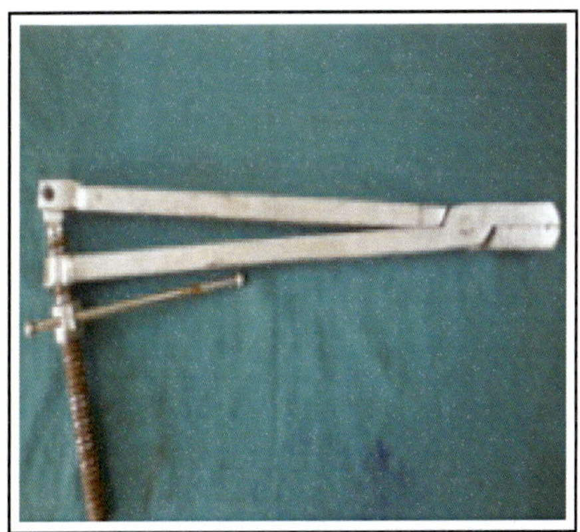

Fig. 7.1: Molar tooth cutter

2. *Tooth rasp* : Usd for rasping the tooth (Fig. 7.2).
3. *Tooth nipper* : It is used to cut the sharp tooth edges in small animals.

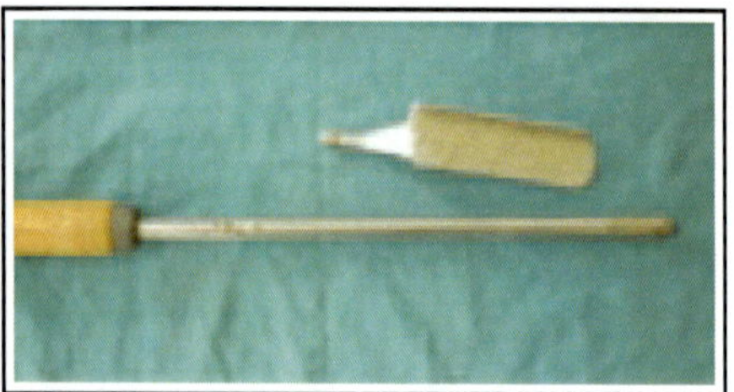

Fig. 7.2 : Tooth rasp

4. *Canine molar extractor* : It is used to remove the molar or premolar teeth in canine (Fig. 7.3).

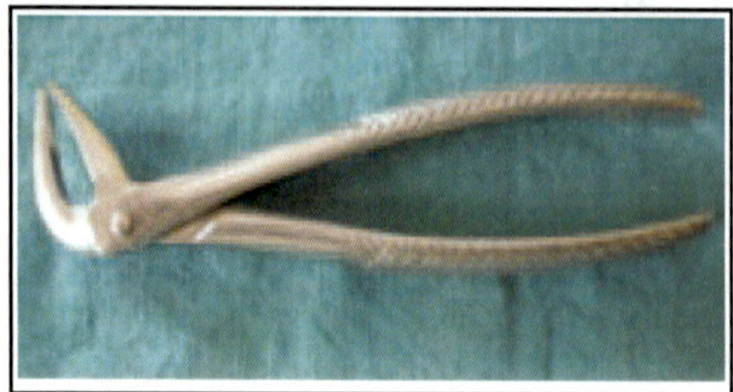

Fig. 7.3 : Tooth extractor

5. *Gray's tooth forceps* : It is used for tempory dental caries in canines and for breaking dental tartar.
6. *Ultrasonic tooth cleaner* : It is used for breaking dental tartars.
7. *Tooth scalar* : It is used to scale the teeth for removal of tartar.
8. *Dental floats* : These are used to rasp the sharp teeth to protect the soft tissues of mouth.
9. *Mouth gags :*
   a. *Varnell's gag* : This gag is used in equines.
   b. *Butler's gag* : This gag is also used in equines.
   c. *Probang gag* : This gag is used for cattle and buffalo.
   d. *Spring gag* : This gag is used in dogs.
   e. *Linton's gag* : This gag is used in sheep.

Exercise 8

Objective : To Study Different Types of Catheters & Their Applications

Catheters are hollow tubes made up of rubber, gum elastic, polyethylene or teflon or metal and are indicated.

1. To evacuate fluid from the body cavity.
2. To collect fluid sample from the hollow organ.
3. To administer medication inside a hollow organ.

S. No.	Type of catheter	Made up of	Length & diameter	End point of catheter	Purpose
1.	Mare catheter	Gum elastic or rubber	≈ 40 inches < 1 inches	Closed, smooth and round	To evacuate urinary bladder
2.	Cattle catheter	Gum elastic or rubber	≈ 8 inches ¾ inches	Beveled	To evacuate urinary bladder
3.	Dog catheter	Gum elastic or Teflon	Different sizes of outer diameter	Closed smooth round, relatively hard and a slit about 4 cm posterior to end.	To evacuate urinary bladder

Contd...

Contd...

4.	Vascular catheter	Teflon	Different sizes of outer diameter	Beveled	To cannulate blood vessels for CPV and MAP
5.	Oesophageal catheter	Teflon	Different sizes of outer diameter		To assess patency of oesophagus from mouth to stomach.
6.	Foley's catheter	Rubber	Different sizes of outer diameter	Inflated cuff and Baloon on the opposite side	To drain bladder and uterine flushing
7.	Uterine catheter (single or double channel)	Metalic	16-18″ less than 1″	Closed, smooth, curved having slit ½ cm posterior to closed end	Draining or infusion of fluid inside uterus.
8.	Endotracheal tube	Rubber, Plastic, Metal	Variable 4-15 mm ID	Beveled like foley catheter	For intubation during anaesthesia or artificial respiration or maintaining positive pressure ventilation
9.	Nasogastric tube/ probing	Metalic, Plastic, rubber			To clear oesophageal passage or to administer drug in to the stomach.
10.	Catheters for CVP and MAP	Plastic, rubber			To observe the central venous pressure or mean arterial pressure.

Question

1. Write the name of artery and vein for catheterization to record the CVP and MAP.

Exercise 9

Objective : Restraining and Positioning of Animals for Surgical Interventions

Restraining means use of strong force or chemical agents to prevent or suppress or to control the action of animal for clinical examination or for prevention of self-injury and for performing surgical interventions.

Restraining can be performed by:

1. Psychic persuasion
2. Physical restraint
3. Chemical restraint

1. Psychic Persuasion

It is suitable in trained companion animals for minor surgical interventions.

2. Physical Restraint

This method is extensively used for restraining of animals. Generally a rope of suitable length and strength is used for this purpose. Common physical restraining methods used in different species of animals are as follows:

Restraining of Equines

1. Twitch
2. Halters
3. Raising of legs
4. Casting (a) Side line method (b) Hobble method.

Restraining of Cattle /Buffalo

1. By holding the tail at is base and raise it upward.
2. By applying a nose lead.
3. Rope is applied in the form of figure of either just above the hock joint of both legs.
4. Casting of animal.
   a. Reuff's method
   b. Country method.

Restraining of Dog

1. Application of temporary muzzle.
2. Elizabethan collar.

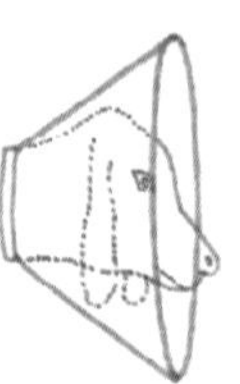

3. Chemical Restraint

Chemical restraining is done with the use of certain drugs to clam down or to anaesthetize the animal. This method is used for zoo or wild animals or furious animals.

Chemical restraining is not a universally accepted means of capturing wild animals. For restaning of animal, drugs can be used by the following methods.

1. *Oral administration* : Drug is mixed with drinking water or feed but this method is not reliable due to improper dosing.
2. *Hand held syringes* : This method can be used only if the animal is in squeeze cage.
3. *Projected syringes or darts* : Palmer capture equipment is used for this purpose. They are of 3 types:
   a. *Short range pistols* : It is a modified pellet gun powered by compressed carbon di-oxide. Its range is about 15 meters.
   b. *Large range rifle* : It is same as pistol but range is about 35 meters.

c. *Extra large range rifle :* It is powered by percussion caps. The maximum range is about 80 meters.

These guns are loaded with syringes containing desired amount of drugs ranging between 1 to 10 ml and fired on animal. The drug delivery system injects full dose of drug into an animal.

4. *Blow guns :* It has silent projection with fewer traumas but has shorter range.

Drugs and doses : Drug selection is based on the following points:

a. Species and breed of animal.

b. Age of the animal.

c. Physical condition of the animal.

d. Purpose of use of chemical restrain.

e. Facilities available and individual choice.

f. Some species can be safely captured in traps e.g. Otters.

g. Chemical immobilization is not safe in some species of animals e.g. deer.

h. Full reversible anaesthetics are preferred in wild animals.

i. Opiod anesthetics (like etorphins) are commonly used in elephants because they are potent and their anaesthetic effects can be reversed.

j. The subcutaneous fat in wild animals like wild bear, hippo etc. are prone to malignant hyperthermia and difficulty in administration of anaesthetics and vein puncture. Ice and cold water should be available to manage hyperthermia. For prevention of hyperthermia, anaesthetic procedures should be planned during coolest part of the day and take advantage of shade.

Dose of HBN* (Hellabrunn mixture) in different species of wild animals

S. No.	Animal/species	Dose (ml)
1.	Lion & Tiger	2-3
2.	Jaguar	1-1.3
3.	Chital / spotted deer	0.6-1.0
4.	Samber	1.5-1.6
5.	Black buck	0.3-0.4
6.	Neelgai	1.7
7.	Sika deer	1.6-1.8
8.	Himalayan black bear	3.0-4.0
9.	Elephant	5.0-6.0

* HBN contains 4.0 ml ketamine (100 mg/ml) in 500 mg xylazine powder vial.

Positioning of Animals for Surgical Interventions

After restraining of animal by physical or chemical methods, they are positioned in sternal or lateral (right/left) or dorsoventral recumbency for efficient working during surgery. The position of animal is maintained by ropes or bandages in small animals or with the help of sand bags in large animals. Positioning of animal can also be done by using different tables e.g. "V" top table for dorsoventral recumbency or flat table for lateral recumbency/ sternal recumbency.

Question

1. Write different factors of failure to inject in wild animals.
2. Write antagonists of
   a. Etorphine
   b. Fentanyl/ carfentanyl
   c. Xylazine
3. Write in detail about restraing of horse and cattle
   a. Twitch
   b. Side line method
   c. Reuff's method

Exercise 10

Objective : Familiarization with Different Apparatuses used for General Anesthesia

General anaesthesia can be induced by parentral anaesthetics or by gaseous or inhalation anaesthetics.

Apparatuses

1. *Syringes* : Disposable plastic syringes of different capacities e.g. 1ml, 2ml, 5 ml, 10 ml, 20 ml and 50 ml.
2. *Hypodermic needles* : They are of different sizes e.g. 16, 18, 20, 22, 24 gauze. They must be sharp with short bevel to reduce risk of transfixing the vein.
3. *Catheters* : They are used for constant infusion of drug or for administration of intermittent small doses of drug.
4. *Infusion apparatus* : They are used for continuous drip infusion of anaesthetic agent and fluid to the animal. The flow rate is controlled by means of clamp and can be estimated by counting the number of drops, which pass through the drip chamber in 1 minute. 1 drop = 0.05 ml.
5. *Endotracheal tubes* : They may be either plane or cuffed. The cuff can be inflated with room air after the tube has passed in to trachea. It allows improved oxygenation and proper ventilation of airways. They are

available in different sizes and lengths depending on the animal for which they are required.

6. *Laryngoscope* : It is used for visualizing the larynx and facilitates endotracheal intubation.
7. *Gags* : Used for inspection of oral cavity and to introduce endotracheal tube in trachea.
8. *Face masks* : They are used for administration of anaesthesia in open system of administration of inhalant anaesthesia.
9. *Boyl's apparatus* : It is a type of breathing circuit used for administration of inhalant anaesthetic to small animals. It consist of :

a. *Cylinders* : These cylinders contain different gases and can be used as anaesthetic combination required. These cylinders are fitted with pressure gauze meter to measure pressure of gas in the cylinder.

b. *Flow meter* :

Gas	Colour of cylinder
Nitrous oxide	Black with white on top
Carbon dioxide	Grey
Cyclopropane ethylene	Orange red

c. *Vaporizer* : It delivers a suitable and accurately known quantity of a volatile anaesthetic agent in the breathing circuit.

d. *One way expiratory values* : During spontaneous breathing these valves should be kept fully open.

e. *Rebreathing bag/ Reservoir* : This is a rubber bag which acts as a reservoir for gases between respiratory excusions. During emergency, this can be used for giving artificial respiration.

f. *Canister with soda lime* : It is used when closed or semi-closed system of anesthesia is adopted. Soda lime absorbs all CO_2 in the system. An indicator like ethyl violet can be used. As the sodalime is exhausted its colour changes from white to pink or violet.

g. *Airways* : These are corrugated pipes used to connect the animal to anaesthetic machine through endotracheal tube.

10. Accessory equipments

    a. Stethoscope

    b. Esophageal stethoscope

c. Pulse oxymeter
d. ECG machine
e. Blood pressure monitors
f. Blood gas analyzer etc.

Question

Make a labell diagram of following equipments :

1. Hypodermic needle and syringe
2. Endotracheal tube
3. Laryngoscope
4. Boyles apparatus

Exercise 11

Objective : Preparation, Calculation and Induction of General Anesthesia

Preparation of Patient for General Anesthesia

1. *Check for feeding status of animal* : Dogs should be kept off feed and off water 8-12 hours ruminants 24-48 hours, and horses 12-24 hours before surgery.

   Advantages

a. To avoid vomition and choking.

b. To avoid respiratory distress due to pressure of full stomach on diaphragm.

c. To avoid gastric rupture.

d. While restraining, there may abdominal rupture.

e. Prevent increase in BMR.

2. Complete blood count like PCV, Hb, DLC and blood chemistry should be undertaken.

3. *Urine analysis* : Physical and gross examination and microscopic examination of urine.

4. *ECG* : In order to rule out cardiac distress and arrhythmia.
5. Radiography of thoracic area.
6. Compensate any dehydration with intravenous fluids.
7. Area of surgery should be shaved one day before surgery.

Induction of Anesthesia

Stages of general anesthesia:

a. Preanaesthetic stage
b. Induction stage
c. Maintenance of anaesthesia
d. Recovery from anaesthesia

a. *Preanesthectic stage* : Refers to preanesthetic drugs given before giving general anesthetic drug so to:
   i. To reduce apprehensions.
   ii. Dose of general anesthetic drug is reduced, so margin of safety is increased.
   iii. Smooth and easy recovery.
   iv. To counter any unwanted effects of general anesthetic drugs e.g. Atropine given to prevent excessive salivation caused by Xylazine.
b. *Induction stage* : It has four stages:
   i. *Stage I or Stage or Voluntary Excitement* : There is transition from conscious to unconscious stage. There is perception of pain. All reflexes like Palpebral, Corneal, Pedal reflexes present and eyeball is central.
   ii. *Stage II or Stage of Involuntary Excitement* : Incoordination, animal is conscious and all above reflexes are present. Perception of pain is reduced. There is increased respiration and tachycardia, pupil slightly dilated, but photomotor reflex is present.
   iii. *Stage III or Surgical stage* : Animal is unconscious, all reflexes absent, respiration decreases and abdominal, heart rate decreases, muscles is relaxed, eye ball rotates ventromedially and partially covered by third eyelid.
   iv. *Stage IV or Stage of Medullary Paralysis or Stage of over dosage* : Complete paralysis of CNS and spinal cord, eyeball central and all reflexes absent especially photomotor reflex.

c. *Maintenance of anesthesia* : After induction, maintenance can be done either by parental or inhalant anesthetics.

d. *Recovery from anesthesia* : Most of postoperative deaths occur in this stage of hypoxia and hypothermia. So to avoid this supplement oxygen through endotracheal tube until recovery or till animal shows coughing reflex.

Question

1. Calculate the dose required (Various anesthetic combinations) for induction of GA in following animals:
   - 20 kg Dog - (Xylazine – Ketamine)
   - 400 kg Horse – (Xylazine – Ketamine)

Exercise 12

Objective : Demonstration, Monitoring of General Anesthesia and Management of Anesthetic Emergencies

The effects of anesthesia need to be monitored to prevent excessive insult to the cardiovascular, respiratory and central nervous system.

1. Evaluation of Central Nervous System (CNS)

Observe reflex activity to monitor degree of CNS depression.

- Eye reflexes
  - i. Palpebral reflex
  - ii. Corneal reflex
  - iii. Position of eye ball
  - iv. Nystagmus
  - v. Lacrimation
  - vi. Pupillary reflex
- Jaw tone
- Anal reflex
- Pedal reflex

2. Evaluation of Cardiovascular System (CVS)

- Auscultation of heart rate and rhythm
- Palpation of pulse
- Evaluation of mucus membrane colour and capillary refill time (CRT)
- Electrocardiogram
- Arterial blood pressure
- Central venous pressure

3. Evaluation of Respiratory System (RS)

- Respiratory frequency and pattern.
- Tidal volume estimation.
- Arterial and venous blood gas analysis.
- Blood pH analysis.

4. Continuous Monitoring of Rectal Temperature

Use of Pulse Oximetry in Monitoring Anesthesia

Pulse oximetry is easy to use, is non-invasive and provides accurate continuous physiological information regarding blood oxygenation and pulse rate. Pulse oximetry can be used on the tongue, lip, ear, prepuce, rectum, and the oral mucosa.

Respiratory Emergency

- Head of the anaesthetized animal should be straight.
- Remove oral, nasal or tracheal foreign material using forceps, suction and postural drainage.
- Endotracheal tube patency. It should not be blocked, kinked or damaged.
- Endotracheal intubation : Endotracheal intubation should be done an earliest, especially in brachycephalic dogs, and it should be kept in place till complete recovery from anaesthesia.
- Respiration rate and depth.

In cases of respiratory or breathing insufficiency i.e. apnea or dyspnea, the following steps should be under taken :

- Stop administration of anaesthetic drugs.
- Perform tracheotomy, if necessary to bypass obstruction.

- Administer pure oxygen through endotracheal / tracheotomy tube.
- Apply local anesthetic sprays to prevent laryngo-spasms in cats associated with endotracheal intrubation.
- Artificial ventilation of the lungs (IPPV) (@ 8-10 ventilations per minute).
- Use of bronchodilators like aminophylline (@ 1-2 mg/Ib, IV).
- Use of analeptic drugs like nikethamide (@ 2-4 mg/Ib, IV, doxapram @ 1-2 mg/Ib, IV in small animals and 0.1-0.3 mg/Ib, IV large animals).
- Administration of sodium bicarbonate (@ 0.5-2.0 mEq/L, IV) or depending upon the base deficit.
- Administration of antagonist(s), if available.
- Supportive care and fluid therapy.

Circulatory Emergency

The following circulatory insufficiencies may occur :

- *Bradycardia* : Give atropine sulpahte or nor-epinephrine, IV.
- *Tachycardia* : Administer Isoproterenol (b-2 adrenergic agonist) IV.
- *Ventricular arrhythmia* : Administer lignocaine hydrochloride, IV.
- *Ventricular fibrillation* : Apply defibrillator on chest.
- *Cardiac arrest* : Chest message
  i. Administration of corticosteroids
  ii. Fluid therapy

Exercise 13

Objective : Hemorrhage and Hemostasis

Hemorrhage is a discharge of blood from the vascular system. Control of bleeding is of great importance because besides anesthetic problems the only disaster befalling the surgeon in the operating room is the result of hemorrhage.

Hemorrhage is Classified as

1. According to Source

Arterial : Blood is bright red and flows in spurts.

Venous : Blood is bluish red and flows freely. Capillary: Blood oozes under low pressure.

2. According to Time of Occurrence

Primary : This occurs immediately after traumatic disruption of blood vessels.

Delayed

i. *Intermediate :* If hemorrhage occurs within 24 h of injury.

ii. *Secondary :* It is the result of ineffective treatment of primary hemorrhage e.g. slipped ligature or necrosis of ligated vessel.

3. According to Extent

Petichial, bruising and deep bruising.

Hemostasis

- Hemostasis is the physiological process to check the hemorrhage. Various surgical methods are used to facilitate the clotting mechanism.
- Hemostasis is essential because of the following reasons :
    i. Blood over the drapes, gloves and operative field increases the chances of infection.
    ii. Extravasated blood delays wound healing.
    iii. Hemorrhage obscures the surgical site.
    iv. Severe hemorrhage may lead to shock, hypoxemia and death of the animal.

Methods Employed to Control Hemorrhage

1. Hemostatic Forceps

- Ends of the bleeding vessels are crushed with haemostatic forceps.
- Halsted mosquito and Kelly forceps are used for small vessels.
- Oshsner and crile forceps are used for large tissue bundles and vessels.
- Tip clamping method : The tip of the forceps is used to grasp the bleeding vessel. (Fig. 13A).
- Jaw clamping method : The jaw of the forceps is used to grasp the bleeding vessel (Fig. 13B).

2. Torsion

Twisting the vessels with forceps before releasing the forceps.

3. Suturing

It also serves to arrest hemorrhage.

4. Pressure

a. Bleeding from small vessels is checked by applying pressure to the bleeding points with gauze sponges or digital pressure.
b. Use of pressure pad hemostasis on large blood vessels is temporary.
c. Hemorrhage after skin incision is controlled by this method. Pressure is applied with gauze sponge over a short period of time.

5. Tourniquet

It should be used for short period only.

6. Cautery

- Cauterization of the vessels is performed by an electrosurgical unit. Intense heat burns the tissue and the resultant scab acts as a haemostatic plug.
- Cauterization is used for hemostasis for arteries upto 1 mm and veins up to 2 mm in diameter.
- An alternate method of cauterization is the direct application of heat, cold or certain chemicals over the vessel.
- Styptics such as silver nitrate and ferric sulfate have astringent action which causes hemostasis.

7. Topical Substances

Styptics have an astringent action on blood vessels. Examples are glacial acetic acid, silver nitrate, ferric sulfate, ferric chloride, alum and tannin. Other topical substances include – Tincture of Benzoin compound, Adrenaline, Gelfoam that is a sponge like substance and Bone wax.

8. Systemic Haemostatic Agents

They are beneficial only when they are deficient in the body. Vitamin K is given preoperatively in conjunction with ascorbic acid. Botropase is also used for hemostasis.

9. Ligatures

Ligatures should be applied certain mm away from the cut ends of the vessel to prevent slippage. Certain ligatures used in veterinary practices are :

i. *Simple ligatures* : The isolated vessel and small vascular pedicles can be occluded by simple ligature. Double ligature is recommended for large isolated vessel/ arteries. (Fig. 13C).

ii. *Halsted transfixation ligatures* : (Fig. 13D).

iii. *Modified transfixation ligature* : (Fig. 13E).

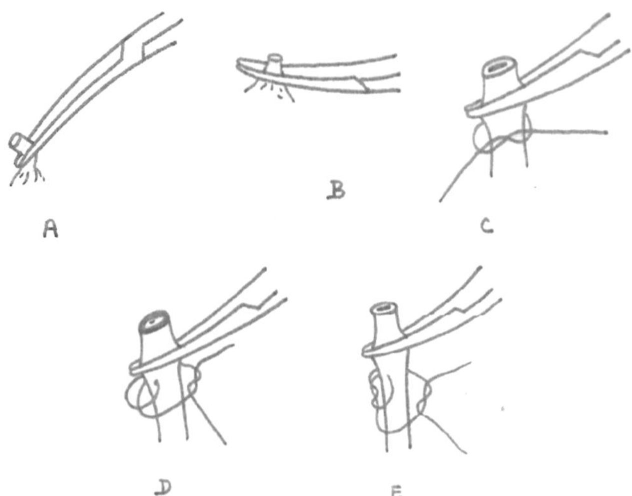

Fig. 13 : Methos employed to control hemorrhage. **A.** By tip clamping methods; **B.** By Jaw Clamping method; **C.** By Simple Ligatures; **D.** By halsted trensfixaction lyatines; **E.** By modified transfixation ligatures.

10. Ligating Clips

- Ligating clips are used for accurate hemostasis during ovario-hysterectomy, splenectomy, intestinal anastomosis, nephrectomy etc.
- Use of ligating clips is limited on vessels that are less than 11 mm in diameter.
- Ligating clips elicited minimal tissue reaction.
- *Advantage* : Advantageous in the area of difficult accessibility.
- *Disadvantages* : Relative instability of the clip in the applicator and permanent presence of metal in the tissue.

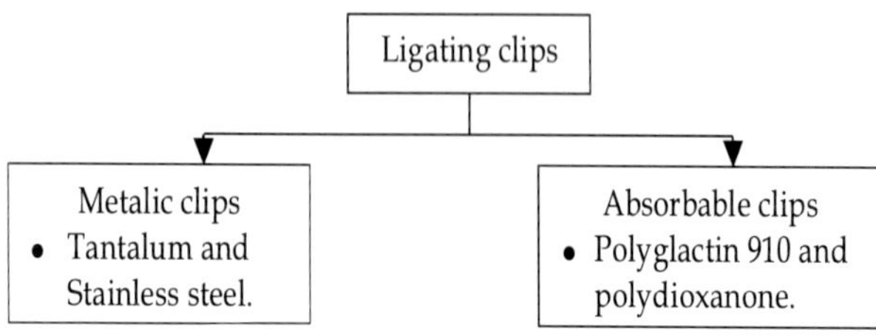

Exercise 14

OBJECTIVE : BANDAGES AND SLINGS

Bandages

- Bandages are used to protect the wound and incisions, as well as support body parts.
- Bandages are also used to immobilize the limbs.
- Bandages are used to promote the wound healing process by :
  - i. Removal of dead and necrosed tissue from the wound (debridement).
  - ii. Application of topical antiseptics.
  - iii. Pressure to reduce the dead space, hemorrhage and edema.
  - iv. Preserving the hemostasis at the wound site.

Bandaging Techniques

- Bandages should be applied evenly and without excessive tightness. If the bandage is applied tightly, it will result in to circulatory impairment and edema distal to bandage.
- Stay sutures are applied to retain the antiseptic soaked bandage over the wound.

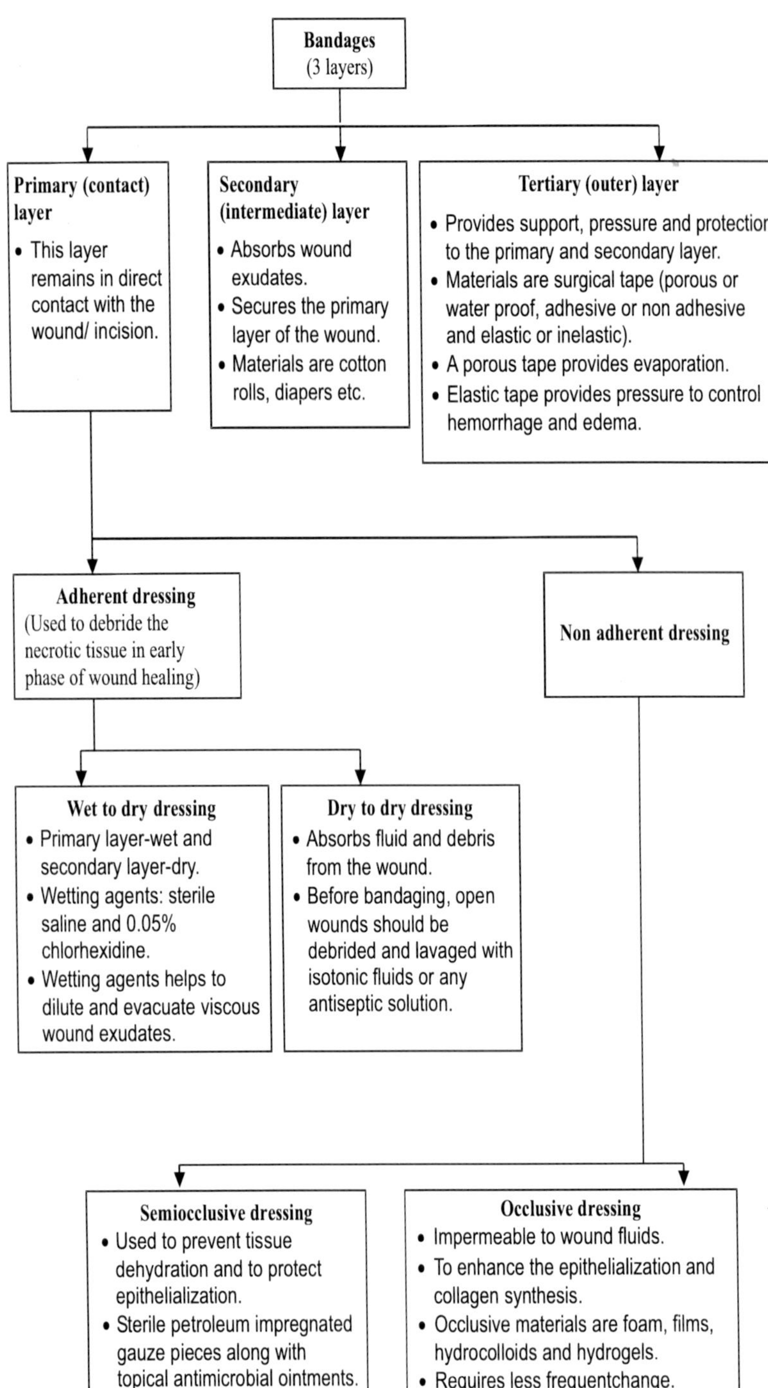
Bandages
(3 layers)
Primary (contact) layer
• This layer remains in direct contact with the wound/ incision.
Secondary (intermediate) layer
• Absorbs wound exudates.
• Secures the primary layer of the wound.
• Materials are cotton rolls, diapers etc.
Tertiary (outer) layer
• Provides support, pressure and protection to the primary and secondary layer.
• Materials are surgical tape (porous or water proof, adhesive or non adhesive and elastic or inelastic).
• A porous tape provides evaporation.
• Elastic tape provides pressure to control hemorrhage and edema.
Adherent dressing
(Used to debride the necrotic tissue in early phase of wound healing)
Non adherent dressing
Wet to dry dressing
• Primary layer-wet and secondary layer-dry.
• Wetting agents: sterile saline and 0.05% chlorhexidine.
• Wetting agents helps to dilute and evacuate viscous wound exudates.
Dry to dry dressing
• Absorbs fluid and debris from the wound.
• Before bandaging, open wounds should be debrided and lavaged with isotonic fluids or any antiseptic solution.
Semiocclusive dressing
• Used to prevent tissue dehydration and to protect epithelialization.
• Sterile petroleum impregnated gauze pieces along with topical antimicrobial ointments.
Occlusive dressing
• Impermeable to wound fluids.
• To enhance the epithelialization and collagen synthesis.
• Occlusive materials are foam, films, hydrocolloids and hydrogels.
• Requires less frequentchange.

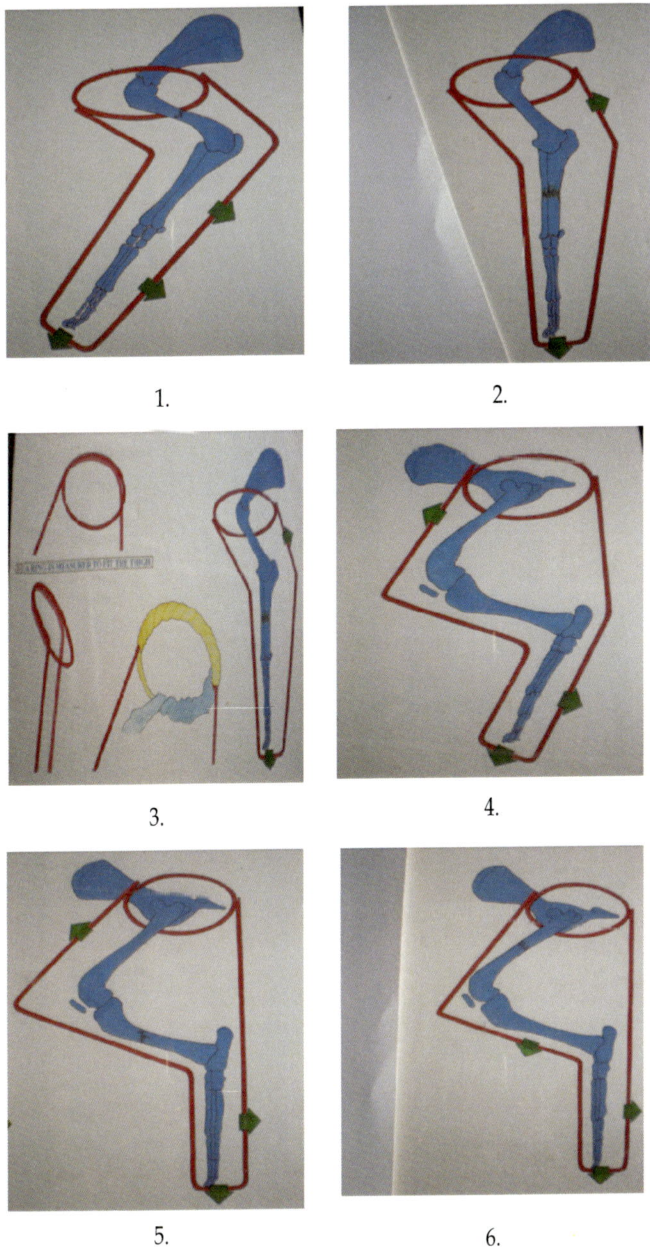

Fig. 1: Thomas splint for fracture of humerus; **2:** Thomas splint for fracture of redius ulina; **3:** Preparction of Thomas splint; **4:** Thomas splint for the management of fracture / dislocation of hock; **5:** Thomas splint for the management of fracture of tibia; **6:** Thomas splint for the management of fracture of femur.

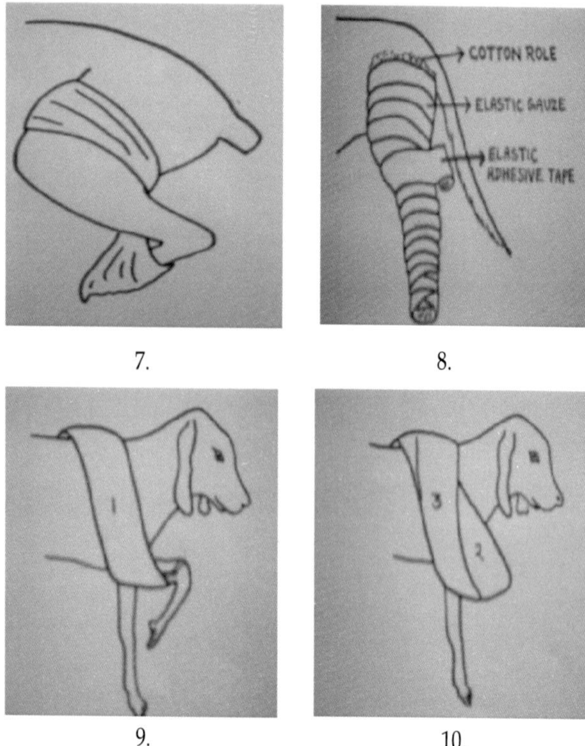

Fig. 7: Ehmer sling; **8:** Modified Robert Jones Bandege; **9:** Velpean sling; **10:** Velpean sling

1. Schroeder-thomas Splint

- Used to immobilize the limbs for the treatment of fractures below the elbow or stifle joint (Fig. 1 to 6).

2. Ehmer Sling

- It provides internal rotation and abduction of the limb.
- This sling is applied to support the limb after coxofemoral luxation.
- A adhesive tape is applied around the stifle and hock joints and to the caudal aspect of abdomen to protect weight bearing on the affected limb (Fig. 7).

3. Limb Bandages

- *Schanz padded limb bandage or modified Robert Jones bandage* : This bandage is used to support the limb in small animals. Bandage extends from the digit to the axillary or inguinal region leaving the middle toes exposed (Fig. 8).

4. Velpeau Sling

- Used to treat the scapulohumeral luxation and scapular fractures.
- Fix the fore limb with padded bandage and held in close apposition to the thorax. (Fig. 9&10).

5. Spica Splint

- Used to support the femoral and humeral fractures.
- A lateral splint is applied that reaches from the digits to the shoulder or hip joint.

6. Robert Jones Bandage

- It provides temporary stabilization of the limbs below the elbow or stifle joints.
- Following adhesive stirrups, cotton roll is applied which is again covered by elastic adhesive tape.

7. Pelvic (Robinson) Limb Sling

- Elastic gauze and adhesive tape are applied around the trunk to form a belly band.
- A tape is applied around the tibia and metatarsal which is attached to the belly band.
- This sling prevents hind limb weight bearing.

Exercise 15

OBJECTIVE : DEMONSTRATION OF MONITORING OF GENERAL ANESTHESIA

General Description of An Animal

1. Age
2. Sex
3. Body weight

S. No.	Parameter	Normal	Preanesthetic medication Atropine/Diazepam	After injection of anaesthesia					
				0 min	5 min	10 min	20 min	30 min	40 min
1.	Heart Rate beats/min								
2.	Rectal temperature (°C)								
3.	Respiration Rate (rate/min)								
4.	Anal reflex								
5.	Palpebral reflex								
6.	Corneal reflex								
7.	Pedal reflex								
8.	Salvation								
9.	Lacrimation								

Preanesthtic - dose and route of administration

General anaesthetic used

- Induction
- Recovery
- Complete recovery

Duration of effect

Exercise 16

OBJECTIVE : ANESTHESIA FOR LABORATORY AND WILD ANIMALS

Many anesthetic drugs are available to immobilize the lab and wild animals. In wild animals, immobilizing agents are usually administered by intramuscular injection.

Common Anesthetic Agents used for Immobilizing Wild Animals

1. Ketamine
2. Telazol
3. Xylazine
4. Medetomidine
5. Carfentanil
6. Etorphine

Precautions During Handling with Immobilizing Agents

- Disposable gloves should be used during handling of these agents. Absorption of such drugs through eyes and mucous membrane of nostril and mouth will result in rapid uptake. Death may occur.
- Darts and needles should be handled carefully.
- After use dispose the syringes and needled properly.
- Antidote should be ready to administer.

Laboratory Animal Anesthesia

- The rodents should be fasted for 1-2 hours only (High metabolic rate of small mammals requires constant supply of food and water).
- Fasting for longer period may cause severe hypoglycaemia.
- The anesthetics can be given by intravenous/ intramuscular or intraperitoneal route.
- During recovery period, the animal should be kept in warm location to prevent hypothermia.
- The lateral ear vein is used for intravenous administration of anesthetics in rabbits.
- **Doses** of certain anesthetic in mg/ kg body weight (IM- Intramuscular, IV-Intravenous, IP- Intraperitoneal).

Anesthetic drugs	Rabbit	Rat	Mice	Guinea pigs
Thiopental (1.25%)	15-30 IV	20-40 IV 40 IP	25-50 IV 50 IP	- -
Ketamine	20-60 IM	50-100 IM	100 IM or IP 50 IV	40 IM
Xylazine	3-9 IM or IV	5-12 IM	2.5 IM	5-40 IP
propofol	7.5-15 IV	7.5-10 IV (For induction) and maintenance @ 44-45 mg/kg/hr	12-26 IV	-

Anesthesia for Reptiles

- Fasting is not necessary in reptiles except in snake (in snake, cardiovascular functions are affected by feed intake prior to anesthesia).
- Sites for intravenous injection in reptiles:
  - i. Lizards - Ventral tail vein and toe nail.
  - ii. Turtles - Brachial plexus and toe nail.
  - iii. Snakes - Ventral tail vein, palatine vein and heart.
- Sites for intramuscular injection:
  - i. Lizards - Front leg and Paravertebral muscles.
  - ii. Turtle or chelonians - Front leg.
  - iii. Snakes - Paravertebral muscles.
- Injectable anesthetics do not provide the adequate analgesia. So inhalant anesthetics should be used for maintenance of anesthesia.

- If injectable anesthetics are used, it should be supplemented with infiltration of local anesthesia at the incision line.
- Because of renal plexus in the caudal half of the body, intramuscular injection should be avoided at this site.
- Induction by inhalant anesthetics can be achieved by placing the snake in the transparent plastic box or aquarium tank in to which 7-10% halothane or isoflurane vapors are supplied.
- After endotracheal intubation (endotracheal tube of size 2-4 I.D. or an I.V. catheter can be used), a non rebreathing circuit is recommended for inhalant anesthetic.
- Doses: In mg/kg body weight
  Xylazine: 0.1-1.25
  Diazepam: 0.2-1.0
  Midazolam: 0.2-2.0
  Medetomidine: 0.1-0.15

Anesthetic drug	Lizard	Snake	Turtle
Ketamine	30-50 IM	20-40 IM	30 IM
Propofol	10 Intraosseous	10 IM	5-10 IM

Anesthesia for Certain Wild Mammals

Animal	Medetomidine	Etorphine (Total dose)	HBN* (Hellabrunn mixture)	Ketamine	Xylazine	Telazol
Black bear	-	-	3.0-4.0 ml	5-9 mg/kg	2.0-4.5	7.0 mg/kg
Axis deer	-	2.0-3.5 mg	0.6-1 ml	-	-	-
Asian elephant	-	14-20 mg	5.0-6.0 ml	-	-	-
Giraffe	-	-		-	-	-
Leopard	-	-		-	-	3.5-6.0 mg/kg
Lion	60-80 µg/ kg	-	2-3 ml	2-3 mg/kg	-	-
Nilgai	-	4-6 mg	1.7 ml	-	-	-
Rhinoceros	-	2-2.5 mg		-	-	-
Tiger	60-80 µg/ kg	-	2-3 ml	2.5 mg/kg	-	4-5 mg/kg
Zebra	-	4.5 mg		-	-	-

* HMB contains 4 ml ketamine (100 mg/ml) in 500 mg xylazine powder vial.

Exercise 17

Objective : Restraining of Animals

Application of various methods of restraints is essential to carry out certain surgical procedures on animals. A particular method of restraint suitable for one animal may proves ineffective for another. Consider the temperament, Age, breed and individual characteristic of the animal as well as purpose of the restraint.

Knots

1. Square Knot : (Fig. 4.37)

- Properly tied square knot will not slip under tension.
- Two separate ropes can be joined by square knot to form a long rope.

2. Granny Knot : (Fig. 4.38)

Granny knot may slip under tension.

3. Slip Knot : (Fig. 17.1)

Slip knot should not be used in the neck region.

4. Bowline Knot : (Fig. 17.2)

- Bowline knot forms a permanent loop that will not slip.
- It can be applied around the neck or limb because it will not affect the respiration and circulation.

5. Hitch

Single half hitch (Fig.17.3), Double half hitch (Fig.17.4) & Clove hitch (Fig.17.5).

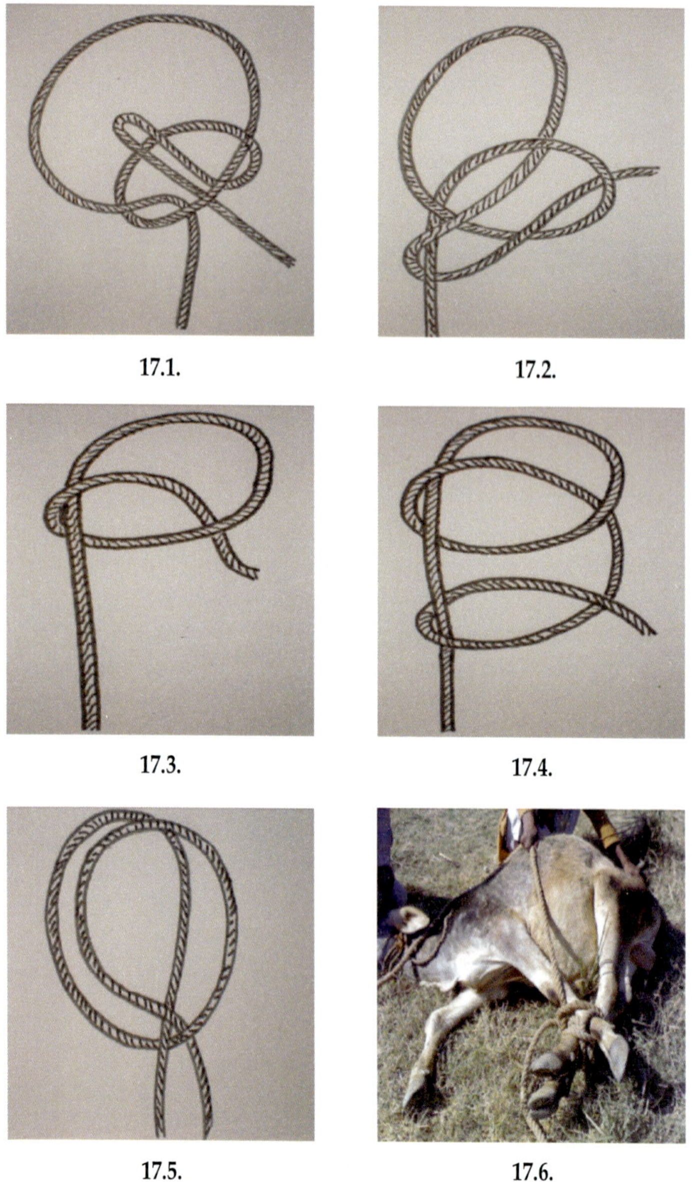

17.1. 17.2. 17.3. 17.4. 17.5. 17.6.

Fig. 17.1: Slip Knot; **17.2:** Bowline Knot; **17.3:** Single Half Hitch; **17.4:** Double Half Hitch; **17.5:** Clove Hitch; **17.6:** Restaining

Restraining of Equines

1. Halter

It is a piece of rope (cotton or hemp) made up in to a particular shape to adjust on the head of the horse for restraining. The halter may be permanent or temporary. Temporary halter can be made as follows :

- Take a rope of about ten feet length and one inch diameter.
- Make a single loop about 2/3 the length of the horse's head on one end of the rope.
- Place this loop over the horse's head with top behind ears and knot under the jaw.
- Pass the rope under the jaw to the offside and bring it forward across the cheek and nose.
- Continue the rope back across the cheek on the near side and tie it to the loop so that the nose is lightly but not tightly encircled.
- Lead the horse by loose end of the rope.

2. Twitch : (Fig. 17.7)

- It is a strong stout wooden stick attached with a rope loop (about 18 inches long) at one end.
- The rope loop can be made from horse's tail hair.
- It is one of the oldest, simplest and most commonly used appliances for restraining of horse.

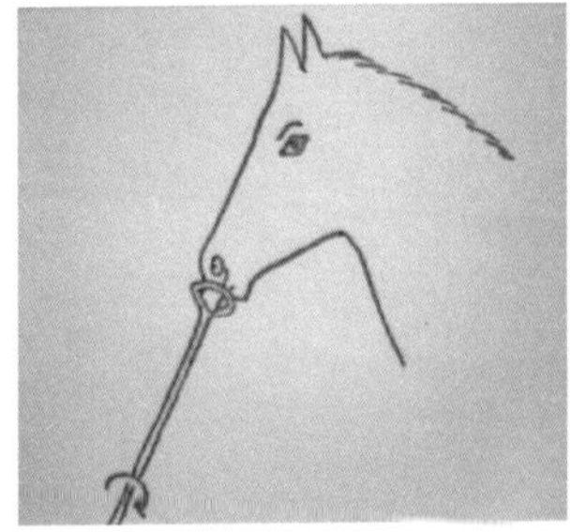

Fig. 17.7: Twitch

- The rope loop is generally applied and twisted on the upper lip but can be applied on the lower lip and base of the ear.
- *Principle* : Pressure is applied to the sensory nerves of the area and the pain produced diverts the horse's attention while less painful work is done elsewhere on the body.

3. Side Sick

- Side stick is also known as side rod and sword stick.
- A side stick can be made from strong smooth piece of wood or from a light metal pipe having holes or straps at each end.

- One end is tightened to the horse's head collar and other to the surcingle or roller pad.
- It prevents the horse from reaching the posterior part of his body with his mouth.
- It restricts the side movements but allows vertical flexion of neck.

4. Neck Cradle : (Fig. 17.8)

- Ten to twelve pieces of wood (About 2 ft long and one inch diameter) having a hole at both ends are threaded along two ropes.
- This cradle is tie around the neck of the animal at the crest.
- The cradle prevents bilateral movements of the animal's head i.e. turning and lowering of neck.
- Neck cradle is usefull in keeping him away from licking a wound on his body or legs.

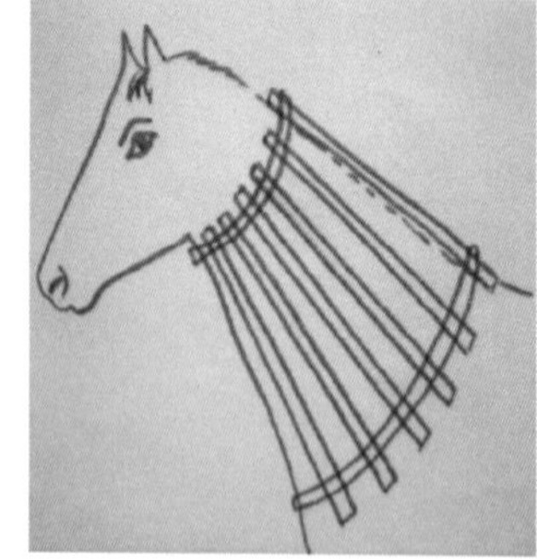

Fig. 17.8: Neck Credle

- Arrangement must be made for raising the feed to the animal's mouth when the cradle is applied.

Casting of horses : Casting of the animal is necessary for major operations.

Precautions to be Taken Before Casting the Animal

- Animal should preferably be kept off fed for 12 hours before casting.
- To minimize struggling, tranquilizers can be given before casting.
- The bit should always be removed before casting to avoid injury to the mouth.
- Apply stable bandages on legs to avoid injury by ropes.
- Valuable horses may have knee caps and hock boots put on.

The ground should be soft, grassy or sandy.

Do not try to cast a horse with fewer men. Arrange for adequate number as follows :

1. A reliable man at the horse's head.
2. Three men on the rope.
3. A man to pull the double rope
4. A leader to supervise and to give signal for casting

Casting by Hobble Method

- The master hobble is attached to the near fore pastern (The leg which will be uppermost after the animal has been cast).
- The fellow of the master hobble goes on to the off hind limb.
- The remaining two hobbles (simple hobbles) are applied on the off fore and near hind limb.
- The buckles must always be on the outside.
- The chain passes from the metal ring of the master hobble on the off fore, off hind, near hind and finally attached by a screw to the master hobble. The screw should be fixed from below upward when the horse is standing.
- A double rope is slipped round the fore arm of the fore leg which is to be uppermost and passed over the withers to an assistant standing on the other side to pull the animal on to the required side.
- At the signal, pull the casting rope and the man at the horse's head is instructed to back the horse. At the same time, the double rope is also pulled by an assistant.
- Backing the horse brings all four feet close together and the horse looses his balance, falls over on his side.
- Man holding the head should sit on the neck and the spare men on the hip when the animal falls down on the ground.
- To release the horse, remove the hobbles while the horse is in recumbent stage.

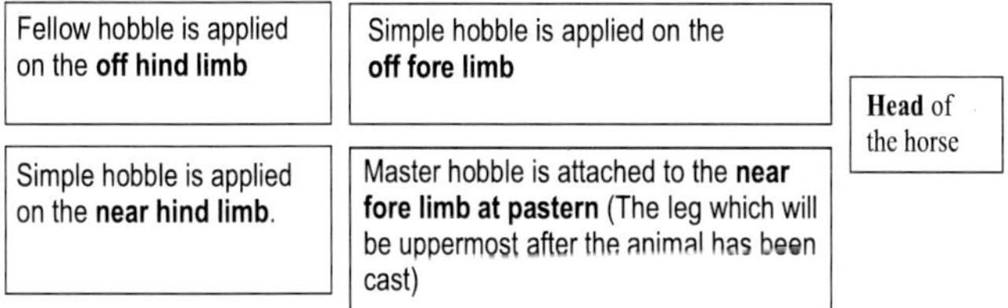

Casting by Side Line Method : (Fig. 17.9)

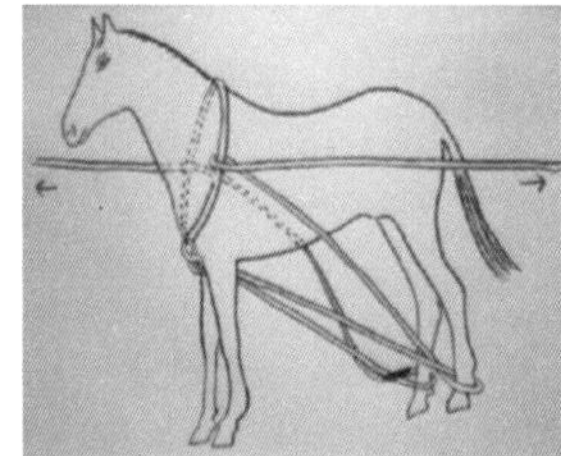

Fig. 17.9: Casting by Side Line Method

- Take a 50 feet long rope and make a loop in the center by applying a figure of "8" knot.
- Place the loop over the animal's head to rest in front of withers.
- Pass the ends of the rope between the forelegs and round the hind limbs to rest over the hocks. (To ensure that if the animal kicks the rope will remain in position).

- The ends of the rope may be passed either from outside inward or from inside outward.
- The ends are then brought forward through the neck loop.
- One end of the rope is held by two men well in front of the horse and the other end by two men well behind him.
- The loops around the hock are slipped down to the pastern.
- At the signal, pull the casting ropes and the man at the horse's head is instructed to back the horse. At the same time, the double rope is also pulled by an assistant to cast the animal on desired side.

Restraining of Bovines

1. *Tailing* : Tail's base is grasped by the hands and lifted directly over the animal's back. Tailing prevents kicking by diverting the attention of the animal.
2. *Twitch* : Rope twitch is applied on the upper lip or at the base of the ear to control the animal.
3. *Nose tong* : Nose tong is applied on the nasal septum through the nostril. Temporary restraining can also be done by grasping the nasal septum between the thumb and middle finger.
4. *Nose ring* : A nose ring is permanently inserted through the nasal septum.
   - **Halter** : Rope halter can be used for minor surgical procedures of head e.g. dehorning, treatment of actinomycosis and actinibacillosis.

Casting of Cattle

Cattle have to cast for surgical operations like upward fixation of patella (Fig. 17.10a), castration (Fig. 17.10b), to trim the overgrown hoof, shoeing of bullocks etc.

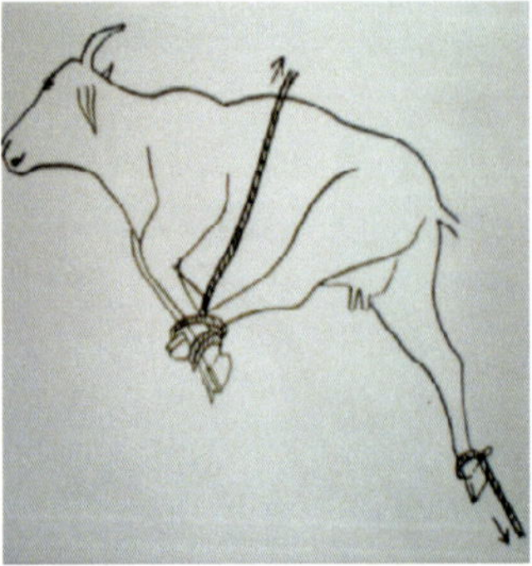

Fig. 17.10a: Casting of animal for medial patellar desmotomy

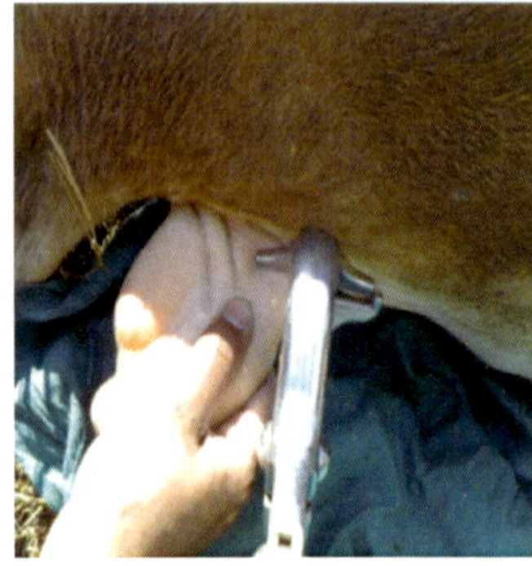

Fig. 17.10b: Castration by burdizzo method

1. Rope Squeeze Method / Reuff's Method : (Fig. 17.11)

- A running noose is made at one end of a rope and passed round the base of the horn. In dehorned cattle the noose can be fixed round the neck.
- A half hitch is made around the chest immediately around the elbows.
- A second half hitch is made around the abdomen in front of the udder or scrotum.
- The rope is pulled by two assistants.
- As soon as the animal falls, one man immediately controls the head and the other pulls the tail under the upper hind leg.

2. Burley's Technique / Alternate Method : (Fig. 17.12)

- Double the thirty feet long rope and pass it over the neck in front of hump.
- Pass the rope between the fore legs and cross both the ends.
- Again cross these separate ends over the loin of the animal.
- Finally pass the both ends between the hind legs on either side of the scrotum or udder.
- Head is controlled by a man and each end of rope is then pulled by two assistant.
- On pulling the rope the animal will sit down.

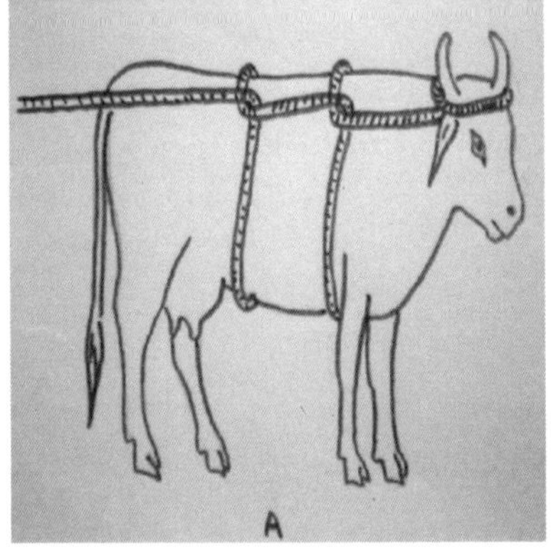

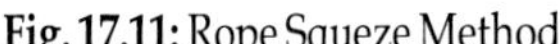
Fig. 17.11: Rope Squeze Method

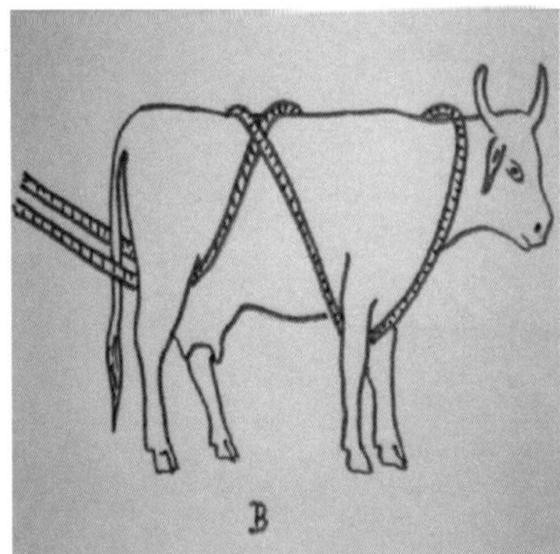

Fig. 17.12: Burley's Technique

Raising the Fore Limb of Cattle : (Fig. 17.13)

- Tie a rope around the pastern of the leg to be lifted.
- Pass the other end of the rope over the wither.
- The attendant on the opposite side of the rope will pull the rope to lift the limb of the animal.
- Lifting of the limb can be assisted by putting the pressure against the shoulder of the animal on the same side as the leg being lifted.

Restraining of Dog and Cat

1. *Tape muzzle :* (Fig. 17.14) Tape muzzle to secure dogs and cats from biting a person while handling. It can be made from ordinary bandage or cord in the following fashion.
   - Make a loop in the center of a one meter cord or bandage using a overhand knot.
   - Slip the loop over the nose of the dog.
   - Tight the loop and bring the ends around the side of the neck.
   - Tie the ends in a reef knot over the crest behind the ears of the dog.
2. *Leather muzzle :* Muzzle of different size should be kept in the clinic for different breeds with variable size of the face.
3. *Restraining in lateral recumbency :* After application of the muzzle, put the animal on the table. The fore limbs are held with one hand and the hind limb with the other. A gentle pressure is applied on the neck and hip of the dog by both the arms.
4. *Restraining in dorsal recumbency :* The animal is restrained in dorsal recumbency for operations like midventral laparotomy, Oariohy-sterectomy etc. and for radiography in vendrodorsal position.

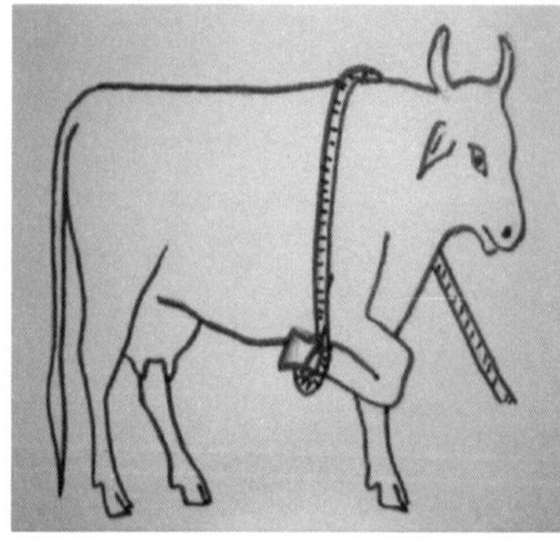

Fig. 17.13: Raising the Fore Limb of Cattle

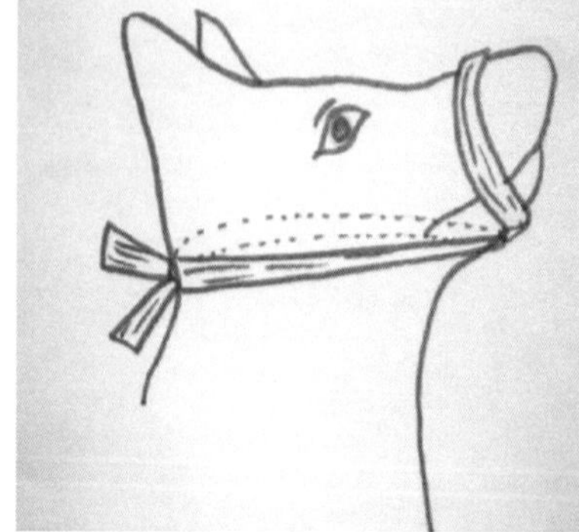

Fig. 17.14: Restraining of Dog and Cat

Restraining of Pig

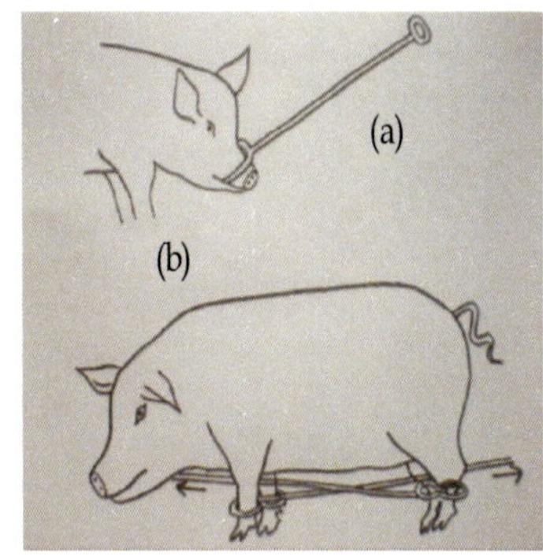

Fig. 17.15: a. Pig Holder **b.** Casting

1. *Twitch or running noose* : Twitch is applied over the upper jaw behind the tusks, twisted tightly and held by an attendant.
2. Pig holder (Fig. 17.15a)
3. *Casting* : (Fig. 17.15b) The fore limbs and hind limbs are tied separately by different ropes. A long rope is fastened in the fore limb and runs backward between the hind legs. Another rope is tightened to the hind limb and runs forward between the fore legs. Both these ropes are pulled, the pig becomes recumbent.

Restraining of Camel

1. For minor surgical interventions, a rope (about 5 meter long 2 cm in diameter) is passed round the pasterns of both the front legs and ends are tied over the neck of the camel (Fig. 17.16a). The attendant of the camel holds his head by a nose rope or halter.
2. For major surgery, another rope is tied round the pastern of hind legs are tied on the back seat of the camel. A soft cushion should be applied on back to prevent the injury caused by the rope. After tying the fore and hind limbs, the camel can be restrained in lateral recumbency (Fig. 17.16b). When the surgery is over, the hind limbs are untied first and forelimbs later. The camel needs a little help to regain his sitting position.
3. *Raising of fore limb* : After flexion of the carpal joint, the cannon and fore arm of the same limb are tied together by a figure of "8" fashion.

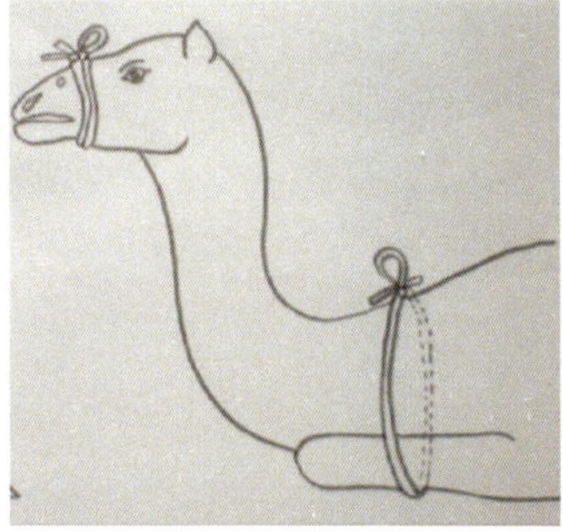
Fig. 17.16a: Restraining of Camel

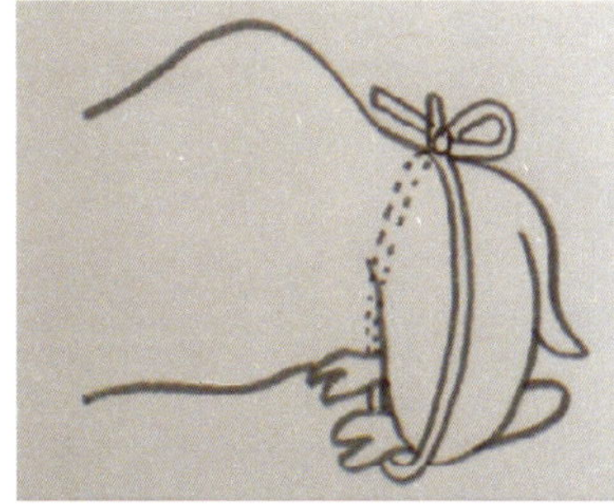
Fig. 17.16b: Restraining of Camel

Exercise 18

Objective :

Miscellaneous Instruments

1. *Trocar and canula* : It is used to remove the gas from the rumen during bloat. It should be inserted by sliding the skin through the left paralumbar fossa. (Fig. 18.1). Sliding of skin decreases the chances the formation of ruminal fistula after its removal.
2. *Probang gag* : It is made of a wooden piece with a hole in the middle and straps on either ends. Wooden block having the hole is fixed in the mouth and straps are fastened behind the horn at the poll. The probing is passed through the hole in to the stomach (Fig. 18.2).

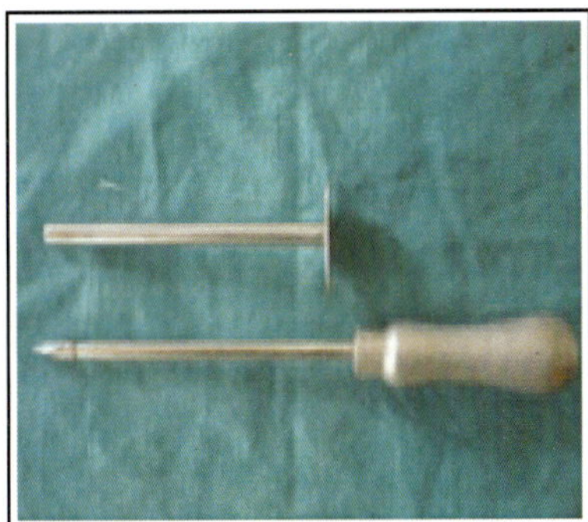

Fig. 18.1: Trocar and canula

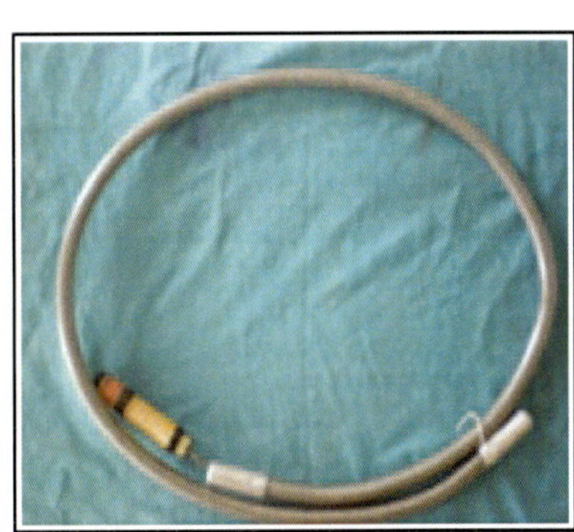

Fig. 18.2: Probang gag

3. *Tracheal tube* : The tube is fixed in the trachea as a temporary or permanent arrangement to provide oxygen in tracheal stenosis for large animals (Fig. 18.3).
4. *Castration clamp* : It is used to clamp the spermatic cord in large animals (Fig. 18.4).

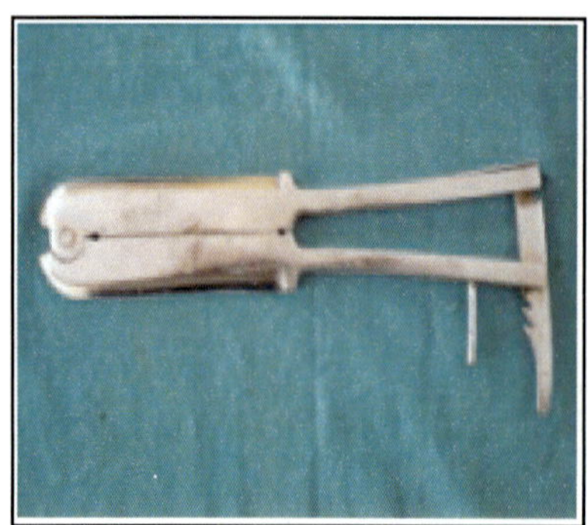

Fig. 18.3: Tracheal Tube

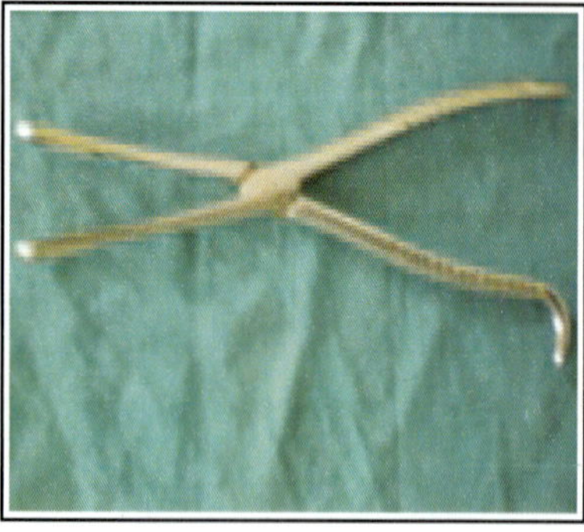

Fig. 18.4: Castration clamp

5. *Burdizzo castrator :* It is used to castrate the bull, ram, buck and boar (Fig. 18.5).
6. *Weingarth's rumenotomy set* : It is used for rumenotomy to check the contamination of peritoneal cavity by rumen fluid (Fig. 18.6). It consist of
   i. Rumen forceps (2)
   ii. A metal ring
   iii. Rumen hooks (6-8)

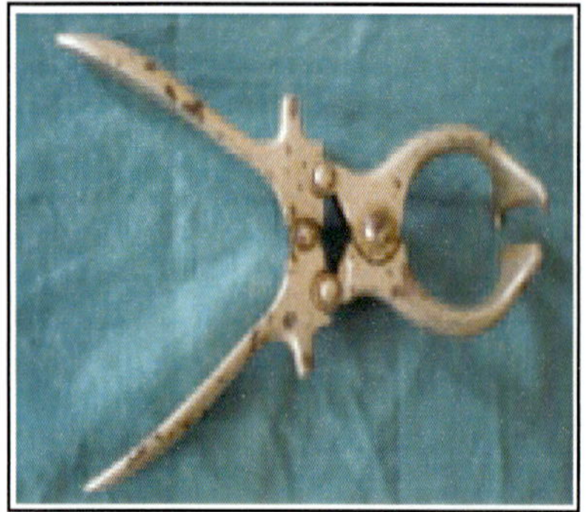

Fig. 18.5: Burdizzo castrator for bull, ram, buck and boar

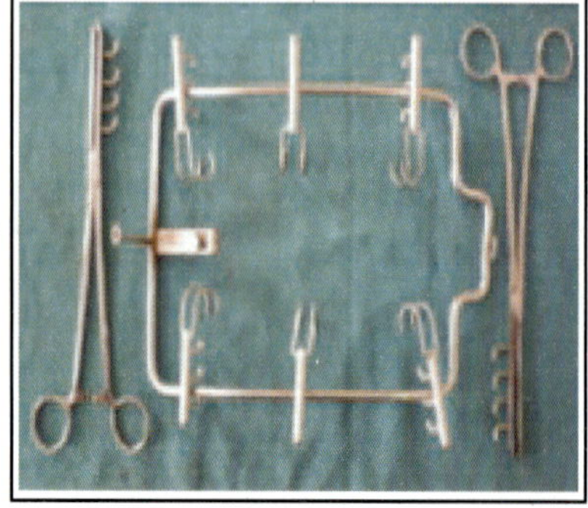

Fig. 18.6: Weingarths set **i.** Rumen forceps **ii.** Metal ring **iii.** Rumen hooks

7. *Nail cutter* : It is used to trim the overgrown nails of canines and felines.
8. *Docking scissors* : It is used for transecting the tail of some breeds of puppies.
9. *Cheatle's sterilizer forceps* : It is used to pick the instruments, sterilized cotton, bandage etc from the sterilizer (Fig. 18.7).
10. *Spring gag* : This gag is used in dogs. The spring between the two arms keeps the jaw apart to the fullest extent.
11. *Suture cutting scissors* : It is used to cut the sutures after wound healing (Fig. 18.8).

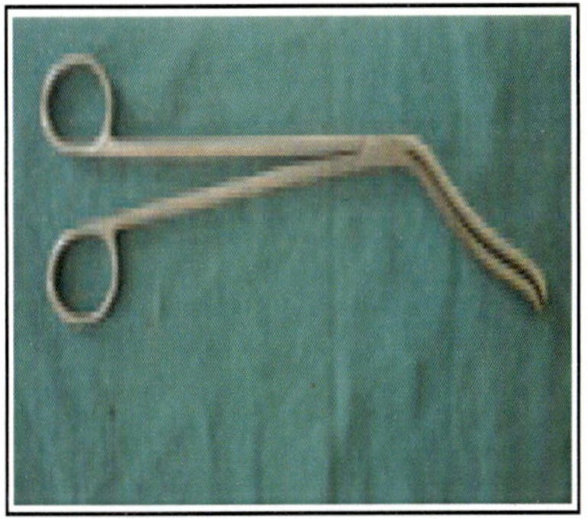

Fig. 18.7: Cheatle's forceps

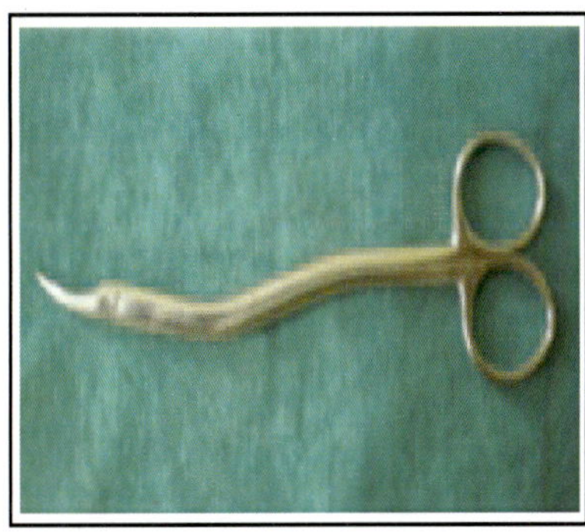

Fig. 18.8: Suture cutting scissors

12. *Tenaculum* : It is used to exteriorize muscles, tendon, ligaments, vessels nerves etc.
13. *Vaginal speculum* : It is used to visualize the vagina (Fig. 18.9).
14. *Doynes intestinal clamp* : It is used to clamp/ hold the cut ends of intestine during enterotomy or enterectomy to prevent the passage of ingesta in to the peritoneal cavity (Fig. 18.10).

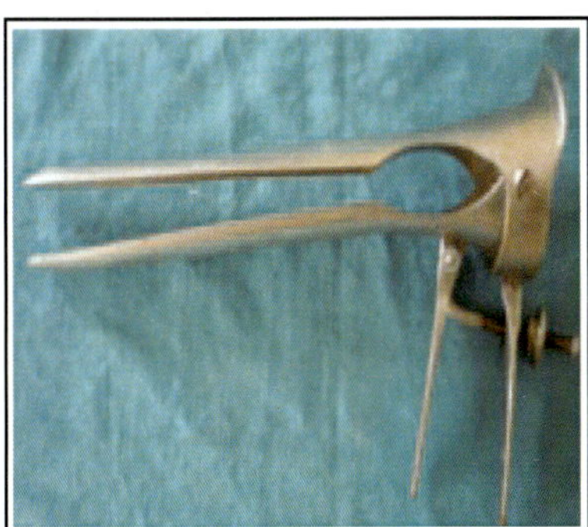

Fig. 18.9: Vaginal speculum

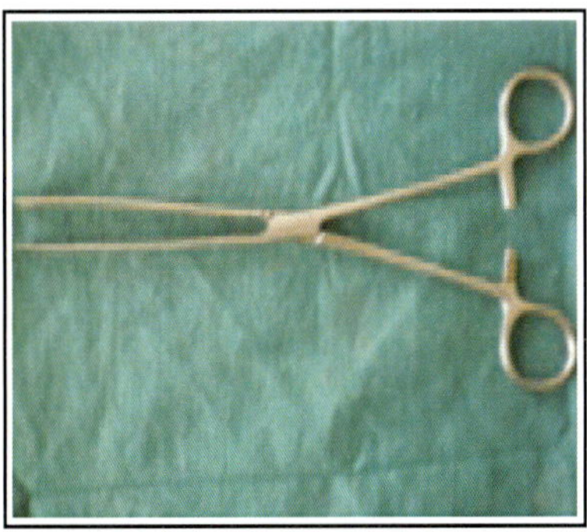

Fig. 18.10: Doynes intestinal clamp

15. *Laryngoscope* : It is used for visualization of larynx. It is also used as an aid for positioning the endotracheal tube (Fig. 18.11 & 18.12).

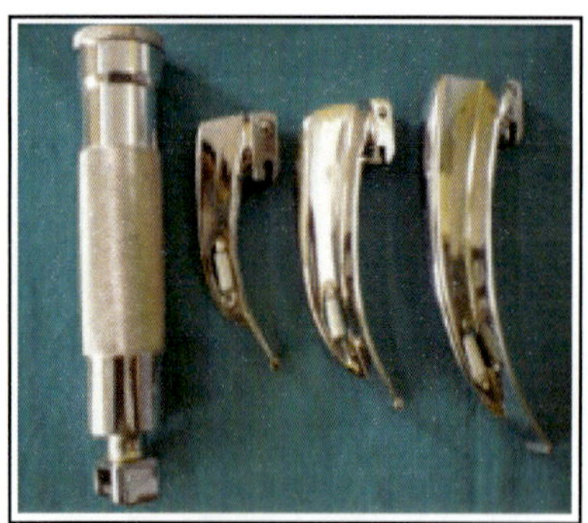

Fig. 18.11: Laryngoscope

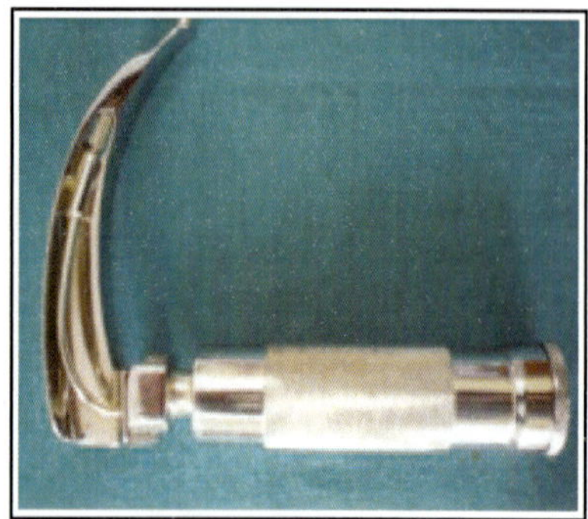

Fig. 18.12: Laryngoscope complete assembly

16. *Volkman wound retractor* : It is used to visualize the deeper tissues during surgical operation.
17. *Firing irons* : Firing irons are used as a highest degree of counter irritant for treatment of chronic inflammatory lesions (Fig. 18.12). Firing irons are of three types :
    - Pin point firing iron
    - Point firing iron
    - Line firing iron

❑❑❑